Recent Results in Cancer Research 136

M. Ponz de Leon

Familial and Hereditary Tumors

With 37 Figures and 16 Tables

Springer-Verlag
Berlin Heidelberg New York
London Paris Tokyo
Hong Kong Barcelona
Budapest

Prof. Dr. M. Ponz de Leon
Università degli Studi di Modena
Istituto di Patologia Medica
Policlinico
Via del Pozzo, 71
41100 Modena, Italy

"Maurizio Ponz de Leon was born in Messina (Italy) in 1948 and graduated at the university of Modena, in 1972.
As Associate Professor (1982) and subsequently Professor (1990) on Internal Medicine at the University of Modena, he published more than 100 papers dealing with various aspects of gastroenterology and oncology. During the past ten years, his publications have entirely been related to colorectal cancer (registration, cell proliferation, and genetic epidemiology).
Dr. Ponz de Leon is a member of the International Collaborative Group on Heriditary Non-polyposis Colorectal Cancer, and in 1993 he was the chairman of a similar study group in Italy."

ISBN-13: 978-3-642-85078-3 **e-ISBN-13: 978-3-642-85076-9**
DOI: 10.1007/978-3-642-85076-9

Library of Congress Cataloging-in-Publication Data. Ponz de Leon, M. (Maurizio), 1948– Familial and hereditary tumors / M. Ponz de Leon. p. cm. – (Recent results in cancer research : 136) Includes bibliographical references and index. ISBN 3-540-57633-9 (alk. paper). – ISBN 0-387-57633-9 (alk. paper) 1. Cancer – Genetic aspects. I. Title. II. Series. [DNLM: 1. Neoplasms – genetics. 2. Neoplastic Syndromes, Hereditary. 3. Neoplasms – etiology. 4. Environmental Exposure – adverse effects. W1 RE106P v. 136 1994 / QZ 200 P819f 1994] RC261.R35 vol. 136 [RC268.4] 616.99'4 s – dc 20 [616.99'4042] DNLM/DLC 94-13711

Softcover reprint of the hardcover 1st edition 1994

Typesetting by Best-set Typesetter Ltd., Hong Kong
SPIN: 10124602 19/3130/SPS – 5 4 3 2 1 0 – Printed on acid-free paper

Preface

For many years the etiology of human tumors has almost exclusively been attributed to environmental factors, which seemed to be involved not only in the induction of neoplasms but also in other phases of tumorigenesis. Cigarette smoking and alcohol are the two best known examples of factors related to our modern lifestyle which have been implicated in the development of cancer of various organs.

From the 1960s onward, the pioneer work of a few investigators clearly showed that hereditary factors were not only related to rare neoplasms, but could also be responsible for the occurrence of a sizeable fraction of tumors that do not usually show features of inheritance (as in the case of breast or colorectal cancer). Thus, the idea that some common human malignancies could be transmitted from one generation to another with features of mendelian genetics became more and more evident. In addition, the veritable explosion of molecular biology in the last 15 years has made a further and substantial contribution to the emerging role of genetics in biomedical research and particularly in cancer.

Despite all this evidence, it is clear that the genetic nature of cancer is not fully appreciated. Thus, for instance, physicians are quite ready to prohibit smoking and to limit alcoholic beverages for their patients (and this is, of course, important), but many of them are surprisingly reluctant to ask for information and to investigate the possible relevance of tumor aggregation in a given family. Similarly, little emphasis is usually given to heritable factors in most of the books dealing with the causes of cancer.

The main purpose of the present book is twofold. First, the volume provides an ample description of the familial and hereditary aspects of either rare or common human malignancies. Second, when possible the genetic background has been compared with the putative role of environmental factors for each specific neoplasm. Thus, chapter after chapter, I have tested the hypothesis that almost invariably cancer develops because of a close interaction between genes and exogenous agents or, in other words, that an inherited condition renders individuals highly susceptible to tumors, but that these usually occur owing to the effect of exogenous factors acting on a predisposed substrate.

The first four chapters form a general introduction in which the most important basic concepts (types of genetic transmission, biomarkers, oncogenes, tumor suppressor genes) are concisely discussed. The other 18 chapters deal with neoplasms of various organs. Sometimes various tumor types have been grouped in a single chapter (i.e., the chapters on "Familial Factors in Cancer of the Genitourinary Tract" and "Familial Tumors of Other Organs"). These final 18 chapters have been structured in the same way; each of them begins with a short introduction highlighting the most relevant aspects and the main biological problems of that specific neoplasm. Then clinical and epidemiologic data are briefly summarized, referring to recent reviews for further details. After this, familial and hereditary aspects are discussed, together with the evidence (if any) of the interaction between environmental and genetic factors in tumor development. The last part of each chapter usually describes the most recent advances in cytogenetics and molecular biology.

Modena, Italy
September 1994

Maurizio Ponz de Leon

Acknowledgments

The author wishes to thank all friends and colleagues who contributed in different ways to the design and the completion of the book, and in particular his collaborators Dr. L. Roncucci, Dr. P. Benatti, Dr. S. De Pietri, and Dr. M. Pedroni at the Istituto di Patologia Medica, Università di Modena and Dr. C. Di Gregorio, Dr. R. Fante, and Dr. L. Losi at the Istituto di Anatomia Patologica, Università di Modena.

Thanks are also due to Dr. E. Buiatti (Centro per lo Studio e la Prevenzione Oncologica, Firenze), Prof. B. Terracini (Dipartimento di Scienze Biomediche, Università di Torino), Dr. G. Lanza (Istituto di Anatomia Patologica, Università di Ferrara), Dr. Doris Hadjistilianou (Istituto di Scienze Oftalmologiche, Università di Siena), Prof. L. Brandi (Dipartimento di Fisiologia Clinica, Università di Firenze), and Prof. G. Emilia (Istituto di Clinica Medica, Università di Modena), who reviewed several chapters, providing many suggestions and helpful criticisms. In addition, the author expresses his gratitude to Dr. L. Losi for her skill in drawing most of the figures appearing in the text.

Finally, the kind and efficient editorial assistance of Mrs. A. Cerri and Dr. M. Hofmann (Springer-Verlag, Ufficio per l'Italia, Milano) is gratefully acknowledged.

Contents

Introduction

> *Cancer is not only a cellular disease, it is basically a genetic disease, as it is stable rearrangements of the genetic material that render the cell neoplastic, i.e., enable it to assume a proliferation pattern outside the boundaries set by normal control mechanisms.*
>
> SVERRE HEIM et al. (1988)

Genetic Epidemiology of Tumors

It is well known that only one out of three or four heavy smokers will develop lung cancer. Similarly, cancer develops only in a fraction of patients or animals exposed to a given carcinogen. Why is this? A possible explanation might be that it is by chance, but only a few of us might be satisfied by this interpretation, especially in the light of the most recent advances in molecular biology [1, 2]. An alternative and more plausible explanation could be that the genetic susceptibility to cancer is different from person to person. Following this line of reasoning we can interpret each cancer as due to a complex interaction between environmental and genetic factors [3]. Thus, we can assume that the genetic background will determine which individuals in the general population are prone to cancer development; subsequently, over the course of many years, environmental factors – and many of these are already well known [4] – may interact with genes in susceptible persons, determining the fraction that will become affected.

There is now evidence that this genetic background is present and plays some role in the pathogenesis of almost all tumors and not only of those neoplasms (colon, breast) whose genetic component has better been characterized in the last two decades [5]. Despite this evidence, there is little doubt that heritable factors have so far received much less attention than environmental factors as a possible cause of cancer. Although on the one hand there is a strong general concern about cigarette smoking and alcohol abuse (the two most common environmental causes of cancer in humans), on the other the attention given by many physicians to the family history of their patients remains limited and, in addition, only quite rarely do first-degree relatives of patients with tumors feel to be at risk of cancer because of a common genetic background. Even more importantly, few efforts have been made to translate an increased knowledge on hereditary and familial cancer into new programs of cancer prevention or surveillance of high-risk individuals.

Many experimental and clinical observations support the existence of a close interaction between genetic and environmental factors in the development of tumors. Mammary carcinogenesis has been particularly informative in this regard. There are strains of genetically susceptible mice in which the administration of low doses of estrogens induces the appearance of many mammary tumors, whereas other strains may tolerate these doses without any tumor development. However, by increasing the dose of estrogens, cancer can be induced even in the apparently resistant mice [6, 7]. In line with these animal observations, there is a recent case report of gastric cancer in two monozygotic twins [8]. Cancer developed simultaneously at the age of 47. One of the twins was a heavy smoker and drank alcoholic beverages; he had an advanced gastric cancer with invasion of the serosa and thus only palliative surgery could be carried out. The other twin did not smoke or drink alcohol; he had an early-stage gastric cancer limited to within the mucosa and curative subtotal gastrectomy was performed. We recently observed a similarly informative family with lung cancer (Fig. 1). Four brothers died of lung cancer during the last 20 years; two of them did not smoke and developed cancer at the age of 70 and 72, respectively, while the other two were heavy smokers and became affected in their fourties.

These examples underscore the importance – in mice as in humans – of the genetic susceptibility to cancer; however, it is clear that the addition of a strong environmental carcinogen or promoter (estrogens in experimental mammary tumors, smoking and alcohol in the case reports) determines the time of appearance and probably the invasiveness of cancer. In its essence, genetic epidemiology is the study of the interaction between genes and environment in the etiology of a given disease. As far as cancer is concerned, evidence of this interaction have been provided for many tumors and can reasonably be hypothesized for almost all neoplasms [5]. Finally, a further element stresses the relevance of genetic epidemiology in tumorigenesis; highly conserved genes have been identified (the best investigated remains p53) in which point mutations at specific codons can be induced by a given chemical carcinogen, such as aflatoxin, or by physical agents [9, 10]; as will be discussed in the following chapters, many of these genes seem to be involved in cancer development.

Genetic Nature of Cancer

Probably the first suggestion of the genetic nature of cancer was given by Theodor Boveri in 1911. The author hypothesized the "presence of definite chromosomes which inhibit division" and "the assumption of the existence of chromosomes which promote cell division" and, more importantly, that

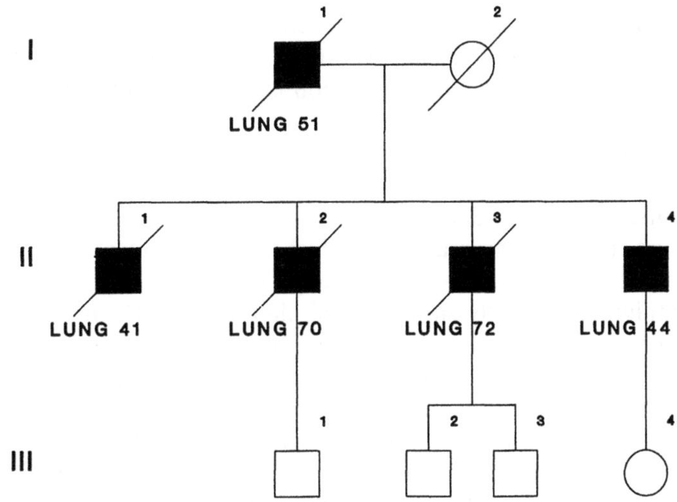

Fig. 1. Genealogical tree of a family with lung cancer aggregation. Patients II-2 and II-3 were nonsmokers and developed cancer at the age of 70 and 72, respectively. Patients II-1 and II-4 were heavy smokers and developed lung cancer at a much earlier age (41 and 44). *Black squares*, affected individuals

"the unlimited tendency to rapid proliferation in malignant tumor cells would be deduced from a permanent predominance of the chromosomes which promote division." If we simply substitute "chromosomes" with "genes," these few sentences may appear suitable for a recent review on the molecular biology of cancer.

There is a general agreement on the concept that cancer is usually initiated by a genetic change (i.e., an abnormality in DNA sequence), presumably in a single cell. This not only appears sound on a logical basis, but it is also supported by many lines of experimental evidence. First, it has been shown that most cancers are monoclonal, i.e., they represent a clone derived from a single abnormal cell. The most cited example remains chronic myelogenous leukemia, in which all neoplastic cells can be distinguished from normal cells by the presence of a translocation between chromosome 22 and 9. Other examples include leukemia and lymphomas which originate from B cells; in these lymphoproliferative disorders, the immunoglobulin genes undergo specific rearrangements which can be used as markers of clonality in Southern blot analysis. Second, there is a close correlation between tumorigenesis and mutagenesis, in the sense that there are chemical compounds and viruses which are known to cause cancer and to induce DNA damage. Finally, genetic abnormalities (point mutations or larger rearrangements leading to activation of oncogenes or to inactivation of tumor suppressor genes) have been reported in almost all human tumors [11, 12].

The problem, however, is much more complex; in fact, we have evidence that a mutation in a single cell may start the process of carcinogenesis, but it is also true that a single mutation is not sufficient to induce cancer. Indeed, other steps, usually referred to as promotion and progression, take place before the full development of the malignant phenotype. Moreover, genetic nature does not imply genetic transmission of cancer, but simply refers to DNA damage, which presumably initiates the process of tumorigenesis. In fact, most of the mutations which occur in cancer cells are somatic events and therefore limited to the neoplasm, while the germ line cells of affected individuals usually show normal alleles, so that cancer-associated genes are not transmitted to the progeny. However, in at least two rare hereditary cancer syndromes – adenomatosis coli and Li-Fraumeni syndrome (see the chapters on "Hereditary Gastrointestinal Polyposis Syndromes" and on "Li-Fraumeni Syndrome") – mutations in the germ line cells have been described [1, 2, 13, 14] which predispose members of these families to an increased susceptibility to cancer of specific sites.

Cancer as a Multistep Process

It is now generally accepted that the development of cancer in many tissues or organs (such as skin or colorectum) is a stepwise process involving populations of altered cells at many steps.

It is improbable that a single mutation (and, thus, a single "event") is sufficient to induce cancer, and this for several reasons. First, the mutational rate is very high, even in an environment which is free of mutagens; it has been calculated that a single gene undergoes mutation on approximately ten separate occasions in a lifetime. Thus, it is likely that some of these mutations may induce changes in the genes responsible for cell replication and differentiation, with the consequence that the mutated cell may escape the control of cell proliferation, giving origin to an autonomous growth. If this were the case, we should expect an extremely high frequency of cancer, presumably in all living cells. Second, tumor development requires that several events (mutations) occur independently in a single cell. Age-specific incidence rates of many cancers have been informative in this regard; in fact, since mutations occur stochastically (i.e., with a fixed probability), the likelihood of developing cancer in a given year should be independent of age. As a matter of fact, however, for most solid tumors the likelihood increases very steeply with age (by the third to fifth power). The mathematical interpretation of age-specific incidence (or mortality) rates suggests that between three and seven events are usually required to transform a normal cell into a neoplastic one. Third, recent studies in molecular biology have pointed out that malignant cells of the most common cancers show a wide range of genetic alterations, including point mutations, larger rearrangements of DNA, frequent allelic deletions, and loss of chromosomal fragments [11, 12, 15].

The multistep process of cancer development implies that a new cell population usually arises in a given organ or tissue as a consequence of mutations; this population functions as a site of origin of another altered population of cells, which are not yet neoplastic. This process is repeated many times and, after each step, there is an increased probability of the population evolving into a malignant one, showing by definition a pattern of growth which is independent of the environment. Thus, multistep tumorigenesis can be viewed as a process of clonal evolution based on the selection of rare cells. The various cell populations which develop in the initial steps of the long precancerous period usually do not show evidence of cancer, while the appearance of cells with invasive properties occurs in the late stages of the process [16].

The various stages of the multistep tumorigenesis can be most easily observed in epithelia such as bladder or colorectal mucosa and the skin. Figure 2 shows very schematically the main steps involved in colorectal cancer development. In normal subjects, cell proliferation is limited to the lower portions of colorectal crypts (stage A); one of the earliest premorphological changes is the appearance of S-phase cells in the upper portions of the crypt (stage B) and their progressive accumulation at the surface (stage C) [17]. The following step is the development of a benign lesion (adenomatous polyp) which grows very slowly and with time may show dysplastic changes (stage D). Although many polyps remain benign or even regress, there is no doubt that most colorectal carcinomas develop from adenomas, especially if these are large, severely dysplastic, or recurrent (stage E) [18]. Colorectal cancer grows independently of the environment, tends to infiltrate the muscular wall and the surrounding organs, and metastatizes mostly to regional lymph nodes, liver, and lung (stage F). The sequence hyperproliferative mucosa–adenoma–carcinoma will be further considered in a later chapter.

Experimental skin cancer is similarly informative; in mice, a single application of a chemical carcinogen to the skin does not induce the appearance of tumors; however, even a single application causes latent genetic damage, since when the skin is reexposed to the same carcinogen, the result is the development of cancer. Moreover, neoplasms may also be induced by the application of other compounds, such as phorbol esters, which are not themselves mutagenic or carcinogenic, but nevertheless can cause cancer if the skin has previously been exposed to strong carcinogens, such as benzopyrene or dimethylbenzanthracene [19].

The two models of colorectal and skin carcinogenesis introduce fairly straightforwardly the concepts of tumor initiation, promotion, and progression. Carcinogens and mutagens are generally considered tumor initiators, since they induce mutations of DNA which represent the first step in cancer development. Phorbol esters, such as tetradecanoylphorbol acetate (TPA), or secondary bile acids (in the case of colorectal tumorigenesis) are called tumor promoters; these compounds can cause cancer only if they are applied after treatment with an initiator. The main effect of promoters is

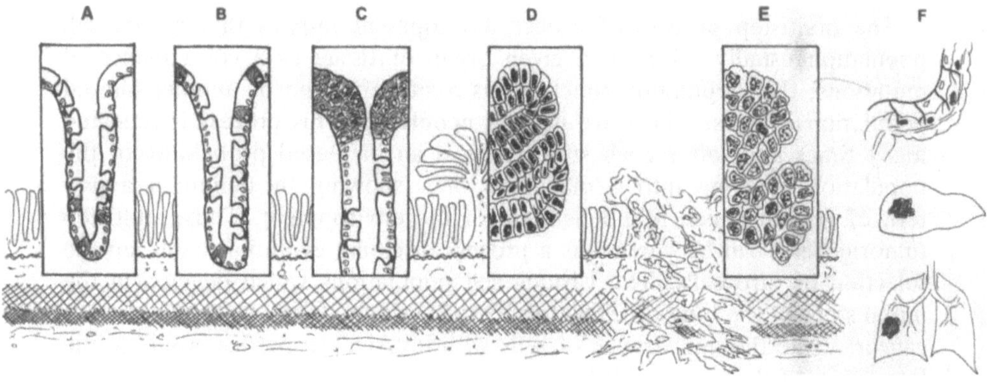

Fig. 2A–F. The main steps involved in colorectal tumorigenesis. For a detailed description, see text

to stimulate cell proliferation or to block terminal differentiation. Thus promoters may selectively expand cell populations that carry an initial mutation; the more cells there are, the greater the chance of a new mutation will be and so the population will move one step towards the fully malignant phenotype. Initiation, therefore, can simply be defined as permanent damage to cellular DNA. Promotion is the process whereby initiated cells are stimulated to grow into polyps, nodules, or other benign neoformations; one of these lesions may behave as a population of origin for the subsequent step, i.e., the development of cancer. Progression is the process by which polyps and other benign lesions evolve into fully malignant phenotypes, with the consequent possible local or metastatic diffusion.

Although extremely useful on theoretical grounds, the subdivision of the process of tumorigenesis into three different stages appears in many cases too rigid and schematic, especially in the light of our increased knowledge about the molecular aspects of diseases. Thus, in Fig. 2 we should expect to find initiated cells along the most actively proliferating crypts of colorectal mucosa; yet only very rarely have DNA mutations or other DNA changes (aneuploidy) been reported in normal mucosa [20]. Although it is entirely possible that at present we are unable to detect these very early events, we cannot exclude the possibility that cellular DNA is still unaltered at this stage and that the abnormal kinetic behavior is due to some undefined epigenetic factor. Moreover, the formation of polyps should be interpreted as a promotional event, due to the stimulatory effect of secondary bile acids (or of other factors) on cell replication. However, many genetic changes have recently been identified in colonic adenomas, including the activation of oncogenes and loss of heterozygosity of tumor suppressor genes [21], that are usually not detectable in normal mucosa. Thus, we cannot exclude the occurrence of initiating events (and not only promotional) even at this stage. Finally, many types of genetic alterations take place during the progression of adenomas to invasive cancer. In summary, the concept of multistep process is probably more suitable than the rigid subdivision into initiation, promotion, and progression to define the complex and still incompletely understood sequence of events which occurs in colorectal carcinogenesis. It is likely that the same reasoning applies to tumorigenesis of several other organs and tissues.

Sporadic, Familial, and Hereditary Tumors

Neoplasms can be defined as sporadic when familial or hereditary factors are apparently absent. For the same reason, it is commonly assumed that sporadic cancers are caused by environmental factors, even when these are not well defined. This reasoning is probably correct in most cases, although one should not forget that a fraction of these sporadic cases may represent new mutations in hereditary cancer syndromes which have escaped our attention, since (a) the phenotype may be indistinguishable from the sporadic counterpart and (b) with a few exceptions [1, 2, 13, 14], there is no genetic biomarker which can be utilized to identify these cases. This is one of the main reasons for the constant underestimation of hereditary tumors.

The definition of familial cancer is similarly vague; rather empirically, these tumors are characterized by the aggregation of cancers within a family. Thus, in familial breast cancer there is a prevalent aggregation of mammary tumors, in familial colorectal cancer of intestinal tumors, and so on. The aggregation of neoplasms might be due to chance alone or it might be the consequence of the exposure of several family members to common environmental factors. Alternatively, it could be due to ill-defined genetic factors; among the various possible interpretations, multifactorial inheritance remains the most likely, whereas monogenic transmission seems improbable.

Finally, in hereditary cancer syndromes there is sufficient clinical and biological information for us to believe that primary genetic factors are of major etiologic importance. In the absence of genetic biomarkers, inspection of the family tree remains of fundamental importance for a proper diagnosis. In the most typical cases, the main features of monogenic dominant transmission – i.e., vertical transmission with a segregation ratio of 0.5 and no skipped generations – are observed. However, late onset of the disease, phenocopies, possible low penetrance, variable expressivity, and above all small families may render the identification of hereditary tumors extremely complex (see the chapter on "Genetic Aspects of Disease: Categories of Genetic Disorders").

References

1. Malkin D, Li FP, Strong LC, Fraumeni JF Jr, Nelson CE, Kim DH, Kassel J et al. (1990) Germ line p53 mutations in a familial syndrome of breast cancer, sarcomas, and other neoplasms. Science 250:1233–1238
2. Li FP (1993) Molecular epidemiology studies of cancers in families. Br J Cancer 68:217–219
3. Taylor JA (1989) Oncogenes and their applications in epidemiologic studies. Am J Epidemiol 130:6–13
4. Doll R, Peto R (1981) The causes of cancer. JNCI 66:1191–1308
5. Lynch HT, Hiroyama T (1989) Genetic epidemiology of cancer. CRC Press, Boca Raton, Florida, pp 1–361
6. Gardner WU (1939) Estrogens in carcinogenesis. Arch Pathol 27:138
7. Loeb L (1940) The significance of hormones in the origin of cancer. J Natl Cancer Inst I:169
8. Matsukura N, Onda M, Tokunaga A, Yoshiyuki T, Shimizu Y, Nishi K, Furukawa K et al. (1988) Simultaneous gastric cancer in monozygotic twins. Cancer 62:2430–2435
9. Hollstein M, Sidransky D, Vogelstein B, Harris CC (1991) p53 mutations in human cancers. Science 253:49–53
10. Makino H, Ishizaka Y, Tsujimoto A, Nakamaura T, Onda M, Sugimura T, Nagao M (1992) Rat p53 gene mutations in primary zymbal gland tumors induced by 2-amino-3-methylimidazol (4,5-f) quinoline, a food mutagen. Proc Natl Acad Sci USA 89:4850–4854
11. Weinberg RA (1991) Tumor suppressor genes. Science 254:1138–1146
12. Strauss BS (1992) The origin of point mutations in human tumor cells. Cancer Res 52:249–253
13. Kinzler KW, Nilbert MC, Su LK, Vogelstein B, Bryan TM, Levy DB, Smith KJ et al. (1991) Identification of FAP locus genes from chromosome 5q21. Science 253:661–665
14. Olschwang S, Laurent-Puig P, Groden J, White R, Thomas G (1993) Germ-line mutations in the first 14 exons of the adenomatous polyposis coli (APC) gene. Am J Hum Genet 52:273–279
15. Sandberg AA, Turc-Carel C, Gemmill RM (1988) Chromosomes in solid tumors and beyond. Cancer Res 48:1049–1059
16. Farber E (1984) The multistep nature of cancer development. Cancer Res 44:4217–4223
17. Lipkin M (1988) Biomarkers of increased susceptibility to gastrointestinal cancer: new application to studies of cancer prevention in human subjects. Cancer Res 48:235–245
18. Morson BC, Whiteway JE, Jones EA, Macrae FA, Williams CB (1984) Histopathology and prognosis of malignant colorectal polyps treated by endoscopic polypectomy. Gut 25:437–444
19. Berenblum I, Shubik P (1947) The role of croton oil applications associated with a single painting of a carcinogen in tumour induction in the mouse's skin. Br J Cancer 1:379–383
20. Hammarberg C, Slezak P, Tribukait B (1984) Early detection of malignancy in ulcerative colitis. Cancer 53:291–295
21. Fearon ER, Vogelstein B (1990) A genetic model for colorectal tumorigenesis. Cell 61:759–767

Genetic Aspects of Diseases: Categories of Genetic Disorders

From the results of a series of straightforward though painstaking experiments, Mendel was able to deduce two fundamental Laws of Genetics. The rediscovery of Mendel's work, and the acceptance of his results, led to the gene mapping techniques that still provide new information about gene structure and organization.

T.A. BROWN (1989)

Introduction: General Aspects

Genetics is the study of heredity, the process by which various characters are transferred from parents to offspring so that human beings, and more generally all living organisms, resemble their ancestors. After the end of the Second World War and the discovery of antibiotics, with the sustained reduction in nutritional and infectious diseases (at least in developed countries) there has been an increasing awareness of the role of genetic factors in human diseases, including neoplasms. At variance with a common belief, genetic disorders are not rare; there are studies indicating that their contribution to total pediatric mortality is in the order of 30%–40% [1, 2], whereas in adults approximately 10% of all hospital admissions are due to genetic diseases. These, however, should be considered as minimum estimates, since the genetic nature of many diseases (in particular neoplasms) is becoming more and more apparent [3].

Genetics as a distinct discipline originated with Gregor Mendel in the middle of the nineteenth century. The central concept of heredity is that the transmission of characters is controlled by specific factors, genes, which are discrete physical entities present in all living organisms. Basically, genes are made up of double-stranded DNA complexed with proteins and packed into chromosomes; it is the DNA sequence that contains the complete genetic information [4]. A *locus* is a specific position or location on a chromosome. Different or alternative forms of a gene at a given locus are known as *alleles*. If both alleles at a specific locus are identical, the individual is defined as *homozygous* for that locus; if they are different, the individual is *heterozygous*. The genetic constitution of a given subject (i.e., the DNA sequence and structure) is called the *genotype*. The *phenotype* is the observable expression of a gene, which results from the interaction of the genotype with environmental factors. A *mutation* is a stable and heritable alteration of the nucleotide sequence of DNA; mutations may be silent, in which case there is no discernible effect on the cell or the organism. Alternatively, they can affect gene transcription and alter gene products, with the consequence of generating an observable change in the phenotype.

A mendelian (or *monogenic*) disease is the result of a single gene mutation that has a visible or measurable effect on the phenotype and that is inherited in a simple pattern, as originally described by Gregor Mendel in garden peas. Disorders caused by single mutant genes can show one of the following three simple patterns of inheritance: (1) autosomal dominant, (2) autosomal recessive, or (3) X-linked. The term "*dominant*" implies that the trait (or disease) will be phenotypically evident when the individual has a single dose of the mutation (i.e., the condition is expressed in heterozygotes). In contrast, "*recessive inheritance*" means that a double dose is necessary for clinical detection (the condition, therefore, will be clinically evident only in homozygotes for the mutant alleles). It is worth noting that dominance and recessivity refer to phenotypes, not to genes; genes are never dominant or recessive (although we often speak of dominant or recessive genes), but their expression produces clinical patterns that can be classified as dominant or recessive. Mendelian diseases are defined as *autosomal* when the mutant gene is located on one of the 22 pairs of autosomes, and X-*linked* when the mutant gene is on the X chromosomes. If a disease shows one of the three mendelian patterns of inheritance, this implies that its pathogenetic events, even if apparently complex, can be attributed to the abnormality of a single protein molecule. This has been shown for sickle cell anemia and cystic fibrosis [5, 6], but the demonstration remains elusive for the large majority of clinical conditions, including familial and hereditary neoplasms.

Gregor Mendel was able to deduce the fundamental laws of genetics through a series of experiments carried out by cross-fertilizing plants of garden peas (*Pisum sativum*). The close observation of the appearance in the progeny plants of various pairs of characteristics (tall or short stem, round or wrinkled peas, violet or white flowers) led to the following conclusions: (a) individual genes are present as pairs of alleles at a single locus; (b) segregation of alleles is a random event; (c) Different pairs of alleles tend to segregate independently. These concepts anticipated several aspects of molecular genetics and still represent the basic knowledge for a proper understanding of monogenic inheritance at a clinical level [7].

Autosomal Dominant Inheritance

Autosomal dominant disorders are clinically manifest in the heterozygous state, i.e., when only one of the two alleles is mutated and the corresponding allele on the homologous chromosome is normal. By definition, the genes

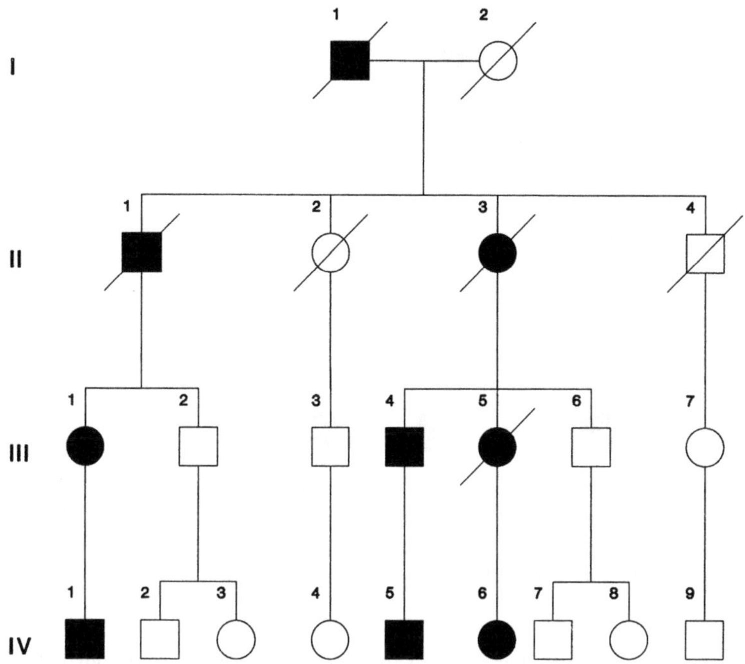

Fig. 1. Representative pedigree of a family with an autosomal dominant disease. *Black squares* indicate affected individuals

responsible for these disorders are located on one of the 22 autosomes. Since homozygous affected individuals are extremely rare in these disorders, the most common mating is that between a normal homozygous subject and a heterozygous affected individual. Since alleles segregate independently at meiosis, there is a one in two chances that the offspring of an affected individual will inherit the mutant or the normal allele. Thus, on average, about half of the progeny will be affected and half will be normal.

The typical pedigree pattern for an autosomal dominant disorder can be seen in Fig. 1. The following characteristics should be noted: (a) males and females are affected approximately in equal proportions; (b) each affected individual has one of the parents similarly affected (with the exception of new mutations); (c) affected individuals should have both normal and affected offspring in equal proportion; (d) normal individuals should have only normal offspring; (e) the disorder can be transmitted with equal probability through male or female individuals.

Thus, the general pattern of inheritance is that of vertical transmission through successive generations (with no skipped generations), especially when the disease does not interfere with the reproductive capacity. This type of genetic transmission, however, is not always as easily detectable as

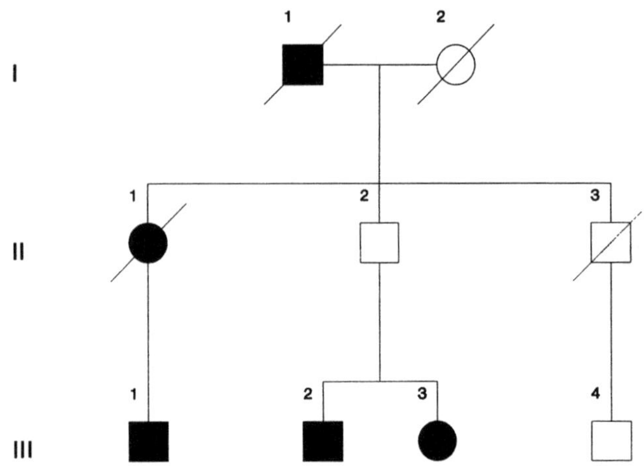

Fig. 2. Example of nonpenetrance in the genealogical tree of a family with an autosomal dominant disorder. Subject II-2 is clinically unaffected, but is an obligate carrier of the mutant allele, since both his offspring are affected. *Black squares* indicate affected individuals

in Fig. 1, and this for several important reasons. First, with the small size of many modern families all the offspring of an affected individual could either be normal or affected just by chance. Second, virtually in every autosomal dominant disorder a certain fraction of affected individuals acquires the disease because of a new rather than an inherited mutation; in this case, affected subjects will have normal parents. In the extreme case in which a dominant mutation induces absolute infertility, all the observed cases are necessarily new mutations, and it would be difficult to prove the genetic nature of the disease. Third, autosomal dominant disorders frequently show variable expressivity, i.e., the same mutated gene can result in phenotypic changes which exhibit a varied degree of severity in different individuals. One of the best example of variable expressivity is observed in neurofibromatosis 1 (see the chapter on "Hereditary Tumors of the Nervous System"), in which clinical manifestations can range from the simple presence of cutaneous spots to disfiguring neurofibromas or severe deformities with functional impairment. Fourth, an affected individual might apparently have normal parents or offspring as the result of reduced penetrance. The degree of penetrance of a gene is given by the proportion of individuals possessing the gene in whom some manifestations of the gene can be found. Thus, a gene will be fully penetrant when all individuals carrying the gene itself show evidence of its expression. At the other extreme, the lack of penetrance of a gene can give origin to skipped generations. While Fig. 1 shows the example of a fully penetrant trait, the pedigree in Fig. 2 illustrates nonpenetrance in an obligate carrier. Although the pattern of inheritance is clearly autosomal dominant, the second member of the second generation (II-2) is at variance with all the others. In fact, II-2 is an obligate heterozygote (and thus carrier of the mutated gene), because he has an affected parent and two affected offspring; however, as a result of reduced penetrance, II-2 had no history and showed no clinical manifestations of the disease. Fifth, autosomal dominant conditions may show a delayed age of onset. This occurs typically in Huntington disease, a degenerative neurologic disorder characterized by choreic movements and progressive dementia. Since the average age of onset is 35–40 years, a gene carrier may have children and die from unrelated causes before showing signs of the disease. Other examples of late onset diseases include polycystic kidney disease and adenomatosis coli (see the chapter on "Hereditary Gastrointestinal Polyposis Syndrome"). Finally, it is worth noting that delayed onset is one of the factors which stabilize or even increase the frequency of some genetic diseases; in fact, the mutant gene may spread within the population, since individuals do not become affected until they have passed the mutant gene to the next generation.

Autosomal Recessive Inheritance

At variance with dominant diseases, autosomal recessive conditions are characterized by clinical manifestations only when the responsible gene is present in double dose (homozygous state). The two sexes will be affected with equal probability. Usually, affected subjects have parents who are heterozygous for the given gene but absolutely healthy; similarly, providing that the affected individual has not married a person heterozygous for the same gene, his or her offspring will be healthy, although all of them are necessarily heterozygous carriers of the gene. In the extremely rare condition of two homozygotes for the same recessive gene having children together, all their offspring will be homozygotes and consequently affected. As far as the offspring of two clinically normal heterozygous individuals are concerned, there are two in four chances that they will be homozygous, either normal or affected, and two in four chances that they will be heterozygous for that gene and therefore healthy carriers like their parents.

A typical pedigree of an autosomal recessive condition is shown in Fig. 3. The pattern of inheritance is markedly different from autosomal dominant disorders, in the sense that there is no vertical transmission and that the presence of affected individuals is limited to one generation, often within one sibship. Of course in extended pedigrees more affected patients in various generations can be detected, but between affected individuals there are necessarily one or more generations of healthy persons (some of them heterozygous carriers of the gene).

The probability that two individuals heterozygous for the same mutant allele will have children together is closely dependent on the frequency of gene carriers (heterozygotes) in the general population. If the mutant gene

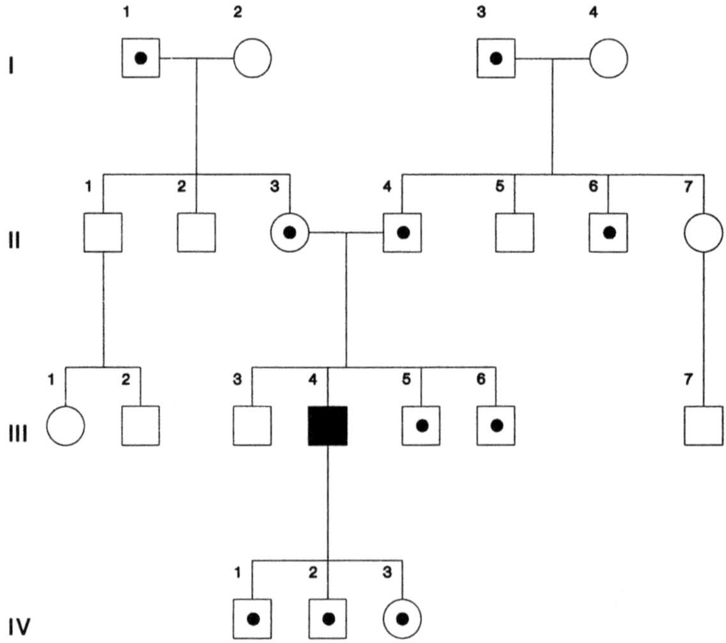

Fig. 3. Representative pedigree of a family with an autosomal recessive trait. The parents of the affected patient are obligate carriers of the mutant allele; similarly, all his offspring are heterozygotes for that specific gene. *Black squares* indicate affected individuals and *black dots* unaffected carriers of the gene

is rare, there will be a low probability of mating between two heterozygous individuals; however, this probability may increase consistently in the case of consanguinity (mating between close relatives, usually cousins), when family members may have inherited the mutant gene from a common ancestor. If, on the other hand, the gene is relatively frequent in a population (as in the case of cystic fibrosis in most Western countries), then mating of individuals heterozygous for that gene will be more common and consanguinity can be found less frequently.

Autosomal recessive disorders are in general less easily detectable than dominant diseases, either because of the features of this kind of genetic disorder (horizontal pattern rather than vertical transmission) or the small size of many modern families. Indeed, since the risk that a child will be affected if both parents are heterozygotes is only one in four, it follows that the large majority of people affected by autosomal recessive disorders appear as sporadic cases, without any family history suggestive of a genetic disease.

The diagnosis and recognition of autosomal recessive diseases is often based on biochemical analysis and, more recently, on biomolecular investigations. In Tay-Sachs disease (an autosomal recessive disorder characterized by blindness, mental retardation, and death in childhood) for instance, the basic defect is the absence in affected persons of the lysosomal enzyme hexosaminidase A. Normal parents of affected individuals have approximately half the normal activity of this enzyme; it follows that the complete or partial enzyme deficiency can be used for diagnosing the homozygous or the heterozygous state and, even more interestingly, may be detected in amniotic fluid cells, thus allowing an accurate prenatal diagnosis. Cystic fibrosis is the most common lethal inherited disorder in the white population of most Western countries. The syndrome is featured by viscous secretions, especially in the pancreas and lung, and by an abnormal electrolyte composition of sweat. Recently, the cystic fibrosis gene was identified and sequenced; it is predicted to encode a 1480-amino acid protein called cystic fibrosis transmembrane conductance regulator [8, 9]. The discovery of naturally occurring deleterious gene mutations not only gave insight into the function of several proteins but, even more relevantly, allows the possibility of detecting heterozygous individuals; these people can now obtain information on their state before starting a family.

X-Linked Inheritance (Recessive or Dominant)

X-linked recessive traits are caused by mutant genes on the X chromosome and become manifest in the homozygous or hemizygous state. Since women have two X chromosomes, if there is a mutant recessive gene in one of them the deleterious effect of the gene can be counterbalanced by the normal allele on the other X chromosome. It follows that women will manifest the trait only in the homozygous state, which is usually a rare event. Much more commonly, women will be healthy carriers of the trait but remain at risk of having affected sons. Men, however, have only one X-chromosome, so that they will always manifest an X-linked mutant gene, even if recessive, owing to the lack of the normal ("wild-type") allele which counteracts its effect. In other words, all male individuals who inherit the mutant X-linked gene are affected.

The transmission of these traits within families is rather peculiar; if the disease is so severe as to cause the death of affected males before the reproductive period, the trait will be transmitted through healthy female carriers (Fig. 4). This is the case, for example, in Duchenne muscular dystrophy and Lesch-Nyhan syndrome. On the other hand, if affected individuals survive into the reproductive period, the disease can be transmitted by both female carriers and affected males (Fig. 5), as occurs in partial color blindness and hemophilia. Considering the example of Figs. 4 and 5, it is clear that all the sons of an affected male will be normal, since they inherit their only X chromosome from the mother. In contrast, all daughters will be obligate carriers, since they inherit one of the two X chromosomes from

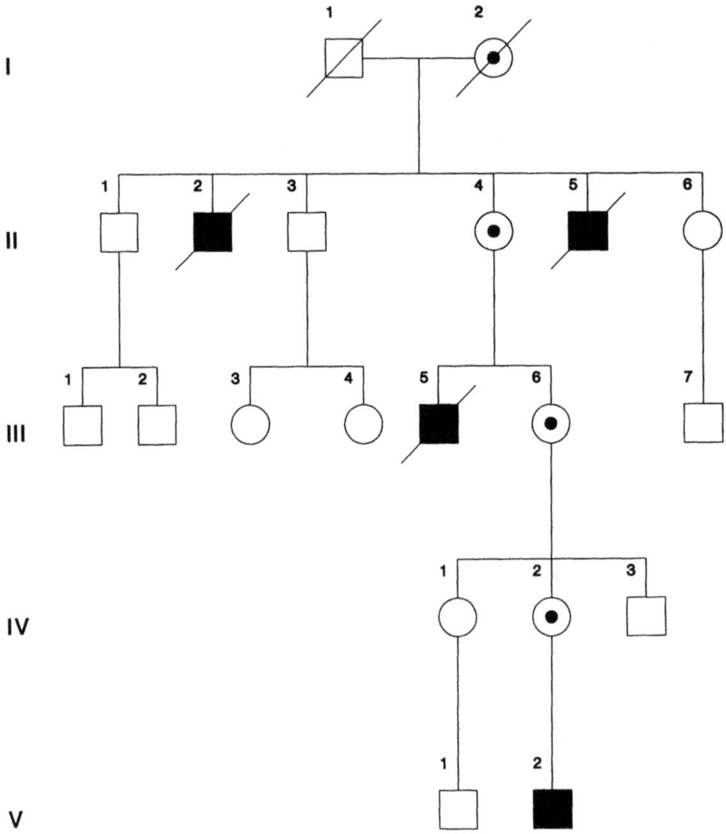

Fig. 4. Genealogical tree of a family with an X-linked recessive trait. The disease is transmitted through healthy female carriers, but only male individuals will be affected. *Black squares* indicate affected individuals and *black dots* unaffected carriers of the gene

their father. If follows that an X-linked trait does not tend to be transmitted from father to son.

On rare occasions, women may show manifestations of a disease thought to be inherited as an X-linked recessive trait. For example, deficiency of the enzyme glucose-6-phosphate-dehydrogenase may be found in about 1% of black women; similarly, some 8% of known carriers of Duchenne muscular dystrophy show symptoms of the disease. There are several possible explanations for this. First, if the mutant allele is common we can expect to find homozygous females with reasonable frequency. Second, a female might be hemizygous for the X chromosome, as in Turner syndrome, in which there are 45 chromosomes and only one X. Third, the expression of an X-linked trait in a woman can be the consequence of rare chromosomal rearrangements, involving translocations between the X chromosome and

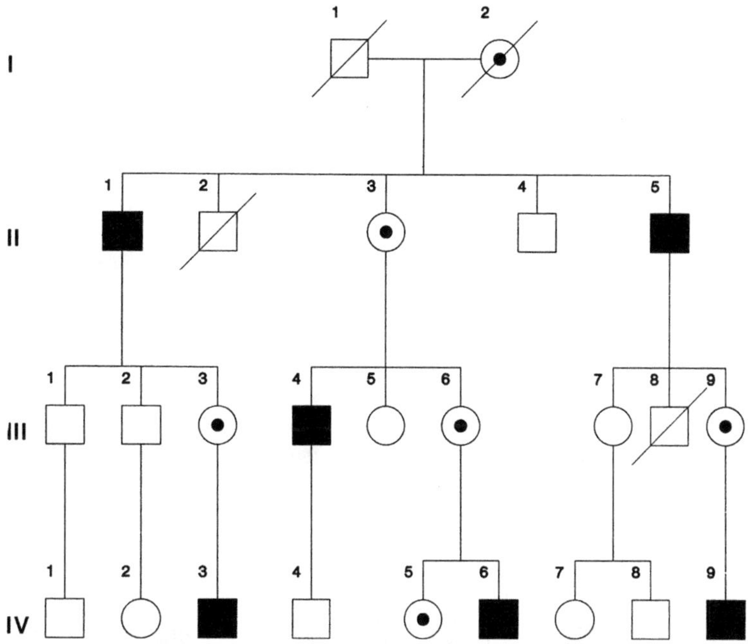

Fig. 5. Representative pedigree for an X-linked condition in which affected individuals reach the reproductive period; the disease can be transmitted by both female carriers and affected males. *Black squares* indicate affected individuals and *black dots* unaffected carriers of the gene

an autosome, thus resulting in loss of X-chromosomal material. Finally, although all cells in human females contain two X chromosomes, only one of them is functionally active, since one of them is randomly and permanently inactivated during embryiogenesis (lyonization) [10]. The manifestation of an X-linked disorder in a female, therefore, might be due to the fact that, by chance, most of the active X chromosomes bear the mutant allele.

Hypophosphatemic (or vitamin D-resistant) rickets and oral–facial–digital syndrome are examples of X-linked dominant inheritance (Fig. 6). A feature of these syndromes is the absolute absence of male-to-male transmission. At variance with the recessive type, in dominant X-linked disorders females are also affected and the ratio of affected males to females is approximately 1:2, reflecting the ratio of X chromosomes in the two sexes. Thus, the mutant gene is transmitted by affected women to half of their daughters and by affected men to all their daughters. Similarly, the disorders are transmitted by affected females to half of their sons, whereas all the sons of affected men will be normal. These pedigrees (Fig. 6) may resemble autosomal dominant family trees; however, the excess of affected

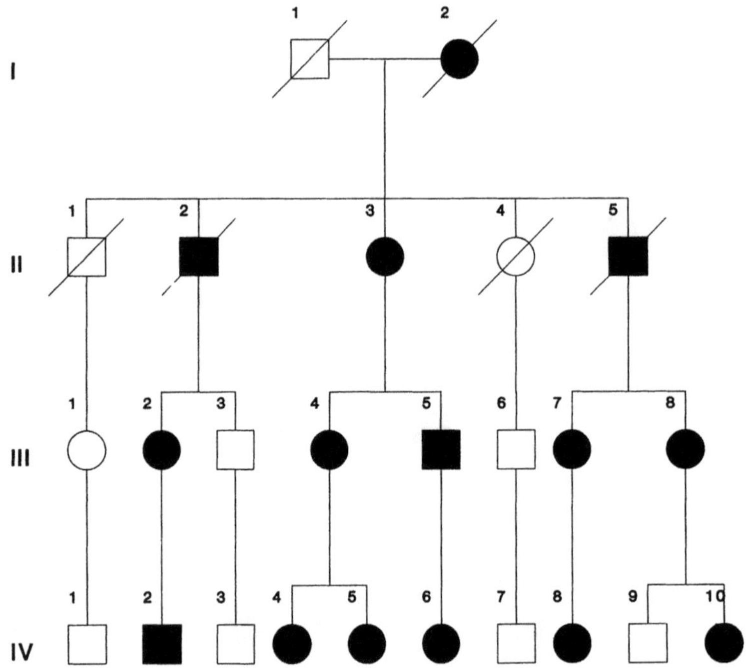

Fig. 6. Example of X-linked dominant inheritance. The resemblance to fully penetrant autosomal transmission (see Fig. 1) is evident. However, there is no male-to-male transmission and the ratio of affected males to females is approximately 1:2. *Black squares* indicate affected individuals

women and the absence of male-to-male transmission can lead to the correct diagnosis of X-linked dominant disorders.

Recessive disorders, either autosomal or X-linked, are often the result of enzymatic defects, and this means that for many enzymes 50% of their activity is compatible with a normal life (heterozygotes are usually asymptomatic) or at least sufficient to prevent the development of diseases. In contrast, autosomal dominant conditions frequently show abnormalities of nonenzymatic proteins, such as hemoglobin or collagen.

Multifactorial Inheritance

Many common diseases occur more frequently among relatives of affected individuals than in the general population. Essential hypertension, coronary heart disease, diabetes mellitus, and peptic ulcer are only a few examples of common disorders which "run in families." In these diseases, however, the genetic component does not manifest itself in an all-or-nothing fashion as in monogenic disorders; instead the familial aggregation has to be attributed to a close interaction between multiple genes and various environmental factors. In monogenic inheritance, the risk to the siblings of an affected individual is in the order of 0.5 (50%) in the case of a fully penetrant dominant trait or 0.25 (25%) in the case of recessive conditions. If the risk of being affected is in the order of 0.01–0.1 (0.1%–10%) for the siblings of various generations, the monogenic model can provide an explanation for the inheritance of the trait only if we assume a greatly reduced penetrance. Alternatively, other types of inheritance should be considered, including the multifactorial model.

In disorders which are considered multifactorial, there is a polygenic component featured by a series of genes cumulatively interacting. By inheriting a given combination of these genes, the individual acquires a certain level of risk for a specific disease; at this point one or more environmental factors (often poorly defined) will determine whether and to what extent the person is affected. If other members of the family inherit the same series of genes and are exposed to the same environmental component, it is likely that they will express the same syndrome. First-degree relatives of affected persons – with whom they share half of the genes and often a series of environmental factors – are all at increased risk of showing the same disease. More distant relatives share, progressively, a smaller fraction of genes; it follows that as the degree of relation becomes more distant, the probability of a relative inheriting the same combination of genes – and thus of being exposed to the risk of the disease – tends to reduce.

The multifactorial model has been of great use for a proper understanding of various familial aggregations which did not fit the mendelian models. It should be noted, however, that this type of inheritance is less "desirable" than monogenic transmission, both for research purposes and genetic counselling. In fact, the multifactorial model presupposes that a given phenotype results from the combined effect of several genes interacting with a series of environmental factors.

It is extremely difficult to unravel this complex interaction in order to define the responsible genes and to characterize the biochemical defect. In contrast, in monogenic disorders a specific locus can be sought through linkage studies and this may lead to the subsequent cloning and sequencing of the gene. Moreover, tests can be developed (either biochemical or biomolecular) and then applied for the identification of heterozygotes and, more generally for the early detection of individuals at risk [8, 9, 11–14]. All this remains elusive for multifactorial disease, where for purposes of counseling the most accurate estimate of the risk for relatives of affected individuals is the use of empirical risks obtained from studying many families and a suitable control group.

For several diseases, multifactorial inheritance and monogenic transmission are not mutually exclusive; in fact, among common phenotypes which are usually considered multifactorial, often a smally proportion of them can be determined by single gene mutations. The best-known example remains coronary heart disease, which is usually considered to be of multifactorial origin; however, approximately 5% of these patients are heterozygous for familial hypercholesterolemia, a monogenic disorder characterized by atherosclerosis and premature myocardial infarction. Similarly, although the large majority of colorectal neoplasms can be considered sporadic or of multifactorial origin, in about 5% of these patients an autosomal dominant disorder has been identified (hereditary nonpolyposis colorectal cancer, or Lynch syndrome, characterized by early onset cancer of the proximal colon, multiple primaries, and frequent association with early onset tumors of other organs; see the chapter on "Hereditary and Familial Colorectal Cancer") [15]. Other examples include peptic ulcer and essential hypertension.

Genetic Heterogeneity

As already discussed, for many common diseases the multifactorial inheritance does not exclude the possible role of monogenic factors, at least in a fraction of affected individuals. This is an example of genetic heterogeneity, an event extremely frequent in human inherited diseases. Basically, genetic heterogeneity implies that different mutations can cause identical or similar phenotypes. More specifically, we can differentiate allelic heterogeneity (different mutations at the same locus) from locus heterogeneity (mutations at different loci). One of the most often cited examples of genetic heterogeneity is the group of Ehlers-Danlos syndromes, disorders of the connective tissue characterized by loose joints, hyperelastic skin, and abnormalities of blood vessels. There are at least six different Ehlers-Danlos syndromes which are inherited with an autosomal dominant type of genetic transmission. This clinical variability is truly genetic, and it is not due to the variable clinical expressivity of a single genotype. Moreover, there are other forms of the syndrome which are transmitted with an autosomal recessive or even X-linked type of inheritance. This extremely variable pattern of transmission clearly indicates that mutations at different loci can produce a similar phenotype. Although less extensively studied, genetic heterogeneity is also common in hereditary tumors; in fact, allelic heterogeneity has been reported in Li-Fraumeni syndrome [16] and in adenomatosis coli [13, 14].

Segregation Analysis

In theory, single-gene disorders should segregate in families according to the predicted mendelian ratios. Thus, for an autosomal recessive disorder one should expect that one in four siblings of two heterozygous parents will be affected. Similarly, for a fully penetrant autosomal disease the expectation is that half of the offspring of an affected individual will carry the mutant gene, thus showing manifestations of the disorder. Finally, in multifactorial inheritance we should be able to document only an increased risk among first-degree relatives. In clinical practice, however, things are much more complex for several reasons: (a) possible reduced penetrance; (b) variable expressivity; (c) late onset of the disease; (d) small size of families; (e) genetic heterogeneity; and (f) inaccuracy of clinical reports. Segregation analyses have been developed in order to solve, at least in part, some of these problems. The main objective of this type of analysis is to test statistically whether a given disease conforms to the expected segregation ratio for a presumed type of genetic transmission. The only way to obtain data for segregation analysis is to find families in which the investigated disease is clinically manifest; however, this search inevitably introduces one of the main problems in this kind of analysis, i.e., to correct for bias which occurs in the selection of families. If the researcher is interested only in the segregation ratio, then simple methods can be used either for dominant or for recessive disorders [17–19]. More complex approaches were developed by Morton, Elston, and coworkers ("maximum likelihood") (20–22).

Chromosomal Disorders

Normal individuals have 46 chromosomes (in each nucleated cell), of which 44 are the 22 pairs of autosomes and the remaining two are the sex chromosomes. Each of the 22 pairs of autosomes and the two sex chromosomes can be distinguished because of their size, localization of the centromere (which divides the chromosome into arms of equal or unequal length), and the characteristic banding pattern (after staining with dyes such as quinacrine hydrochloride or Giemsa). Human chromosomes can be divided in seven groups (A–G) in relation to the length of the arms and the position of centromeres. The long arm is designated q, the short arm p. If the centromere lies in the middle of the chromosome (so that the two arms are of equal length), this is called metacentric. In submetacentric chromosomes, the centromere is somewhat distant from the center (arms of unequal length); in acrocentric chromosomes, the centromere is near the end, so that p arms are very short ("satellites"). By convention, the banding pattern of each chromosome is numbered from the centromere to the terminal portion of the two arms. In the karyotype, chromosomes are arranged according to the above-mentioned criteria. When describing a karyotype, we first list the number of autosomes, followed by the sex chromosome constitution and then by various abnormalities (if any). Thus, the normal male or female karyotype will be designated as 44, XY and 44, XX, respectively. Haploid (n) is the number of chromosomes in a nurmal gamete, diploid (2n) is the number of chromosomes in a normal somatic cell and euploid refers in general to any exact multiple of n. The term "aneuploid" indicates any deviation from euploidy and often refers to extra copies of one chromosome (trisomy) or to the lack of a single chromosome (monosomy).

Chromosomal abnormalities may be numerical or structural. Numerical abnormalities include trisomy, monosomy, and other changes of euploidy; aneuploidy is a consequence of nondisjunction or failure of two homologous chromosomes to separate normally during mitosis. Structural abnormalities may be of various types and involve either one or more chromosomes. Thus, there are deletions (loss of chromosomal material), duplications of a portion of the chromosome, inversion of a chromosomal fragment, and translocations (i.e., breakage and reunion of pieces of chromosomes).

There is an increasing interest in chromosomal abnormalities in human cancer. Neoplastic transformation and tumor progression have been associated with a series of genetic changes that in many cases are secondary events. At a cytogenetic level, chromosomal translocations, deletions, and other changes have frequently been reported, and there is an urgent need to integrate these findings in the molecular events of carcinogenesis. As an example, in adenomatosis coli, it was a cytogenetic observation [23], followed by a series of biomolecular studies [24], which led to the identification of the adenomatosis coli gene.

References

1. Roberts DF, Chavez J, Court SDM (1970) The genetic component in child mortality. Arch Dis Child 45:33–38
2. Carter CO (1956) Changing patterns in the causes of death at the Hospital for Sick Children. Great Ormond St J 11:65–68
3. Ponz de Leon M, Scapoli C, Zanghieri G, Sassatelli R, Sacchetti C, Barrai I (1992) Genetic transmission of colorectal cancer: exploratory data anlysis from a population based registry. J Med Genet 29:531–538
4. Albert B, Bray D, Lewis J, Raff M, Roberts K, Watson JD (1989) Molecular biology of the cell. Garland, New York
5. Boat TF, Welsh MJ, Beaudet AL (1989) Cystic fibrosis. In: Scriver CL, Beaudet AL, Dly WS, Valle D (eds) (1989) The metabolic basis of inherited disease, 6th edn. McGraw-Hill, New York, pp 264–280
6. Quinton PM (1990) Cystic fibrosis: a disease in electrolyte transport. FASEB J 4:2709–2717
7. McKusick VA (1969) Human genetics, 2nd edn. Englewood Cliffs, Prentice-Hall
8. Rommens JM, Iannuzzi MC, Kerem B et al. (1989) Identification of the cystic fibrosis gene: chromosome walking and jumping. Science 245:1059–1065
9. Riordan JR, Rommens JM, Kerem B et al. (1989) Identification of the cystic fibrosis gene: cloning and characterization of complementary DNA. Science 245:1066–1073
10. Grant SG, Chapman VM (1988) Mechanisms of X-chromosome regulation. Annu Rev Genet 22:199–233
11. Goldstein JL, Brown MS (1989) Familial hypercholesterolemia. In: Scriver CR, Beaudet AL, Sly WS, Valle D (1989) The metabolic basiss of inherited diseases, 6th edn. McGraw-Hill, New York, pp 1215–1250

12. Gusella JF, Wexler NS, Conneally PM, Naylor SL, Anderson MA, Tanzi RE et al. (1983) A polymorphic DNA marker genetically linked to Huntington's disease. Nature 306:234–238
13. Kinzler KW, Nilbert MC, Su LK, Vogelstein B, Bryan TM, Levy DB et al. (1991) Identification of FAP locus genes from chromosome 5q21. Science 253: 661–665
14. Groden J, Thilveris A, Samowitz W, Carlson M, Gelbert L, Albertsen H et al. (1991) Identification and characterization of the familial adenomatous polyposis coli gene. Cell 66:589–600
15. Lynch HT, Smyrk TC, Watson P et al. (1993) Genetics, natural history, tumor spectrum, and pathology of hereditary non-polyposis colorectal cancer: an updated review. Gastroenterology 104:1535–1539
16. Srivastava A, Tong YA, Devadas K, Zou ZQ, Sykes VW, Blattner WA et al. (1992) Detection of both mutant and wild-type p53 protein in normal skin fibroblasts and demonstration of a shared "second hit" on p53 in diverse tumors from a cancer-prone family with Li-Fraumeni syndrome. Oncogene 7:987–991
17. Gart JJ (1967) A simple nearly efficient alternative to the simple sib method in the complete ascertainment case. Annu Hum Genet 31:283–291
18. Li CC, Mantel N (1968) A simple method of estimating the segregation ratio under complete ascertainment. J Hum Genet 20:61–68
19. Fisher RA (1934) The effects of methods of ascretainment upon the estimation of frequencies. Annu Eugen 6:13–25
20. Morton NE (1959) Genetic tests under incomplete ascertainment. Am J Hum Genet 11:1–6
21. Morton NE, Yee S, Lew R (1971) Complex segregation analysis. Am J Hum Genet 23:602–611
22. Elston RC (1979) Major locus analysis for quantitative traits. Am J Hum Genet 31:655–663
23. Herrera L, Kakati S, Gibas L, Pietrzak E, Sandberg AA (1986) Brief clinical report: Gardner syndrome in a man with an interstitial deletion of 5q. Am J Med Genet 25:473–476
24. Bodmer WF, Bailey CJ, Bodmer J, Bussey HJR, Ellis A, Gorman P (1987) Localization of the gene for familail adenomatous polyposis on chromosome 5. Nature 328:614–619

Biomarkers of Increased Susceptibility to Cancer

The ability to detect markers of biologic activity that reflect not evidence of, but the potential for, neoplastic progression, may help clinicians to predict individual cancer risk and devise rational strategies to reduce or eliminate that risk.

PETER GREENWALD et al. (1992)

Introduction

Tumor markers can be defined, in general terms, as biological indicators of the presence of cancer. These markers can be found in the tumor itself – and revealed using biochemical, immunologic, or histochemical techniques – or, more often, can be detected in excessive quantities in the blood of patients with cancer. Carcinoembryonic antigen, α-fetoprotein, acid phosphatase, and polyamines are well-known examples of tumor markers frequently used in clinical practice. Moreover, in recent years several other compounds (CA-19-9, CA-125, and many others) of potential interest have been investigated [1, 2]. Though sometimes of value in evaluating the extent of the disease and in monitoring the response to treatment, tumor markers are of little or no value in the early detection of cancer and in the definition of the risk profile of unaffected individuals.

At variance with classical tumor markers, biomarkers of increased susceptibility to cancer are specifically related to the earlier stages of tumorigenesis, including premorphologic and preneoplastic changes. Investigation in this area basically consists in the identification of biological factors or functions whose changes parallel the evolution of neoplasms from the initial, often premorphologic, derangement of cell replication, maturation, and organization to the frank neoplastic phenotype. It follows that the evaluation of these biomarkers might allow us to define a risk profile, at least in certain tumors; moreover, genetic susceptibility to the development of tumors, especially of the digestive organs, can be revealed and assessed with the proper use of some of these biological markers [3, 4]. Several commonly used markers of susceptibility to cancer refer to various aspects of cell biology, and will be reviewed in this chapter; the emerging role of molecular biology and molecular genetics in the field of cancer susceptibility will be discussed in the following chapter 4.

Many morphologic abnormalities should be included by definition among biomarkers of increased susceptibility to cancer. These include dysplastic and metaplastic changes, chronic inflammatory conditions, and various types of polyps. Conventionally, however, these lesions have been referred to as pathologic changes more than biomarkers. The role of precancerous conditions in hereditary and familial tumors will be discussed separately for neoplasms of various organs.

Cell Proliferation

Since cancer is basically a disorder of cell growth and differentiation, it is not surprising that in the search of biomarkers of increased susceptibility to neoplasms, cell replication has been one of the most extensively investigated areas. Figure 1 outlines the main events of the cell cycle. Proliferating cells move clockwise around the cycle; just after division, the cell which is committed to a further division enters the G-1 stage, whereas other cells enter a resting phase called G-0. A cell in G-1 subsequently moves to the S phase, during which its DNA is duplicated, and then through a G-2 phase to mitosis. In the last few years, a general model of cell cycle control in eukaryotic cells has been proposed [5].

There are several techniques currently available for measurement of cell replication in human tissues, including: (a) mitotic count; (b) assessment of thymidine or bromodeoxyuridine incorporation during the S phase; (c) the evaluation of S-phase fraction by flow cytometry; (d) Ki-67 or PCNA (proliferating cell nuclear antigen) labeling index; and (e) measurement of nucleolar organizer regions (AgNors) [6–10]. Although all these techniques have drawbacks and limitations, they have contributed significantly to our increased knowledge of the modifications of cell proliferation and differentiation that occur in disorders or conditions which predispose to cancer.

One of the best models of cell replication as a biomarker of increased susceptibility to cancer is given by the digestive organs; the model was first described by Lipkin, Deschner, and coworkers [11, 12] and subsequently evaluated by many other authors [13–16]. In esophageal, gastric, and colonic mucosa, undifferentiated precursor cells proliferate in the deep portions of

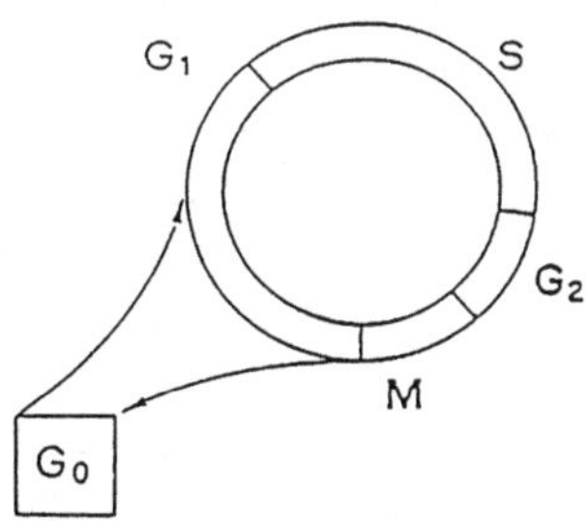

Fig. 1. The four successive phases of a typical eukaryotic cell cycle. The duration of a cell cycle may vary from less than 8 h to several days or months in adult animals. Most of the variability is in the length of the G-1 phase

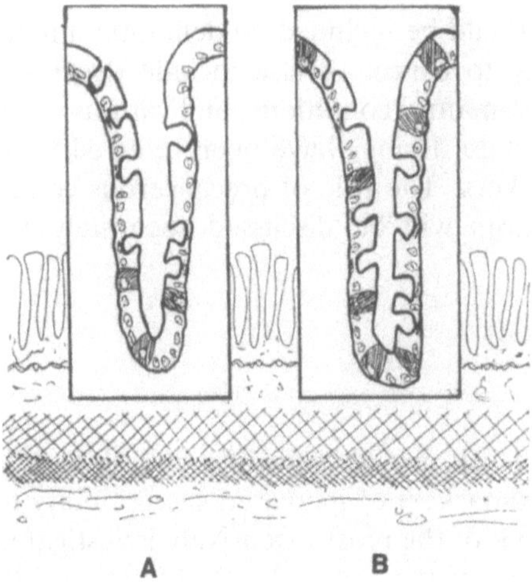

Fig. 2A,B. Cell replication in colorectal mucosa. **A** Replicating cells (darkly stained) are limited to the lower portion of the crypt. **B** There is an expansion of the proliferative compartment to the whole gland and the luminal surface

the epithelium; as these cell migrate to the most superficial (luminal) portions of the crypts, they undergo morphological and functional differentiation, stop their replication, and eventually are extruded in the lumen. In disorders that predispose to gastrointestinal cancer, this process is no longer as strictly regulated and the cell cycle control mechanisms are somehow modified; this leads to a continued synthesis of DNA in maturing cells and to a delayed terminal differentiation.

One of the consequences is the expansion of the proliferative zone, which is no longer confined to the deep regions of the gastrointestinal mucosa (Fig. 2). Thus, immature S-phase cells appear at the surface of the mucosa and directly contact the luminal content. As replicating cells are particularly susceptible to the mutational effect of various agents, this process might ultimately lead to cancer development.

In accordance with this model, various acquired diseases of the esophagus or stomach which are clinically related to an increased risk of carcinoma show an absolute increase in replicating cells with an expansion of the proliferative compartments [17, 18]. Similar changes can be observed in apparently normal colonic mucosa of patients with sporadic adenomas or with inflammatory bowel diseases [19, 20]. Moreover, the same extension of the proliferative zone of colorectal mucosa to the most superficial portions of the crypt has also been reported in familial polyposis [3, 4, 21], an autosomal dominant disorder in which the responsible gene (adenomatous polyposis coli, APC) has recently been isolated [22, 23] (see later chapter). It is tempting to speculate that the APC gene function might be related to the control of cell replication in the large bowel mucosa and that mutations of the gene could lead to loss of this function with consequent derangement of cell replication, expansion of the proliferative zone, and early development of polyps disseminated in the various intestinal segments. Finally, these premorphologic changes are not limited to large bowel mucosa; thus, in precancerous lesions of the cervix, a similar increase of cell replication with expansion of the proliferative zone has been observed [24].

In addition to epithelia, cell replication may also be a useful biomarker of increased susceptibility to cancer in different tissues; for example, a recent report suggests that cirrhotic livers showing a high proliferative rate are more prone to develop hepatocellular carcinoma than livers with the same architectural changes but with a relatively low replicative activity [25].

A new biomarker of increased predisposition to colorectal cancer has recently been characterized in animal and human intestine. In experimental colonic tumorigenesis, shortly after treatment with a given carcinogen, darkly stained (with methylene blue), enlarged, and slightly elevated crypts can be observed against the background of normal crypts on the mucosal surface (Fig. 3). These lesions have been referred to as aberrant crypts and, when associated to dysplasia, as microadenomas [26]. In normal colonic mucosa of patients with familial polyposis, the average number of aberrant crypt foci per cm^2 is significantly higher than in normal mucosa of unaffected individuals [27], thus suggesting that these lesions might be precursors of adenomatous polyps (and colorectal carcinoma) and a valuable mucosal marker of an increased risk for these neoplasms.

Flow Cytometric Analysis of Nuclear Ploidy

Flow cytometry has become the technique of choice for a rapid DNA analysis of normal, precancerous, and cancerous cells. Basically, flow cytometers measure and record fluorescence after suspending cells or intact nuclei and staining with an appropriate fluorochrome. Among these, propidium iodide and ethidium bromide are the most commonly used for DNA analysis; moreover, fluorescent molecules, such as fluorescein isothiocyanate, can be attached to virtually any antibody, thus rendering possible the cytometric evaluation of many cellular antigens (and hence specific cell types).

When only a single parameter is evaluated (i.e., DNA content), the results are usually displayed as frequency histograms, in which the absolute number of stained cells (or nuclei) is plotted versus the fluorescence energy (expressed in channel numbers), which in turn is dependent on the amount of DNA. The flow cytometric analysis of DNA content of normal tissues usually shows a major peak, representing cells in G-1, and a smaller second peak, which includes cells in G-2 and M phases; cells in the S phase of the cycle are between the two peaks (Fig. 4A). When an aneuploid cell population is analyzed, this will be visualized by the appearance of one or more "new" peaks (Fig. 4B). Nuclear ploidy is commonly expressed as the DNA

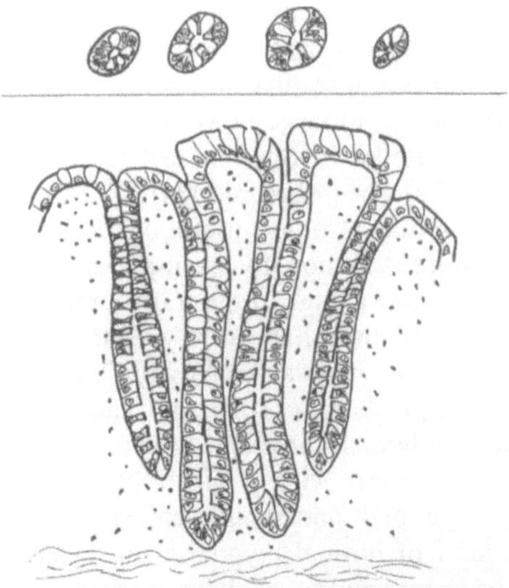

A

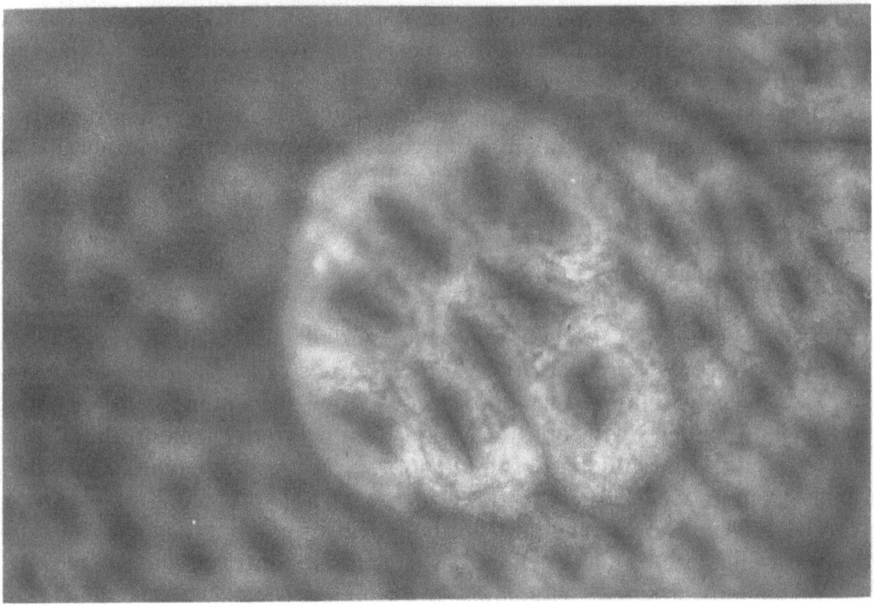

B

Fig. 3. A Aberrant crypt foci in colorectal mucosa; two crypts appear longer than the others and protrude into the lumen. **B** Colonic mucosa observed at low magnification after staining with methylene blue; enlarged and elevated crypt foci are easily recognized against the background of normal crypts

index, a formula which defines the position of histogram peaks in reference to that of the normal diploid peak [28]. Thus, normal tissues and diploid tumors should have a DNA index of 1, whereas aneuploid malignancies usually have DNA indices between 1 and 2.

An abnormal DNA content is frequent in human neoplasms; in solid tumors the fraction of cases showing aneuploidy is in the order of 60%–80%, whereas lymphoproliferative disorders show a more variable pattern

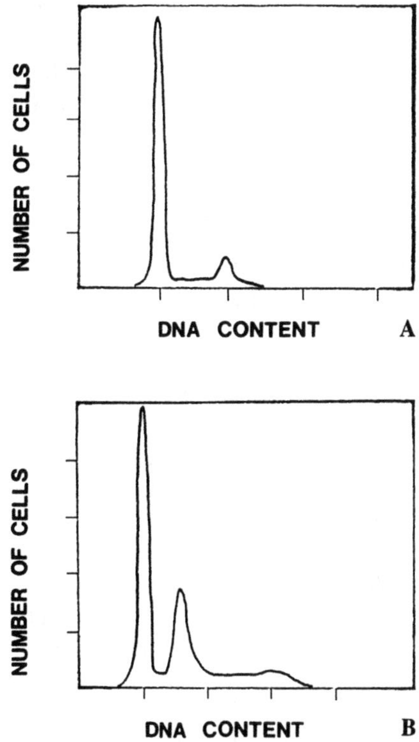

Fig. 4. A Flow cytometric analysis of DNA of human normal (diploid) cells. The major peak corresponds to G-0/G-1 cells and the second peak to G-2/M cells. Cells replicating their DNA (S phase) are between the two peaks. **B** DNA analysis of an aneuploid cell population. A third peak is present, immediately after the G-0/G-1 peak, corresponding to a DNA content between 2n and 4n

[29]. DNA index is usually evaluated as a biological indicator of the clinical outcome; although in most instances aneuploid tumors tend to have a worse prognosis, this is not a general rule, and there are malignancies in which nuclear ploidy does not seem to be related to survival. Moreover, it is still unclear – at least for the most common neoplasms – whether flow cytometric parameters (DNA index and S-phase fraction) provide additional information which can be translated into a more appropriate management of cancer patients [30]. Finally, DNA ploidy might also be of help for the identification of tumors of different etiology: two recent reports suggest that the diploid pattern tends to be more frequent in hereditary colorectal tumors than in sporadic cases (70%–79% versus 20%–30%) [31, 32].

The role of DNA ploidy as a biomarker of increased susceptibility to cancer is still undefined. Aneuploidy, however, is not only a feature of malignant tissue; in fact, some 20%–30% of colonic adenomas show an abnormal DNA index [33, 34], which tends to be correlated to the degree of dysplasia. Moreover, in long-standing quiescent ulcerative colitis or in Crohn disease, aneuploidy has been detected without any apparent relation to dysplasia, thus suggesting the possible use of this variable as an early marker of malignant transformation of the mucosa [35, 36].

DNA Repair

The environment in which we live contains a myriad of physical (ionizing or ultraviolet radiation), chemical (polycyclic aromatic hydrocarbons, aliphatic nitrosamines and many others), and biological (free radicals) factors with a well-defined cancer-inducing activity. The main effect of these agents in tumorigenesis can be attributed to their ability to interact with biologically relevant molecules and, in particular, to cause structural alterations of cellular DNA. Carcinogens usually induce a broad spectrum of DNA lesions, including single- and double-strand breaks, DNA cross-links, substitutions, degradation, and liberation of bases. Ionizing radiations, for example, probably produce more than 100 chemically distinct changes in the four bases and in the sugar moiety of DNA. Similarly, alkylating agents attack specific nucleophilic centers of DNA, leading to several reaction products. Moreover, ultraviolet radiation also induces DNA damage, although the spectrum of these alterations is relatively narrow when compared to other agents [37].

If one considers the importance of DNA integrity for all living organisms, then it is not surprising that cells should possess several enzymatic activities that "repair" the various types of structural modifications in the genetic material. Several DNA repair processes have been described in different cellular systems; some kinds of damage can be repaired directly, i.e., the altered site is returned to normal in situ, without any further modification of DNA. Excision repair, probably the most versatile system, can deal with a large variety of DNA lesions; this process involves several steps, which can be summarized as follows: (a) recognition of the damaged fragment of DNA; (b) incision, near the lesion, by a damage-recognizing endonuclease; (c) excision of a short stretch of nucleotides containing the damaged bases; (d) repair synthesis of the gap formed in one strand using the undamaged complementary strand as a template; and (e) ligation of the newly synthesized DNA with the preexisting DNA termini. A third, more complex and poorly understood repair process is called postreplication repair [38]. Recently, a group of rare hereditary diseases was defined in which a particular susceptibility to the development of tumors seems to be correlated with abnormalities in the DNA repair processes. These disorders – which include xeroderma pigmentosum, ataxia-telangiectasia, Fanconi's anemia, and Bloom's and Cockayne's syndromes – will be discussed in more detail in the chapter on "Cancer-Prone Hereditary Diseases Associated with Abnormalities of DNA Repair."

DNA repair synthesis can also be used as a biomarker of increased susceptibility to cancer. Pero and coworkers recently showed that peripheral blood mononuclear cells from patients with familial polyposis or with sporadic colorectal polyps had significantly lower unscheduled DNA synthesis (i.e., DNA repair) than asymptomatic controls [39]. In this series of experiments, DNA damage was induced by incubating cells with 1μ*M* *N*-acetyl-*N*-2-fluorenil acetamide, whereas the repair was assessed by evaluating labeled thymidine incorporation into DNA. The authors suggested that patients with adenomatous polyps may have a genetic predisposition which makes them more susceptible to environmental carcinogens, since they cannot repair DNA damage as adequately as normal individuals. Moreover, since adenomatous polyps are considered a precursor lesion of colorectal cancer, this deficiency of DNA repair might be a sensitive biomarker of possible value in studying mechanisms of genetic predisposition to malignancies. Similarly, Kovacs et al. evaluated ultraviolet light-induced DNA repair synthesis in peripheral blood lymphocytes of patients with breast cancer [40]; a significant reduction in unscheduled DNA synthesis was found as compared to lymphocytes of normal controls. Finally, Licastro et al. reported a reduced DNA repair synthesis in peripheral blood T lymphocytes from normal individuals of advanced age (77–104 years) [41]. Since aging is by far the most common condition associated with cancer development, we are led to hypothesize that a reduction in the normal capability to adequately repair the cumulative DNA damage might play a role in human tumorigenesis. All these examples stress the importance of DNA repair measurements as a biomarker of increased susceptibility to cancer.

Immune System and Major Histocompatibility Complex

While immunotherapy of human cancer has become an issue of active investigation [42], the basic immunologic characterization of patients with cancer remains unsatisfactory and, consequently, immunologic biomarkers of increased susceptibility to cancer are virtually lacking. The only promising area seems to be that of the human major histocompatibility complex (HLA). This is a cluster of genes localized on the short arm of chromosome 6 occupying approximately 3000 kb of DNA. The proteins encoded by HLA genes are of three main classes (I, II, and III); in general, class I and II protein products are critical for the recognition of foreign antigens and are responsible for the ability of skin graft to survive after transplantation. It follows that the main practical use of HLA typing is the characterization of donors and recipients for tissue and organ transplantation: if there is a good match of antigens, the probability of success is higher. In other words, products of the HLA genes are proteins that are formed on cell membranes and that enable the immune system to distinguish between its own cells and those of other individuals [43].

Class I and II genes are extremely polymorphic and this explains their frequent use in linkage studies. One of the most frequently cited examples is idiopatic hemochromatosis. The gene responsible for this autosomal recessive disease is localized on the short arm of chromosome 6, between the A and the B genes of the class I cluster of HLA. Although the hemochromatosis gene has not yet been cloned and sequenced, when an individual is found to be affected, the risk for siblings can be assessed by studying the linkage to HLA. This is particularly important in this disease, since the identification of unaffected homozygotes (through linkage studies) can be followed by an early treatment of iron overaccumulation in the liver (the main metabolic defect). If untreated, iron overload usually leads to chronic liver disease and eventually to hepatocarcinoma.

For many disorders usually termed autoimmune, a close association has been found between the presence of particular HLA antigens and the risk of the disease itself. Thus, for example, HLA DR3 is particularly frequent (about 50%) in patients with Graves' disease, systemic erythematous lupus, and insulin-dependent diabetes mellitus; similarly, HLA DR2 is closely associated with multiple sclerosis. However, the most striking association is that between the B 27 allele (at the HLA B locus) and ankylosing spondylitis. It has been estimated that if this allele is inherited by an individual, this subject has a 100-fold greater chance of being affected by the disease than a person without the allele. However, ankylosing spondylitis remains a typical multifactorial disease, since the presence of B 27 is not sufficient for the development of the syndrome, other unknown factors being necessary. As a matter of fact, less than 15% of individuals who inherit the allele will develop the disorder.

Despite the fact that some of these associations may appear impressive, their meaning is at present only hypothetical. If the protein encoded by the HLA gene is directly responsible for the increased susceptibility to the disease, then the study of these antigens might be of interest in elucidating the intimate mechanisms of cancer predisposition. If so, the HLA genes (and their expression products) might become valuable biomarkers.

References

1. Torosian MH (1988) The clinical usefulness and limitations of tumor markers. Surg Gynecol Obstet 166:567–579
2. Kane RA, Littrup PJ, Babaian R et al. (1992) Prostate-specific antigen levels in 1965 men withouth evidence of prostate cancer. Cancer 69:1201–1207
3. Deschner E, Lewis CM, Lipkin M (1963) In vitro study of human rectal epithelial cells. I. Atypical zone of H^3-thymidine incorporation in mucosa of multiple polyposis. J Clin Invest 42:1922–1928
4. Deschner EE, Lipkin M (1975) Proliferative patterns in colonic mucosa in familial polyposis. Cancer 35:413–418
5. Kirschner M (1992) The cell cycle then and now. TIBS 17:281–285

6. Quinn CM, Wright NA (1990) The clinical assessment of proliferation and growth in human tumours: evaluation of methods and applications as prognostic variables. J Pathol 160:93–102
7. Hitchcock CL (1991) Ki-67 staining as a means to simplify analysis of tumor cell proliferation. Am J Clin Pathol 96:444–446
8. Jain A, Filipe MI, Hall PA et al. (1991) Prognostic value of proliferating cell nuclear antigen in gastric carcinoma. J Clin Pathol 44:655–659
9. Egan MJ, Crocker J (1992) Nucleolar organiser regions in pathology. Br J Cancer 65:1–7
10. Lacy ER, Kuwayama H, Cowart KS et al. (1991) A rapid, accurate, immunohistochemical method to label proliferating cells in the digestive tract. Gastroenterology 100:259–262
11. Lipkin M (1974) Phase 1 and phase 2 proliferative lesions of colonic epithelial cells in diseases leading to colonic cancer. Cancer 34:878–888
12. Deschner EE, Winawer SJ, Lipkin M (1972) Patterns of nucleic acid and protein synthesis in normal human gastric mucosa and atrophic gastritis. J Natl Cancer Inst 48:1567–1574
13. Bleiberg H, Mainguet P, Galand P (1972) Cell renewal in familial polyposis: comparison between polyps and adjacent healthy mucosa. Gastroenterology 63:240–245
14. Terpstra OT, VanBlankenstein M, Dees M et al. (1987) Abnormal pattern of cell proliferation in the entire colonic mucosa of patients with colon adenoma or cancer. Gastroenterology 92:704–748
15. Ponz de Leon M, Roncucci L, Di Donato P et al. (1988) Pattern of epithelial cell proliferation in colorectal mucosa of normal subjects and of patients with adenomatous polyps or cancer of the large bowel. Cancer Res 48:4121–4126
16. Scalmati A, Roncucci L, Ghidini G et al. (1990) Epithelial cell kinetics in the remaining colorectal mucosa after surgery for cancer in the large bowel. Cancer Res 50:7937–7941
17. Herbst JJ, Berenson MM, McCloskey DW et al. (1978) Cell proliferation in esophageal columnar epithelium (Barrett's esophagus). Gastroenterology 75:683–687
18. Lipkin M, Correa P, Mikol Y et al. (1985) Proliferative and antigenic modifications in epithelial cells in chronic atrophic gastritis. J Natl Cancer Inst 75: 613–619
19. Cole JW, McKalen A (1963) Studies on the morphogenesis of adenomatous polyps in the human colon. Cancer 16:998–1002
20. Biasco G, Lipkin M, Minarini A et al. (1984) Proliferative and antigenic properties of the rectal cells in patients with chronic ulcerative colitis. Cancer Res 44:5450–5454
21. Iwama T, Utsunomiya J, Sasaki J (1977) Epithelial cell kinetics in the crypt of familial polyposis of colon. Jpn J Surg 7:230–234
22. Kinzler KW, Nilbert MC, Su LK et al. (1991) Identification of FAP locul genes from chromosome 5q21. Science 253:661–665
23. Groden J, Thliveris A, Samowitz W et al. (1991) Identification and characterization of the familial adenomatous polyposis coli gene. Cell 66:589–600
24. Schubert B, Kunz J, Banaschak A (1983) Labelling patterns of carcinomas of the cervix and their precancerous stages after ^{3}H-thymidine incorporation. Acta Histochem 27:111–115
25. Tarao K, Shimizu A, Harada M et al. (1989) Difference in the vitro uptake of bromodeoxyuridine between liver cirrhosis with and without hepatocellular carcinoma. Cancer 64:104–109

26. Tudek B, Bird RP, Bruce WR (1989) Foci of aberrant crypts in the colons of mice and rats exposed to carcinogens associated with foods. Cancer Res 49: 1236–1240
27. Roncucci L, Pedroni M, Fante R et al. (1993) Cell kinetic evaluation of human colonic aberrant crypts. Cancer Res 53:3726–3729
28. Shapiro HM (1989) Flow cytometry of DNA content and other indicators of proliferative activity. Arch Pathol Lab Med 113:591–597
29. Barlogie B, Raber MN, Schumann J et al. (1983) Flow cytometry in clinical cancer research. Cancer Res 43:3982–3997
30. Williams NN, Daly JM (1990) Flow cytometry and prognostic implications in patients with solid tumors. Surg Gynecol Obstet 171:257–266
31. Kouri M, Laasonen A, Mecklin JP et al. (1990) Diploid predominance in hereditary nonpolyposis colorectal carcinoma evaluated by flow cytometry. Cancer 65:1825–1829
32. Frei JV (1992) Hereditary nonpolyposis colorectal cancer (Lynch syndrome II). Cancer 69:1108–1111
33. Van den Ingh HF, Griffioen G, Cornelisse CJ (1985) Flow cytometric detection of aneuploidy in colorectal cancer adenomas. Cancer Res 45:3392–3397
34. Sciallero S, Bruno S, Di Vinci A et al. (1988) Flow cytometric DNA ploidy in colorectal adenomas and family history of colorectal cancer. Cancer 61:114–120
35. Löfberg R, Caspersson T, Tribukait B et al. (1989) Comparative DNA analyses in longstanding ulcerative colitis with aneuploidy. Gut 30:1731–1736
36. Löfberg R, Broström O, Karlén P et al. (1991) Carcinoma and DNA aneuploidy in Crohn's colitis: a histological and flow cytometric study. Gut 32:900–904
37. Paterson MC, Gentner NE, Middlestadt MV et al. (1984) Cancer predisposition, carcinogen hypersensivity, and aberrant DNA metabolism. J Cell Physiol 3:45–62
38. Cleaver JE (1980) DNA damage, repair systems and human hypersensitive diseases. J Environ Pathol Toxicol 3:53–68
39. Pero RW, Ritchie M, Winawer SJ et al. (1985) Unscheduled DNA synthesis in mononuclear leukocytes froma patients with colorectal polyps. Cancer Res 45:3388–3391
40. Kovacs E, Stucki D, Weber W et al. (1986) Impaired DNA-repair synthesis in lymphocytes of breast cancer patients. Eur J Cancer Clin Oncol 22:863–869
41. Licastro F, Franceschi C, Chiricolo M et al. (1982) DNA repair after gamma radiation and superoxide dismutase activity in lymphocytes from subjects of far advanced age. Carcinogenesis 3:45–48
42. Rosenberg SA (1992) The immunotherapy and gene therapy of cancer. J Clin Oncol 10:180–199
43. Auffray C, Strominger JL (1986) Molecular genetics of the human major histocompatibility complex. Adv Hum Genet 15:197–247

Oncogenes and Tumor Suppressor Genes

The striking advances in cancer genetics during the past fifteen years have made it clear that the root causes of this disease are linked to malfunctioning genes.

R.A. WEINBERG (1992)

Introduction

During the last 20–30 years, a large body of epidemiologic, cytogenetic, and experimental studies have supported the hypothesis that tumors are caused by genetic damage. The recent advances in molecular biology have definitively proved that this hypothesis was correct, and at present there is no doubt that the basic lesion of the malignant cell is an abnormality in the DNA structure or sequence which results in uncontrolled growth. Two particular classes of genes have been identified – oncogenes and tumor suppressor genes – which are of major importance in the initiation and progression of human malignancies [1].

Oncogenes can be defined as mutated alleles of wild-type genes (proto-oncogenes) with the new and aberrant ability to promote cancer development. Proto-oncogenes are normal cellular genes which appear to exert an essential role in controlling cell proliferation and differentiation. This can also be deduced by the conservation of the DNA sequence of many proto-oncogenes during the evolution from lower vertebrates to humans. However, despite their role in normal cell growth, there is evidence that these genes, when abnormally expressed, can also be involved in cancer induction [2]. As expected, the proteins encoded by proto-oncogenes exert their function in many intracellular processes, acting as protein kinases (*jun* oncogene), growth factors (*sis* oncogene), growth factor receptors (*erbB1* oncogene), or membrane-associated signal transducers (*ras* oncogene).

While oncogenes act in a dominant way, i.e., they are activated by a mutation of a single allele, another class of cancer-associated genes requires the inactivation of both alleles. These are called tumor suppressor genes and their main function is to restrain neoplastic growth, so that the lack of normal protein product consequent to their inactivation will contribute to the development of cancer. Although Rb (retinoblastoma), Wt (Wilms' tumor), and p53 remain the best characterized among tumor suppressor genes, many other recessive oncogenes have recently been identified or localized in almost all chromosomal arms.

Role of Oncogenes in Tumor Development

The first step towards the study of the molecular basis of neoplasms was made by Peyton Rous in 1911, who showed that sarcoma could be transmitted from one bird to another by injecting a cell-free, filtered extract of the tumor [3]. Further studies led to the identification of the retrovirus (Rous sarcoma virus) which is responsible for this avian tumor, and acute transforming RNA viruses were subsequently found in many other species, including humans. However, it is now clear that tumor viruses are responsible for only a small proportion of human cancers, usually through complex pathogenetic mechanisms (as in the case of liver cancer) which involve the concomitant effect of one or more associated factors (in hepatocarcinoma, alcohol abuse, drug consumption, and chronic liver damage). It follows that the pathogenesis of most human neoplasms cannot be ascribed to viral genes, but should be related to factors that are intrinsic to the cell itself. Several lines of research indicate that mutations or aberrant expression of proto-oncogenes, the cellular homolog of viral oncogenes, are intimately correlated with cancer development.

If mutations of specific genes are capable of inducing a malignant phenotype, and if these mutations are dominant at the cellular level, then the transfer of DNA from a malignant cell to a normal cell should result in transformation to the neoplastic phenotype. This type of assay was successfully carried out in 1981 by transfecting DNA from a human bladder carcinoma into a nonmalignant mouse fibroblast cell line (NIH 3T3) [4, 5]. When the transforming gene was absorbed and expressed by 3T3 cells, these piled up on the plate, forming visible foci of transformation. Moreover, transformed cells were also able to generate tumors when injected subcutaneously into nude mice, a property not shown by untransfected 3T3 cells. The results of this kind of experiment strongly suggest that the investigated bladder cancer contained a DNA sequence acting as a dominant cancer gene. In this specific case, the responsible gene was homologous to the transforming sequence of the Harvey sarcoma virus and differed from the human proto-oncogene by a single point mutation at codon 12, converting a glycine at that position to a valine. This oncogene was named H-*ras* (for Harvey *ras*) and belongs to a family which includes others closely related genes (K-*ras* and N-*ras*). Activated *ras* genes contain point mutations in either codon 12, 13, or 61, suggesting that these positions are of critical importance for the normal control of cell replication.

Besides point mutations there are other plausible mechanisms for "activation" (i.e., altered function, leading to or favoring cancer development) of proto-oncogenes. Thus, if a normal proto-oncogene is inappropriately expressed, the excessive amount of normal protein products can be related to the appearance of the malignant phenotype [6]. A frequent cause of overexpression is gene "amplification", i.e., an increase in the number of copies of the gene in the cell. This occurs for the N-*myc* gene in neuroblastoma and in small cell lung carcinoma [7], for the c-*myb* gene in colonic cancer, and for c-*erbB2* in human breast tumors [2]. Oncogene activation can also be consequent to genetic rearrangements, as it occurs in chromosomal translocation near a proto-oncogene locus. The two best-investigated models are the 8;14 translocation observed in Burkitt lymphoma and the 9;22 translocation involving the c-*abl* gene in chronic myelogenous leukemia [2, 8]. In Burkitt lymphoma, the translocation involves the *myc* oncogene (which maps to 8q24) and the immunoglobulin heavy-chain locus (14q32); it follows that the *myc* locus is juxtaposed downstream from a gene that is being actively transcribed in B cells, resulting in a markedly increased expression of the oncogene.

Proteins encoded by proto-oncogenes are all members of a few functional groups, and at present there is evidence of three main biochemical mechanisms by which these genes act [9]: (1) phosphorylation of proteins, with serine, tyrosine, and threonine as substrates; (2) transmission of signals by GTPases, as firstly shown with the *ras* oncogenes, which encode a previously unknown type of GTPase; and (3) regulation of DNA transcription, as for the products of *myc* and *fos* genes, which take part in the replication of DNA. Proto-oncogenes involved in common human tumors and the most probable mechanisms of their activation are shown in Table 1.

Table 1. Main proto-oncogenes investigated in human tumors

Proto-oncogene	Type of cancer	Genetic damage	Reference
ras family (H, K, and N)	Colon, lung, thyroid and genitourinary tract carcinoma, melanoma, leukemia	Point mutations at codons 12, 13, and 61	4, 5
myc	Burkitt lymphoma	Translocation	2, 8
L-*myc*	Lung carcinoma	Amplification	7
N-*myc*	Neuroblastoma, non-small-cell lung carcinoma	Amplification	7
abl	Chronic myelogenous leukemia	Translocation	2, 8
erbB1	Squamous cell	Amplification	2
erbB2	Breast, ovary, and gastric carcinoma	Amplification	2
gip	Ovary and adrenal gland carcinoma	Point mutation	52
gsp	Thyroid carcinoma	Point mutation	52
ret	Multiple endocrine neoplasia type 2	Point mutation	56
bcl-2	Lymphomas, lung carcinoma	Abnormal expression	57

Tumor Suppressor Genes

The other group of genes that are important in tumorigenesis seem to operate in normal cells to restrain their replication. At variance with proto-oncogenes, these genes are lost from the genome during cancer induction and progression, and it is their absence, and not the activation, that allows the development of tumors. One of the first documentations of the existence of tumor suppressor genes was provided by a series of experiments which examined the malignant behavior of cell hybrids constructed between normal and cancer cells [10]: when malignant cells were fused with normal cells, the resulting hybrid population was usually nontumorigenic. The most likely interpretation for this phenomenon is that genes from normal cells may restore a defective function in cancer cells, so that these become responsive to the factors controlling cell replication and differentiation. In accordance with this contention, cytogenetic and molecular studies showed that specific losses of chromosomal material are often associated with human cancer. By coupling these two lines of evidence, we can hypothesize the existence of genes with the precise role of inhibiting the development of cancer that must be inactivated or lost before a cell can become malignant [11, 12].

The results of somatic cell hybridization and restriction fragment length polymorphism studies strongly suggest the existence of tumor suppressor genes, but cannot be taken as definitive proof. This has recently been provided by the identification of the gene responsible for retinoblastoma (see also the relevant chapter in this volume). This is a pediatric eye tumor which occurs in both hereditary and sporadic form. Hereditary retinoblastoma shows an autosomal dominant type of transmission and is usually bilateral and multifocal. In 1971, Alfred Knudson proposed a model – based on the statistical analysis of retinoblastoma incidence – which might provide an explanation for both types of tumors [13]. In hereditary retinoblastoma, one mutant allele should be inherited from a parent and would be present in all cells of the individual, including the germ line cells. Subsequently, a second mutation in the other allele in the target organ (retina) would induce the development of the neoplasm. In the sporadic form of the tumor, mutations of both alleles should occur somatically in the same cell, and this explains the more frequent unifocal and unilateral lesions.

Further experimental studies led to the identification and cloning of the Rb gene [14, 15] and definitively showed that the "two-hits" hypothesis was correct, which is the most likely explanation for the development of this rare disease. The following points should be further considered: First, in affected individuals the inherited presence of only one normal Rb allele occurs in all cells of the body; consequently, nonretinal tissues might also develop tumors if a second mutation alters this allele. This is actually the case, since osteosarcoma and other tumors frequently occur in patients affected by inherited retinoblastoma (but not in the sporadic cases). Second, although we commonly refer to Rb as the gene responsible for retinoblastoma, it should be noted that it is not the gene itself, but rather its loss or inactivation which are associated with cancer occurrence. Third, the Knudson model leads to the paradoxical conclusion that while the inheritance of the susceptibility to retinoblastoma is dominant, the actual mechanism of tumor induction in a specific cell appears to be recessive, since both the alleles have to be inactivated for the appearance of the neoplastic phenotype. It follows that the use of the classical mendelian terminology in this specific aspect of tumor biology can be confusing.

The elegant investigations which provided definitive evidence for the tumor suppressor gene hypothesis can be summarized as follows: cytogenetic analysis showed an interstitial deletion of the long arm of chromosome 13 in some patients with Rb associated with mental retardation and birth defects. In all cases this deletion included region 13q14, which therefore seemed to be a possible candidate for the location of the gene; in the same region of chromosome 13, a gene was mapped which encodes for esterase D, a polymorphic enzyme suitable for linkage studies. When families with retinoblastoma were assessed with this type of analysis, a close linkage was found between Rb and esterase D genes, thus suggesting that the same gene (Rb) was mutated in familial retinoblastoma and deleted in patients with the interstitial deletion of chromosome 13 [16, 17].

In the Knudson model, mutations in both alleles of a specific gene are associated with the formation of tumors; however, the fundamental event in cancer development is the inactivation (not necessarily mutational) of a tumor suppressor gene. Thus, the term "mutation" should be used in a broad sense to refer to either a point mutation at a specific locus or the loss of a locus by various mechanisms. In retinoblastoma, besides independent mutations of the two Rb alleles, analysis of tumor tissue has showed that cancer induction frequently involves loss of the normal allele of Rb gene. This could either be accomplished by the loss of the entire chromosome 13, by loss and duplication of the chromosome, or, finally, by more complex mechanisms involving the exchange of genetic material during mitosis between homologous chromosomes (mitotic recombination) [18]. Loss of the normal allele when the other is mutated is commonly referred to as reduction to homozygosity and can be considered a paradigm of tumor suppressor gene activity.

The Rb gene is a 190-kb fragment of DNA in chromosome 13q14 [13, 14, 19] which is ubiquitously expressed and conserved in the evolution of vertebrates. The gene is expressed in normal retinal cells, while its transcripts are absent or abnormal in retinoblastoma cells; moreover, mutations of Rb have also been reported in several other tumors, including osteosarcoma, breast, prostate, and lung carcinoma [18]. The gene encodes a 105-kDa phosphoprotein which is a substrate of the *cdc*2 (cell division cycle) kinase and which might be involved in the control of cell cycle progression, though the intimate mechanisms of action remain unclear. Finally, recent studies have showed that the Rb gene plays an essential role in the normal mouse development and that its action does not seem to be limited to a barrier against tumor formation [20, 21].

Another extensively investigated tumor suppressor gene – p53 – has been localized on the short arm of chromosome 17 (17p13). Point mutations of p53 are probably the most common genetic alteration in sporadic human neoplasms; moreover, germ line mutations of p53 have been found in Li-Fraumeni syndrome and in patients with osteosarcoma or multiple tumors [22–24]. The p53 gene was initially discovered as a 53-kDa phosphoprotein which coprecipitated with the large T antigen of simian virus 40 (SV40) and was classified as a tumor antigen. Subsequent studies showed that p53 could immortalize cells in culture and cooperate with oncogenes in inducing the transformation of rat embryo fibroblasts; accordingly, the gene was then considered a dominant oncogene. However, this transforming effect is only observed with mutant forms of p53, whereas the wild-type gene conversely suppresses the transformation induced by mutant p53 or *ras* oncogene; thus, the gene is now classified as a tumor suppressor gene, negatively regulating cell proliferation and requiring inactivating mutations for tumor formation [25].

Although several lines of evidence support the tumor suppressor activity of p53, the biology of this gene remains unclear and rather controversial. In a large fraction of common tumors (colon, breast, and lung tumor and leukemia in particular), both p53 alleles are inactivated, usually one by point mutation and the other through deletion. This is in accordance with the general paradigm of tumor suppressor genes and suggests that mutations of p53 are recessive to the wild type, thus contributing to the development of the malignant phenotype only when the wild-type gene is inactivated [26, 27]. However, sequencing data showed that in many tumors both the mutant and the wild-type allele can be present and, in addition, the two proteins simultaneously expressed [28]. In this specific case, a "dominant negative" effect has been postulated, by which the mutant p53 product binds to the wild-type product, generating an inactive oligomeric complex [29]. Another possibility is that certain mutant forms of p53 behave as dominant oncogenes (i.e., require only mutation in one allele to induce cancer) [30, 31]. This hypothesis is also supported by studies in which a mutant form of the gene was introduced into cell lines not expressing p53: the expression of the mutant p53 protein enhanced the ability of these cells to induce tumors when injected in animals [25].

In human cancers, the large majority of p53 mutations are not randomly scattered in the gene, but localized in four regions of the protein which are highly conserved in the evolution of vertebrates from *Xenopus laevis* to human beings [32]. Several "hot spots" for mutations have been identified in different types of cancer; thus, mutations at codons 175, 194, 273, and 280 are particularly frequent in breast cancer [28], mutations at codons 175, 248, and 273 in colorectal tumors, and at codons 157, 176, 248, and 273 in non-small-cell lung carcinoma cell lines [33]. Moreover, a specific mutation at codon 249 has been reported by several investigators in hepatocellular carcinoma from China and South Africa; since the mutation was not seen in the same cancer type from Western countries, the authors suggested that this mutation specificity could reflect the exposure to a well-defined carcinogen. The most likely candidates are aflatoxin (which is a common food contaminant in some regions of Africa and Asia) and the hepatitis B virus [34–36]. Finally, although the large majority of p53 mutations are clustered in exons 5–9, corresponding to amino acid residues 117–285, recent reports suggest that point mutations can also be recorded outside this highly conserved region and, more specifically, in exons 1–4 and in introns 3–7 and 9 [28]. These observations may account for the frequently observed discrepancy between sequencing data (which are usually restricted to exons and often to the fragment 5–9) and immunohistochemistry, which utilizes a panel of monoclonal and polyclonal antibodies to various mutated forms of p53 protein and can detect mutations in the whole gene [37]. However, it is still unclear whether biomolecular studies underdetect or antibody-staining methods tend to overdetect p53 mutations [28]. As for the type of point mutation, transitions are prevalent in colorectal, breast, brain, and lymphoproliferative tumors, whereas transversions are the most frequent substitutions seen in lung and liver cancer [38].

The most relevant effect of wild-type p53 is the suppression or inhibition of cell transformation in culture by either viral or cellular oncogenes. The physiological role of p53 remains unclear, although there is little doubt that the gene should be involved in the cell cycle control. The p53 protein is phosphorylated in a cell cycle-dependent pattern (with maximum level of phosphorylation during mitosis) by the *cdc*2 kinase. Within the cell, p53 proteins accumulate in the cytoplasm during G-1 and then migrate to the nucleus at the beginning of the S phase. Transformed cells which were transfected with wild-type p53 gene are usually arrested in G-1 [25]. In a recent experiment, a null mutation of p53 was introduced into the rat genome by homologous recombination in embryonic stem cell [39]. Mice homologous for the mutated allele developed normally, but they became susceptible to the spontaneous occurrence of tumors (particularly sarcomas and lymphomas) by 6 months of age. The heterozygous progeny, which carried a single copy of the wild-type gene, did not tend to develop spontaneous tumors. This study underscores the following points: (a) p53 gene is not indispensable for normal growth and development of mouse; (b) the loss of both normal alleles of p53 renders these animals at particular risk of specific neoplasms; (c) the presence of one normal allele is sufficient to prevent cancer occurrence, and (d) an oncogenic point mutation of p53 in not necessarily required for tumor induction (in these animals it is the lack of the gene and of its transcription products which is associated with an increased susceptibility to cancer).

A concise outline of the most extensively investigated tumor suppressor genes in human malignancies is shown in Table 2.

Table 2. Tumor suppressor genes with a documented or postulated activity in the development of human tumors

Suppressor gene	Chromosomal locus	Type of cancer	Reference
Rb	13q14	Retinoblastoma, osteosarcoma, breast, bladder, lung cancer	14, 15
p53	17p13	Li-Fraumeni, sarcoma, multiple tumors of young adults, many other tumor types	25, 39
Wt-1	11p13	Wilms' tumor	11, 19
Wt-2	11p15	Wiedemann-Beckwith syndrome	11, 19
APC	5q21	Adenomatosis coli	45, 46
MCC	5q21	Colorectal cancer	47, 54
DCC	18q21	Colorectal cancer	11, 55
NF-1	17q11	Neurofibromatosis-1	11, 19
MEN-1	11q13	Multiple endocrine neoplasia	53
nm23	17q21	Melanoma, colorectal cancer	50, 58
NF-2	22q	Neurofibromatosis-2	59

Cooperation Between Oncogenes and Tumor Suppressor Genes in Tumor Development

Since there is now convincing evidence that most tumors arise through a multistep process (see the "Introduction"), it is unlikely that a single genetic event may be responsible for the full development of the neoplastic phenotype. In accordance with this contention, biomolecular studies of many common neoplasms (especially colon, breast, and stomach) have invariably shown that several genetic abnormalities – including alterations of DNA methylation, oncogene activation, and loss of tumor suppressor genes – can be found in the same cancer cells [18, 40]. This evidence leads to the concept of interaction and cooperation between genes in the induction and progression of cancer; two or more genes cooperate when they act in concert in order to convert a normal cell a neoplastic one. One example of this "collaboration" has been described for *ras* and *myc* oncogenes: when introduced independently into rat embryo fibroblasts, neither *ras* nor *myc* was able to induce transformation; however, the simultaneous transfection with both genes induced the neoplastic phenotype [41]. More generally, oncogene products that act in the nucleus seem to cooperate with those that exert their action in the cytoplasm. The nuclear oncogenes include c-*myc*, N-*myc*, L-*myc*, *fos*, *jun*, and several viral genes, such as papillomavirus E7 and SV40 large T antigen. The cytoplasmic oncogenes include the *ras* family, *src*, *erbB*, and polyomavirus middle T antigen. According to this hypothesis, therefore, the conversion of a normal cell into a tumor cell

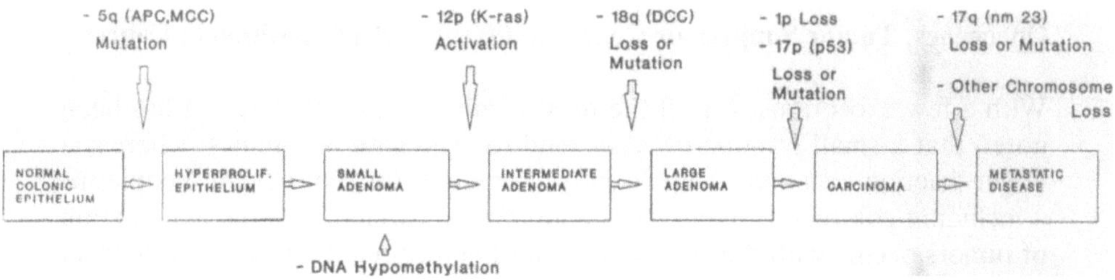

Fig. 1. The molecular basis of colorectal tumor development (for discussion see text and [11, 12, 44])

requires at least two types of changes in the control of cell replication, one occurring in the nucleus and the other in the cytoplasm; *ras* and its analogs would induce the cytoplasmic changes and *myc*, *fos*, or the other nuclear oncogenes would be responsible for changes in the nucleus [40].

Similar types of cooperation seem to occur between oncogene activation and tumor suppressor gene inactivation. Various mutated forms of p53 can cooperate with *ras* genes in the transformation of rat embryo cells; in contrast, wild-type p53 suppresses the transformation induced by dominant oncogenes, thus confirming its inhibitory role in cell replication [42, 43]. At present, however, the paradigm of gene interaction and cooperation in tumor development is represented by the "genetic model of colorectal tumorigenesis" proposed by Vogelstein and coworkers [11, 12, 44] (Fig. 1). According to this model, the first genetic event would be a mutation on chromosome 5 at locus 5q21, where the APC (adenomatous polyposis coli) and the MCC (mutated in colorectal carcinoma) genes have been located and characterized [45–47]. The consequence of this alteration is an uncontrolled cell replication along the colonic crypt with an upwards expansion of the proliferative compartment [48, 49]. Subsequent changes include hypomethylation of DNA and K-*ras* mutations, which might be associated with the development of adenomas. Allelic deletions of chromosome 18q (DCC locus, see Table 2) and 17p (p53) occur at a later stage of tumorigenesis and seem to be associated with the growth of small adenomas to large polyps and to the appearance of carcinomatous changes. Deletions in other chromosomes (1p, 17q) can be observed in the most advanced stages of colorectal cancer [50]. Although a preferred order for these genetic alterations seems to exist, the observed data suggest that the progressive accumulation of genetic damage, rather than the order of the various events, is the major determinant of tumor progression and is responsible for the biologic properties of these tumors.

Oncogenes, Tumor Suppressor Genes, and Genetic Predisposition to Cancer

With a few exceptions, for all the most common types of cancer it has been noted that a small fraction of cases tend to aggregate in families, whereas a larger fraction occur in an apparently sporadic form. For several neoplasms – including colorectal, breast, and endometrial carcinoma – the aggregation of tumors occurs with the typical pattern of autosomal dominant inheritance, although in many cases the multifactorial model of genetic transmission has also been considered. In hereditary tumors the disease is usually absent at birth and develops only after several years or decades; it appears, therefore, that a single mutation is probably insufficient to induce cancer, but rather predisposes the carrier of the mutated gene to an increased risk of malignancy. This is clearly observed in adenomatosis coli (see later chapter), an autosomal dominant condition in which the risk of colorectal cancer approaches 100% by the age of 40–50 years [51].

In theory, either oncogenes or tumor suppressor genes might be responsible for the increased susceptibility to cancer observed in hereditary and familial tumors. In practical terms, however, the activation of a dominant oncogene during fetal life would appear incompatible with a normal development, so that it is much more likely that oncogenes become involved in cancer induction only after a complete embryologic development. In contrast, tumor suppressor genes are recessive at the cellular level, and in heterozygosity their presence can be masked by the wild-type allele; it follows that the allele can be transmitted through the germ line cells. A cell with a mutated tumor suppressor allele can be phenotypically normal and will take part in normal fetal development. During adult life, however, mutation or loss of the normal allele can completely inactivate the gene, resulting in uncontrolled growth and cancer occurrence in one or more target organs. Since somatic gene loss is not rare in normal cells, it appears that germ line null alleles for tumor suppressor genes are a major congenital determinant of cancer predisposition [1]. This sequence of events has been extensively documented for retinoblastoma [16–19] and is the most plausible explanation for the pathogenetic interpretation of more complex cancer family syndromes, such as adenomatosis coli and Li-Fraumeni syndromes [18, 19] (see the chapters on "Hereditary Gastrointestinal Polyposis Syndromes" and "Li-Fraumeni Syndrome").

References

1. Weinberg RA (1992) The integration of molecular genetics into cancer management. Cancer 70:1653–1658
2. Slamon DJ (1987) Proto-oncogenes and human cancers. N Engl J Med 317: 955–957
3. Rous PA (1911) A sarcoma of the fowl transmissible by an agent separable from the tumor cells. J Exp Med 13:397–411

4. Santos E, Tronik SR, Aaronson SA et al. (1982) T24 human bladder carcinoma oncogene is an activated form of the normal human homologue of BALB and Harvey-MSV transforming genes. Nature 298:343–347
5. Reddy EP, Reynolds RK, Santos E et al. (1992) A point mutation is responsible for the acquisition of transforming properties by the T24 human bladder carcinoma oncogene. Nature 300:149–152
6. Stacey DW, Kung HF (1984) Transformation of NIH 3T3 cells by microinjection of Ha-ras p21 protein. Nature 310:508–511
7. Little GD, Nau MM, Carney DN et al. (1983) Amplification and expression of the c-myc oncogene in human lung cancer cell lines. Nature 306:194–196
8. Dalla-Favera R, Bregni M, Erikson J et al. (1982) Human c-myc onc gene is located on the region of chromosome 8 that is translocated in Burkitt lymphoma cells. Proc Natl Acad Sci USA 79:7824–7827
9. Bishop JM (1991) Molecular themes in oncogenesis. Cell 64:235–248
10. Harris H, Klein G (1969) Malignancy of somatic cell hybrids. Nature 224: 1314–1316
11. Stanbridge EJ (1990) Identifying tumor suppressor genes in human colorectal cancer. Science 247:12–13
12. Fearon ER, Vogelstein B (1990) A genetic model for colorectal tumorigenesis. Cell 61:759–767
13. Knudson A (1977) Genetics and the etiology of human cancer. Adv Hum Genet 8:1–66
14. Lee WH, Bookstein R, Hong F et al. (1987) Human retinoblastoma susceptibility gene: cloning identification, and sequence. Science 235:1394–1399
15. Friend SH, Bernards R, Rogeli S et al. (1986) A human DNA segment with properties of the gene that predisposes to retino-blastoma and osteosarcoma. Nature 323:643–646
16. Benedict WF, Srivatsan ES, Mark C et al. (1987) Complete or partial homozygosity of chromosome 13 in primary retinoblastoma. Cancer Res 47:4189–4191
17. Bunin GR, Beverly SE, Meadows AT et al. (1989) Frequency of 13q abnormalities among 203 patients with retinoblastoma. J Natl Cancer Inst 81:370–374
18. Weinberg RA (1989) Oncogenes, antioncogenes and the molecular bases of multistep carcinogenesis. Cancer Res 49:3713–3721
19. Weinberg RA (1991) Tumor suppressor genes. Science 254:1138–1146
20. Lee EYHP, Chang CY, Hu N et al. (1992) Mice deficient for Rb are nonviable and show defects in neurogenesis and haematopoiesis. Nature 359:288–294
21. Jacks T, Fazeli A, Schmitt EM et al. (1992) Effect of an Rb mutation in the mouse. Nature 359:295–300
22. Eeles AE (1993) Predictive testing for germline mutations in the p53 gene: are all the questions answered? Eur J Cancer 29A:1361–1365
23. Malkin D, Jolly KW, Barbier N et al. (1992) Germline mutations of the p53 tumor-suppressor gene in children and young adults with second malignant neoplasms. N Engl J Med 326:1309–1315
24. Toguchida J, Yamaguchi T, Dayton SH et al. (1992) Prevalence and spectrum of germline mutations of the p53 gene among patients with sarcoma. N Engl J Med 326:1301–1308
25. Levine AJ, Momand J, Finlay CA (1991) The p53 tumour suppressor gene. Nature 351:453–456
26. Nigro JM, Baker SJ, Presinger AC et al. (1989) Mutations in the p53 gene occur in diverse human tumour types. Nature 342:705–708
27. Baker SJ, Fearon ER, Nigro JM et al. (1989) Chromosome 17 deletions and p53 gene mutations in colorectal carcinomas. Science 244:217–221
28. Coles C, Condie A, Chetty U et al. (1992) p53 mutations in breast cancer. Cancer Res 52:5291–5298

29. Nigro JM, Baker SJ, Presinger AC et al. (1989) Mutations in the p53 gene occur in diverse human tumor types. Nature 342:705–708
30. Hinds P, Finlay CA, Quartin RS et al. (1990) Mutant p53 DNA clones from human colon carcinomas cooperate with ras in transforming primary rat cells: a comparison of the "hot spot" mutant phenotypes. Cell Growth Differ 1:571–580
31. Dittmer D, Pati S, Zambetti G et al. (1993) Gain of function mutations in p53. Nature Genetics 4:42–45
32. Soussi T, Caron de Fromentel C, May P (1990) Structural aspects of the p53 protein in relation to gene evolution. Oncogene 5:945–952
33. Mitsudomi T, Steinberg SM, Nau MM et al. (1992) p53 gene mutations in non-small-cell lung cancer cell lines and their correlation with the presence of ras mutations and clinical features. Oncogene 7:171–180
34. Bressac B, Kew M, Wands J (1991) Selective G to T mutations of p53 gene in hepatocellular carcinoma from southern Africa. Nature 350:429–431
35. Ozturk M (1991) p53 mutation in hepatocellular carcinoma after aflatoxin exposure. Lancet 358:1356–1359
36. Scorsone KA, Zhou YZ, Butel JS et al. (1992) p53 mutations cluster at codon 249 in hepatitis B virus-positive hepatocellular carcinomas from China. Cancer Res 52:1635–1638
37. Cunningham J, Lust JA, Schaid DJ et al. (1992) Expression of p53 and 17p allelic loss in colorectal carcinoma. Cancer Res 52:1974–1980
38. Hollstein M, Sidransky D, Vogelstein B et al. (1991) p53 mutations in human cancer. Science 253:49–53
39. Donehower LA, Harvey M, Slagle BL et al. (1992) Mice deficient for p53 are developmentally normal but susceptible to spontaneous tumours. Nature 356: 215–221
40. Hunter T (1991) Cooperative between oncogenes. Cell 64:249–270
41. Land H, Parada LF, Weinberg RA (1983) Tumorigenic conversion of primary embryo fibroblasts requires at least two cooperating oncogenes. Nature 304: 596–602
42. Levine AJ, Momand J (1990) Tumor suppressor genes: the p53 and retinoblastoma genes and gene products. Biochim Biophys Acta 1032:119–136
43. Finlay CA, Hinds PW, Levine AJ (1989) The p53 protooncogene can act as a suppressor of tranformation. Cell 57:1083–1093
44. Hamilton SR (1993) The molecular genetics of colorectal neoplasia. Gastroenterology 105:3–7
45. Kinzler KW, Nilbert MC, Su LK et al. (1991) Identification of FAP locus genes from chromosome 5q21. Science 253:661–665
46. Groden J, Thilveris A, Samowitz W et al. (1991) Identification and characterization of the familial adenomatous polyposis coli gene. Cell 66:589–600
47. Kinzler K, Nilbert MC, Vogelstein B et al. (1991) Identification of a gene located at chromosome 5q21 that is mutated in colorectal cancers. Science 251:1366–1370
48. Deschner EE (1988) Cell proliferation and colonic neoplasia. Scand J Gastroenterol 23 [Suppl 1]:94–97
49. Ponz de Leon M, Roncucci L, Di Donato P et al. (1988) Pattern of epithelial cell proliferation in colorectal mucosa of normal subjects and of patients with adenomatous polyps or cancer of the large bowel. Cancer Res 48:4121–4126
50. Cohn KH, Wang F, DeSoto-LaPaix F et al. (1991) Association of nm23-H1 allelic deletions with distant metastases in colorectal carcinoma. Lancet 338: 722–724
51. Bülow S (1989) Familial adenomatous polyposis. Ann Med 21:299–307
52. Lyons J, Landis CA, Harsh G et al. (1990) Two G protein oncogenes in human endocrine tumors. Science 249:655–659

53. Brandi ML (1991) Multiple endocrine neoplasia type 1: general features and new insights into etiology. J Endocrinol Invest 14:61–72
54. Scott N, Quirke P (1993) Molecular biology of colorectal neoplasia. Gut 34: 298–292
55. Itoh F, Hinoda Y, Ohe M et al. (1993) Decreased expression of DCC mRNA in human colorectal cancers. Int J Cancer 53:260–263
56. Mulligan LM, Kwok JB, Healey CS et al. (1993) Germ-line mutations of the RET proto-oncogene in multiple endocrine neoplasia type 2A. Nature 363: 458–460
57. Pezzella F, Turley H, Kuzu I et al. (1993) bcl-2 protein in non-small-cell lung carcinoma. N Engl J Med 329:690–694
58. Wang L, Patel U, Ghosh L et al. (1993) Mutation in the nm23 gene is associated with metastasis in colorectal cancer. Cancer Res 53:717–720
59. Kinzler KW, Vogelstein B (1993) A gene for neurofibromatosis 2. Nature 363:495–496

Genetic Factors in Solid Tumors of Childhood

... nor there is any better way to advance the proper practice of medicine than to give our mind to the discovery of the universal low of nature by careful investigation of cases of rare forms of diseases.

WILLIAM HARVEY (1657)

Introduction

Childhood cancer is relatively rare in all Western and developed countries. In the United States, approximately 4000 new cases of malignant solid tumors are diagnosed each year [1], while data from cancer registries in Europe indicate that the fraction of all pediatric malignancies (i.e., diagnosed between 0 and 14 years of age) is in the order of 0.8% of all registered tumors [2]. Despite the relative rarity, there are several reasons for interest in these tumors. First, for many cancers of childhood a genetic nature has been suspected, and then documented, by observing the striking familial aggregation and vertical transmission of uncommon tumors; retinoblastoma (Rb), Wilms' tumor (WT), and Li-Fraumeni syndrome are examples of well-defined hereditary neoplastic diseases of infancy. Second, some of these neoplasms (Rb and WT, in particular) have become a paradigm for interpreting tumor development as being due to the sequential inactivation of the two alleles in a tumor suppressor gene (see the previous chapter). This model, initially suggested for Rb [3], is applicable to many other clinical conditions which are at present under active investigation (adenomatosis coli, hereditary breast and colonic cancer). Third, the distribution of childhood cancer is rather peculiar and markedly different from that of adult malignant tumors, as shown in Fig. 1. In fact, tumors of the lymphohematopoietic system represent 50% of all malignancies developed before the age of 15, brain tumors 22%, and sarcoma 11%; all together, carcinomas do not reach 6% of total pediatric tumors. Cancer distribution is entirely different in adults, where carcinomas represent the large majority (89% of total), and altogether the most frequent neoplasms of childhood do not reach 12% of all registered tumors. The reasons for this striking difference in cancer distribution are unclear, though rather intuitively one may suspect that genetic factors affect pediatric tumors more than the adult types, which in turn should be more closely dependent on the cumulative effect of environmental factors.

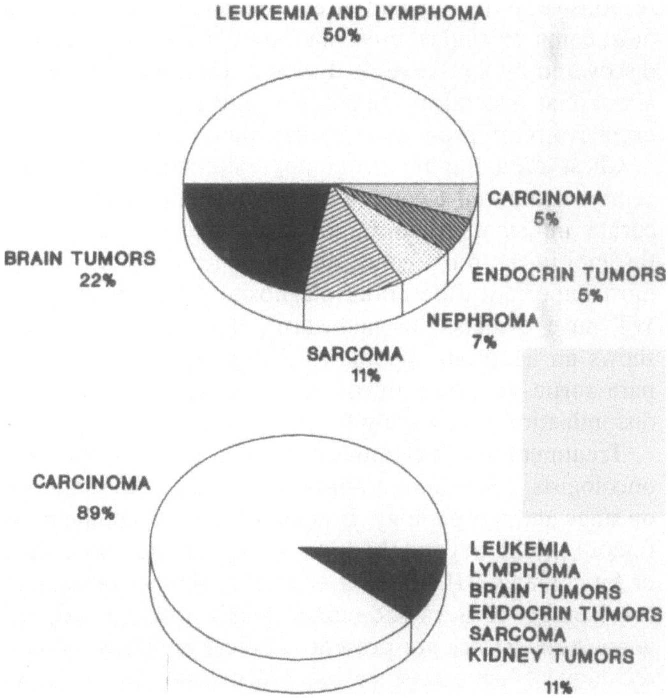

Fig. 1. Prevalence of malignant tumors in childhood (*top*) and in adulthood (*bottom*)

Several neoplasms of childhood (Rb, Li-Fraumeni syndrome, leukemia, lymphomas) will be discussed in later chapters in this book; the main focus of this chapter will be on WT, Wiedemann-Beckwith syndrome (WBS), and neuroblastoma (NB).

Wilms' Tumor (Nephroblastoma)

Morphology and Clinical Aspects

WT accounts for approximately 5%–6% of all pediatric malignancies. The prognosis of the disease has changed radically over the last 50 years; at the beginning of the century, virtually all children with WT died, but by 1950 about 50% of these young patients survived, and at present more than 90% are cured by a combination of medical and surgical treatments [4]. The prognosis, however, is strongly dependent on tumor stage and morphologic features. There are three main histologic variants of WT: (1) mesoblastic nephroma (usually curable by nephrectomy alone), (2) nephroblastomatosis, and (3) focal or diffuse anaplastic tumor. These anaplastic WT are much less responsive to therapy and often associated with a poor clinical outcome. The most common clinical presentation of WT is with a painless abdominal mass, discovered by a relative or during a routine examination; symptoms include abdominal distension, hematuria, and high blood pressure (related to the excessive renin production by the tumor cells).

Chest radiography, urography, abdominal ultrasounds, and, more recently, computed tomography or magnetic resonance imaging provide accurate information on tumor size, extent of local infiltration (including thrombi in the renal vein), and presence of metastases [1]. NB remains the most important differential diagnosis. Approximately 20% of patients with WT have evidence of metastasis at diagnosis, especially when histology shows an anaplastic neoplasm. Nodal spread occurs predominantly to the para-aortic or other intra-abdominal lymph nodes, while hematogenous dissemination is relatively frequent to the lung, brain, and bones.

Treatment of WT requires a close cooperation between surgeons, pediatric oncologists, and radiotherapists. Moreover, management is closely dependent on stage and morphology. In stage I, tumor is confined to the kidney; stage II tumors extend beyond the kidney and penetrate into the perirenal soft tissue or fat; in stage III, there is a residual tumor confined to the abdomen and involvement of intra-abdominal lymph nodes; finally, in stage IV hematogenous metastases are present. Radical or simple nephrectomy remains the technique of choice; since bilateral tumors are particularly frequent (5%–10% of all cases), the controlateral kidney should always be explored, which requires a transabdominal approach. Preoperative chemotherapy or irradiation have been favored in Europe, since these treatments may reduce the size of the tumor or even eliminate thrombi in the vena cava, thus allowing surgeons to reconsider for operation children with tumors inoperable at the first presentation. In America, the preoperative approach is less popular, owing to possible errors in preoperative diagnosis and the importance of surgical staging in planning subsequent treatment [1, 4–6]. Postoperative chemotherapy can be given to patients of all stages, although probably many stage I WT patients would have an excellent prognosis with surgery alone. Combination chemotherapy with vincristine, actinomycin D, and doxorubicin seems to provide the best clinical results [5]. Postoperative irradiation is usually given to all patients, often immediately after surgery; the dose is closely dependent on the age of the child and ranges between 1000 and 4000 cGy [4]. Bilateral disease is difficult to treat; one common procedure consists of total nephrectomy of the more severely affected kidney with partial nephrectomy on the other side.

Genetic Epidemiology

The incidence of WT is approximately 1 in 10000 newborn [7]. Like Rb, WT occurs in either hereditary or sporadic forms, although the latter probably accounts for more than 90% of these tumors. Moreover, a subset of WT – in the order of 2% of the total [7] – occurs in association with a series of other abnormalities, often referred as WAGR syndrome (WT, aniridia, genito-urinary abnormalities, mental retardation) [4].

Familial clusters of WT have been described by several authors, and because of the rarity of this neoplasm it is unlikely that these aggregations are due to chance alone. Knudson and Strong [8] reviewed three pedigrees all consistent with a fully penetrant autosomal dominant inheritance. In one of these families, the proband was a 14-month-old female with bilateral tumors; one out of two sisters had unilateral WT at the age of 6 months; their father had undergone a nephrectomy at the age of 4 for a tumor of the right kidney. In this family, a very rare cancer developed in three members of two successive generations, which clearly suggests an autosomal dominant transmission. A pedigree of a family segregating for WT was described by Grundy et al. [9]; in this large kindred there were five unilateral and two bilateral WT in two successive generations; there was no family history of consanguinity or clinical features of WAGR. The autosomal dominant pattern of transmission was considered the most likely, though with reduced penetrance. Finally, there are reports of WT in identical twins [8, 10].

Using simple statistics and observing the age at diagnosis of WT in different subgroups of patients, Knudson and Strong suggested a "two-hit" mutational model similar to that previously proposed for Rb [3, 8]. The two hit model predicts that a fraction of total cases are hereditary, are often bilateral, and develop at an early age, since they arise from a mutation of a germ line cell and a second random somatic mutation. Another fraction of cases are nonhereditary and frequently unilateral, occur on average at an older age, and arise from two random somatic mutations. When this hypothesis was tested with the available data, the authors found further confirmation of their theory. In a series of 103 WT patients, hereditary cases occurred earlier than sporadic ones and were more often bilateral; the mean age at diagnosis was around 2 years for hereditary cases, but 3–4 years in the whole series. Finally, the fraction of cases not yet diagnosed at any given age decreased exponentially in both familial and bilateral WT, but this did not occur with unilateral or total cases. The authors concluded that:

> . . . as for retinoblastoma, this finding is compatible with the belief that bilateral cases are all hereditary, that each tumor develops in a hereditary case as a result of a single somatic event, and that tumors develop in non-hereditary cases as a result of two somatic events [8].

These pioneering observations were subsequently followed by cytogenetic and biomolecular studies which led to the isolation and characterization of the WT locus on the short arm of chromosome 11 (11p13, WT-1); however, despite the similarities between Rb and WT models of carcinogenesis and the tumor suppressor activity of both genes, it now appears that there are also differences, that loss of function of other genes may be associated with

WT development, and, more generally, that there are still questions, in the case of WT, regarding the applicability of the two-hit model of tumorigenesis [9].

Molecular Biology

A small fraction (approximately 2% of total) of WT cases occur in association with aniridia (a defect in iris development), urogenital abnormalities, and mental retardation [4, 11]. This complex of disorders (WAGR syndrome) has provided valuable clues regarding the molecular mechanisms of WT. In fact, WAGR syndrome has been associated with a constitutional deletion of DNA on the short arm of chromosome 11 (band 11p13) [12]. Further studies with sensitive gene-probing techniques showed loss of genetic material from 11p13 in tumors which did not show the deletion on karyotypic analysis [13], thus suggesting that in WT the absence of genetic material from the short arm of chromosome 11 is a rather frequent event. This line of investigation led to the conclusion that at least in a subset of WT the inactivation or loss of a gene in 11p13 may play a key role in tumor development. In analogy with the Rb model, this phenomenon might represent the loss of a cancer suppressor gene, which allows an uncontrolled progression of the disease. This contention was further confirmed by a different approach: the introduction of a normal chromosome 11 segment into cultured cells of WT markedly reduced the aggressiveness of these cells, thus suppressing their capability to induce tumors when injected into nude mice [14]. Further studies defined the physical map of the WAGR region and localized the putative WT gene on the short arm of chromosome 11 band 11p13 [11]. The WT locus has been limited to a region of less than 345 kb; the gene is expressed at high levels in the embryonic kidney and in a subset of hemopoietic cells, whereas its expression is very low or absent in other tissues and organs. The structure of the predicted protein encoded by the gene suggests that it may function as a transcription factor. Finally, mutations at this locus have recently been identified in tumors from patients with WT [15, 16].

The biology of WT, however, is undoubtedly more complex than that of Rb; in the latter, both sporadic and hereditary tumors can be attributed to the inactivation of a gene at a single locus; in contrast, WT tumor development is associated with the functional inactivation of other loci. In sporadic WT, recent studies have revealed loss of heterozygosity in the 11p15 region in the absence of detectable alterations of the 11p13 region [17, 18]. Moreover, other investigations have showed that in WT, allelic deletions at 11p13 are not necessarily related to WT-1 mutations [19]. These observations suggest the existence of a second genetic locus involved in the etiopathogenesis of WT; this gene – named WT-2 and localized on 11p15.5 – has been related to the WBS (which is frequently associated with the development of WT) [20]. In addition, linkage studies carried out in two large families with multiple cases of unilateral and bilateral WT [9, 21] excluded the possibility that the gene responsible for WT is localized on the short arm of chromosome 11, thus indicating the existence of a third genetic locus. Taken together, these observations suggest a genetic heterogeneity for WT, i.e., that multiple genetic pathways may lead to the same disease, and further emphasize the differences between WT and Rb models. These can be summarized as follows: (a) in WT, mutations of the responsible genes do not seem to be associated with the development of tumors in other organs (as they are in the case of Rb; see following chapter); (b) in contrast to Rb, WT are histologically heterogeneous; (c) according to the available experimental evidence, more than two loci seem to be involved in the pathogenesis of WT; and (d) WT-1 gene is expressed only in a limited range of cell types, more specifically kidney and hematopoietic cells (in contrast to Rb, which is ubiquitously expressed) [22].

Wiedemann-Beckwith Syndrome

WBS is a sporadic or hereditary clinical condition characterized by multiple congenital abnormalities and by an increased risk of childhood cancer. WBS was first reported independently and almost simultaneously by Beckwith, in an autopsy series, and by Wiedemann, who described three affected siblings [23, 24]. Approximately 400 cases of WBS have been reported from the time of its original description to 1983; the prevalence of the disease seems to be 0.07 per 1000 births [20]. Clinical features of WBS include macroglossia (82% of all patients), umbilical anomalies (75%), increased birth weight (38.5%), craniofacial dysmorphia (38.5%), earlobe anomalies (38%), post-natal gigantism (32.7%), hepatomegaly (32%), genitourinary abnormalities (24%), nephromegaly (23%), cardiac alterations (15%), and mental retardation (12%). Abnormal blood tests such as hypoglycemia, polyglobulia, hypocalcemia, and dyslipidemia are also part of the symdrome [20].

WBS is associated with an increased risk of certain specific tumors of childhood [25, 26]. Among these, the most frequent are WT (approximately 45%, or 14 out of 32 tumors in a recent series) [26], followed by adrenal carcinoma, hepatoblastoma, pancreatic cancer, and NB [20]. All tumors reported in WBS are diagnosed in early childhood and in no case after the age of 10 years. The fact that various tumors of embryonal origin often occur in the same patient strongly suggests that a constitutional mutation predisposes several organs to the development of specific neoplasms. The clinical association between WBS and WT has further been confirmed by genetic studies showing a close linkage between locus WT-2 (11p15) and WBS [27]. If the tumor suppressor model of Rb and WT is applied to WBS, then one might hypothesize that a germ line predisposing mutation is responsible for the constitutional abnormalities of various organs and that a second mutational event (i.e., inactivation of the wild-type allele in a given organ) would then give origin to the neoplasm [20].

Although sporadic cases of WBS are frequently observed, familial forms have also been described and are usually interpreted as autosomal dominant. Niikawa et al. described four families with WBS in which vertical transmission through two or three generations was observed [28]. The presence of individuals affected by this rare disease in different generations, the calculated segregation ratio of 0.57 (close to the value expected for dominant inheritance), the sex ratio of affected individuals close to unity, and the broad spectrum of clinical manifestations all strongly indicated the autosomal dominant model, with variable expressivity, as the most plausible type of genetic transmission.

Neuroblastoma

NB accounts for approximately 7% of all pediatric neoplasms, and the large majority of cases develop before the age of 4. These tumors originate in the neural-crest cells of the sympathetic nervous system; adrenal medulla and retroperitoneal nervous tissue are therefore the most common primary sites of appearance. Their origin renders NB closely related to pheochromocytomas, and in fact both tumors are characterized by the secretion of adrenal medullary hormones and of their metabolites (valillyl mandelic acid). One common clinical presentation is that of a painless abdominal mass associated with aspecific symptoms (fever, anemia). About 20% of affected individuals present with localized disease, but the majority have involved regional lymph nodes or show metastasis in more distant organs (especially liver, bones, and skin); subcutaneous metastases often show a characteristic bluish color. In addition to biopsy, the diagnosis of NB is based on measurement of urinary catecolamines and of their metabolites; moreover, radiological investigations (including computed tomography and scintiscan), abdominal ultrasounds, and bone marrow aspiration are of value for establishing the extent of the disease. For differential diagnosis, WT, Ewing's sarcoma, neurofibroma, medulloblastoma, and other tumors of the nervous system should be considered.

Since treatment is mainly based on the extent of disease, an accurate preoperative staging appears to be of great clinical relevance. Stage I tumors are confined to the site of origin, whereas in stage II the neoplasm extends beyond the primary site, but does not cross the midline (ipsilateral lymph nodes may be involved). In stage III, tumors extend across the midline or show bilateral lymph nodes involvement; finally, in stage IV, distant metastases are present. Although the clinical management of NB is still unsatisfactory, progress in treatment has doubled the rate of cure over the last 20 years [1]. Stage I and II tumors are usually treated by surgery with or without irradiation; some authors discourage the "heroic" removal of large or invasive neoplasms, but rather recommend "second look" operations – after chemotherapy or radiotherapy – in order to remove the residual tumor

[1, 29]. Stage III and IV NB are usually treated with a combination of antineoplastic agents (cyclophosphamide and doxorubicin, with or without cisplatin, but other combinations seem to be similarly effective) [1]. The prognosis is good for localized tumors, with survival rates of 80% or more, but remains poor for patients with lymph node involvement or metastasis at presentation [30].

Although most NB are apparently sporadic, familial cases have also been reported. Kusher et al. reviewed 23 familial aggregations of NB, including several cases with possible vertical transmission (tumors in two successive generations) and four couples of identical twins [31]. In one of these families, NB was diagnosed in four out of four siblings [32]. Familial cases were characterized by an increased frequency of multiple tumors (including four bilateral adrenal gland tumors) and by the tendency to develop earlier than the sporadic forms (average age of diagnosis, 9 months versus 2.5 years). The authors concluded that familial cases of NB conform to an autosomal dominant type of genetic transmission and that the observed findings could be interpreted with a "two-hit" model of carcinogenesis as previously proposed for Rb and WT [3, 8, 31]. According to this model [31, 33], two events are postulated to affect a pair of alleles in a tumor suppressor gene locus; the first event is a germ line mutation, and the second is the somatic inactivation or deletion of the other allele. Further cytogenetic and biomolecular studies, however, showed that the pathogenesis of NB is undoubtedly more complex and cannot simply be reduced to the paradigm of tumor suppressor gene inactivation.

Cytogenetic analysis showed that in NB the short arm of chromosome 1 is frequently deleted [34, 35]; using chromosome-1-specific DNA probes, a common region of loss of heterozygosity was found at the distal end of this arm (1p36.1–3) [36, 37]. It is likely, therefore, that loss or inactivation of a tumor suppressor gene at this site play a certain role in cancer development. However, deletions and other rearrangements at chromosomes 11, 14, and 17 were also found to occur with increased frequency in NB [38–41]. Another genetic abnormality of NB is the amplification of N-*myc* proto-oncogene; at a cytogenetic level this is manifested by the appearance of either extrachromosomal double minute chromatin bodies or chromosomal homogeneously staining regions [42, 43]. Interestingly, N-*myc* amplification seems to be associated with a rapid tumor progression and with a poor clinical outcome; thus, together with an advanced stage, this genetic change might reveal a useful marker of adverse prognosis [43]. Various defects of the nerve growth factor receptor have recently been found in NB cell lines [34]. Since nerve growth factor is required for differentiation and maturation of sympathetic neurons, the authors hypothesized that alterations of its receptors might be responsible for induction and maintenance of the indifferentiated state of neuroblasts. Being in a relatively uncontrolled state, the cell might acquire further genetic changes – such as N-*myc* amplification or allelic deletions at various chromosomal loci – which ultimately induce the development of the malignant phenotype. In line with this contention, recent studies reported high levels of expression of the TRK gene (which encodes for a component of the nerve growth factor) in the majority of NB, especially in those of individuals in the earlier stages of the disease [44]. Finally, Leone et al. [45] found various molecular alterations to the nm23 gene (i.e., overexpression and point mutations) in NB; moreover, an increased expression of the gene was closely related with a poor clinical outcome.

Other Solid Tumors of Childhood

Other pediatric solid tumors include astrocytoma, medulloblastoma, rhabdomyosarcoma, osteosarcoma, Ewing's sarcoma, and undifferentiated sarcoma. Most of these neoplasms develop as sporadic forms, with a low tendency to aggregate in families; some of these tumors, however, may occur in the spectrum of neoplasms of more complex cancer family syndromes (i.e., osteosarcoma in Li-Fraumeni symdrome) and will be discussed in the following chapters.

References

1. Young JL, Ries LG, Silverberg et al. (1986) Cancer incidence, survival and mortality for children younger than age 15 years. Cancer 58 [Suppl 2]:598–602
2. Berrino F, Crosignani P, Gatta G et al. (1986) Incidenza di tumori e cause di morte in Lombardia. Notizie Sanità 10:1–95
3. Knudson AF (1986) Genetics of human cancer. Annu Rev Genet 20:231–251
4. National Wilms' tumor study Committee (1991) Wilms' tumor: status report, 1990. J Clin Oncol 9:877–887
5. D'Angio GJ, Breslow N, Beckwith JB et al. (1989) Treatment of Wilms' tumor: results of the third National Wilms' tumor study. Cancer 64:349–360
6. Tournade MF, Com-Nouguè C, Voute PA et al. (1993) Results of the sixth international society of pediatric oncology Wilms' tumor trial study. J Clin Oncol 11:1014–1023
7. Matsunaga E (1981) Genetics of Wilms' tumor. Hum Genet 57:231–246
8. Knudson AG, Strong LC (1972) Mutation and cancer: a model for Wilms' tumor of the kidney. J Natl Cancer Inst 48:313–324
9. Grundy P, Koufos A, Morgan K et al. (1988) Familial predisposition to Wilms' tumor does not map to the short arm of chromosome 11. Nature 336:374–376
10. Hewitt D, Lashof JC, Stewart AM (1966) Childhood cancer in twins. Cancer 19:157–161
11. Call MK, Glaser T, Ito CY et al. (1990) Isolation and characterization of a zinc finger polypeptide on the human chromosome 11 Wilms' tumor locus. Cell 60:509–520
12. Riccardi VM, Sujansky E, Smith AC et al. (1978) Chromosomal imbalance in the aniridia–Wilms' tumor association: 11p interstitial deletion. Pediatrics 61:604–610

13. Fearon ER, Vogelstein B, Feinberg A (1984) Somatic deletion and duplication of genes on chromosome 11 in Wilms' tumours. Nature 309:176–178
14. Weissman BE, Saxon PJ, Pasquale SR et al. (1987) Introduction of a normal human chromosome 11 into a Wilms' tumor cell line controls its tumorigenic expression. Science 236:175–180
15. Baird PN, Groves N, Haber DA et al. (1992) Identification of mutations in the WT-1 gene in tumours from patients with WAGR syndrome. Oncogene 7:2141–2149
16. Gessler M, Konig A, Moore J et al. (1993) Homozygous inactivation of WT-1 in a Wilms' tumor associated with WAGR syndrome. Genes Chromos Cancer 7:131–136
17. Dowdy SF, Fasching CL, Araujo D et al. (1991) Suppression of tumorigenicity in Wilms' tumor by the p15.5–p14 region of chromosome 11. Science 254:293–295
18. Reeve AE, Sa S, Raizis AM et al. (1989) Loss of allelic heterozygosity at a second locus on chromosome 11 in sporadic Wilms' tumor. Mol Cell Biol 9:1799–1803
19. Cowell JK, Groves N, Baird P (1993) Loss of heterozygosity at 11p13 in Wilms' tumours does not necessarily involve mutations in the WT-1 gene. Br J Cancer 67:1259–1261
20. Engstrom W, Lindham S, Schofield P (1988) Wiedemann-Beckwith syndrome. Pediatrics 147:450–457
21. Huff V, Compton DA, Chao LY et al. (1988) Lack of linkage of familial Wilms' tumor to chromosomal band 11p13. Nature 336:377–378
22. Slater RM, Mannens MMAM (1969) Cytogenetics and molecular genetics of Wilms' tumor in childhood. Cancer Genet Cytogenet 61:111–121
23. Beckwith JB (1969) Macroglossia, omphalocele, adrenal cytomegaly, gigantism and hyperplastic visceromegaly. Birth Defects 5:188–196
24. Wiedemann HR (1964) Complex malformatif familial avec hernie ombilicale et macroglossie. Un syndrome noveau? J Genet Hum 13:223–232
25. Sotelo-Avila C, Crooch WM (1976) Neoplasms associated with the Beckwith-Wiedemann syndrome. Perspect Pediatr Pathol 3:255–272
26. Wiedemann HR (1983) Tumor and hemihypertrophy associated with Wiedemann-Beckwith's syndrome. Eur J Pediatr 141:129–131
27. Ping AJ, Reeve AE, Low DJ et al. (1989) Genetic linkage of Wiedemann-Beckwith syndrome to 11p15. Am J Hum Genet 44:720–723
28. Nikawa N, Ishikariyama S, Takahashi S et al. (1986) The Wiedemann-Beckwith syndrome. Pedigree studies of 5 families with evidence for autosomal dominant inheritance with variable expressivity. Am J Med Genet 24:41–55
29. Smith EI, Krous HF, Tunell WP et al. (1980) The impact of chemotherapy and radiation therapy on secondary operations for neuroblastoma. Ann Surg 191:561–569
30. Rosen EM, Cassady JR, Frantz CN et al. (1984) Neuroblastoma: the joint center for radiation therapy/Dana Farber cancer Institute/Children hospital experience. J Clin Oncol 2:719–732
31. Kushner BH, Gilbert F, Helson L (1986) Familial neuroblastoma. Cancer 57:1887–1893
32. Chatten J, Voorhess ML (1967) Report of a kindred with multiple disorders, including neuroblastomas in four siblings. N Engl J Med 277:1230–1236
33. Knudson AG, Strong LC (1972) Mutation and cancer: neuroblastoma and pheochromocytoma. Am J Hum Genet 24:514–532
34. Brodeur GM, Fong CT (1989) Molecular biology and genetics of human neuroblastoma. Cancer Genet Cytogenet 41:153–174

35. Peter M, Michon J, Vielh P et al. (1992) PCR assay for chromosome 1p deletion in small neuroblastoma samples. Int J Cancer 52:544–548
36. Fong CT, Dracopoli NC, White PS et al. (1989) Loss of heterozygosity for the short arm of chromosome 1 in human neuroblastoma. Proc Natl Acad Sci USA 86:3753–3757
37. Weith A, Martisson T, Cziepluch C et al. (1989) Neuroblastoma consensus deletion maps to 1p36 1–2. Genes Chromos Cancer 1:159–166
38. Suzuki T, Yokota J, Mugishima H et al. (1989) Frequent loss of heterozygosity on chromosome 14q in neuroblastoma. Cancer Res 49:1095–1098
39. Srivastan ES, Lin Ying K, Seeger RC (1993) Deletions of chromosome 11 and of 14q sequences in neuroblastoma. Genes Chromos Cancer 7:32–37
40. The I, Murthy AE, Hannigan GE et al. (1993) Neurofibromatosis type 1 gene mutations in neuroblastoma. Nature Genet 3:62–66
41. Tonini GP (1993) Neuroblastoma: a multiple biological disease. Eur J Cancer 29A:802–804
42. Schwab M, Alitalo K, Klempnauer KH et al. (1983) Amplified DNA with limited homology to myc cellular oncogene is shared by human neuroblastoma cell lines and a neuroblastoma tumor. Nature 305:245–248
43. Brodeur GM, Azar C, Brother M et al. (1992) Neuroblastoma: effect of genetic factors on prognosis and treatment. Cancer 70:1685–1694
44. Nakagawara A, Arima-Nakagawara M, Scavarda NJ et al. (1993) Association between high levels of expression of the TRK gene and favorable outcome in human neuroblastoma. N Engl J Med 328:847–854
45. Leone A, Seeger RC, Hong CM et al. (1993) Evidence for nm23 RNA overexpression, DNA amplification and mutation in aggressive childhood neuroblastoma. Oncogene 8:855–865

Retinoblastoma

One reason for the intense interest in the retinoblastoma (Rb) gene on humal chromosome 13 is that mutations in both alleles of this gene induce tumor formation in the retina. The apparent simplicity of this model system suggests that understanding the function of the Rb gene may provide important insights into the regulation of cell proliferation.

P.A. HAMEL et al. (1992)

Introduction

Retinoblastoma (Rb) is a tumor of the retina that appears in children younger than 3–4 years of age. Despite its rarity (approximately one case per 15000–20000 live births throughout the world), this tumor has been extensively investigated in the last 20 years for several important reasons: First, Rb represents the best example, at a clinical level, of the "two-hit" hypothesis of carcinogenesis proposed by Knudson nearly 20 years ago [1, 2]. Second, there is ample experimental evidence indicating that Rb is the first heritable tumor induced by the inactivation of a tumor suppressor gene which has precisely been localized and characterized [3]. Third, the Rb model may account for both hereditary and sporadic cases of the disease. Finally, the available evidence suggests that as well as in Rb, the Rb gene might also play a major role in the pathogenesis of other tumors (in particular, osteogenic sarcoma, breast cancer, bladder and small cell lung carcinoma) with different histology and embryologic origin [4]. Although the Rb gene has already been discussed in the chapter on "Oncogenes and Tumor Suppressor Genes" as a tumor suppressor gene, we will now review in more detail the most relevant clinical and biological aspects of the disease.

Clinical Features

Although rare in absolute terms, Rb represents about 3% of all pediatric malignancies; it can occur in both hereditary and nonhereditary forms. Approximately 40% of all cases are genetically determined and are characterized by multiple foci of tumor growth, often in both eyes; the mean age of

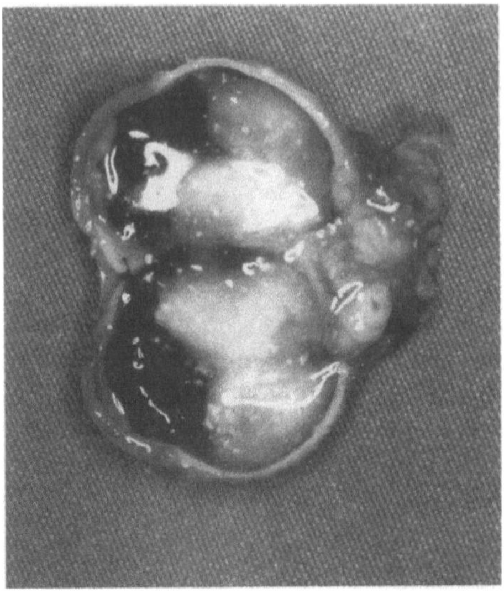

Fig. 1. Endophytic bilobate retinoblastoma occupying more than half of the vitreus

onset is 15 months. Sporadic Rb represents 60% of the total; the tumor is usually unilateral and unifocal, and the diagnosis is reached significantly later, between the second and the third year of life. Hereditary Rb follows an autosomal dominant type of genetic transmission [4, 5]. The main clinical sign of Rb is a white pupil ("cat's eye reflex"); less frequently, these children may show strabismus, glaucoma, or inflammatory changes within the eye. The diagnosis is based on an accurate ophthalmological examination, whereas bone scintiscan, computed tomography, and magnetic resonance are of great help in assessing the diffusion of disease. Tumors initially spread into the vitreous humor, and subsequently the sclera, optic nerve, and periglobal structures can be involved; distant metastases may develop in the liver, brain, lung, and bone marrow. The tumor seems to originate from a retinal precursor cell, called a retinoblast, and at histologic examination consists of small, round cells with large hyperchromatic nuclei and scant cytoplasm (Figs. 1, 2) [4]. Other retinal lesions, designated retinomas, have recently been found in approximately 2% of adult relatives of children with Rb. Since the adult retina does not develop Rb, it has been proposed that retinomas appear in nearly fully differentiated retina, when the replicative activity of retinoblasts is declining [6]. The origin and clinical significance of these lesions remain unclear.

In recent years the therapeutical approach to Rb has changed from an immediate enucleation of the affected eye to a more conservative attitude; this policy is based on the particular sensitivity of Rb to radiation and on the development of new techniques, such as cryotherapy and photocoagulation. As a matter of fact, in localized Rb, eradication of tumors with preservation of vision has now become feasible; in contrast, large or locally invasive

A

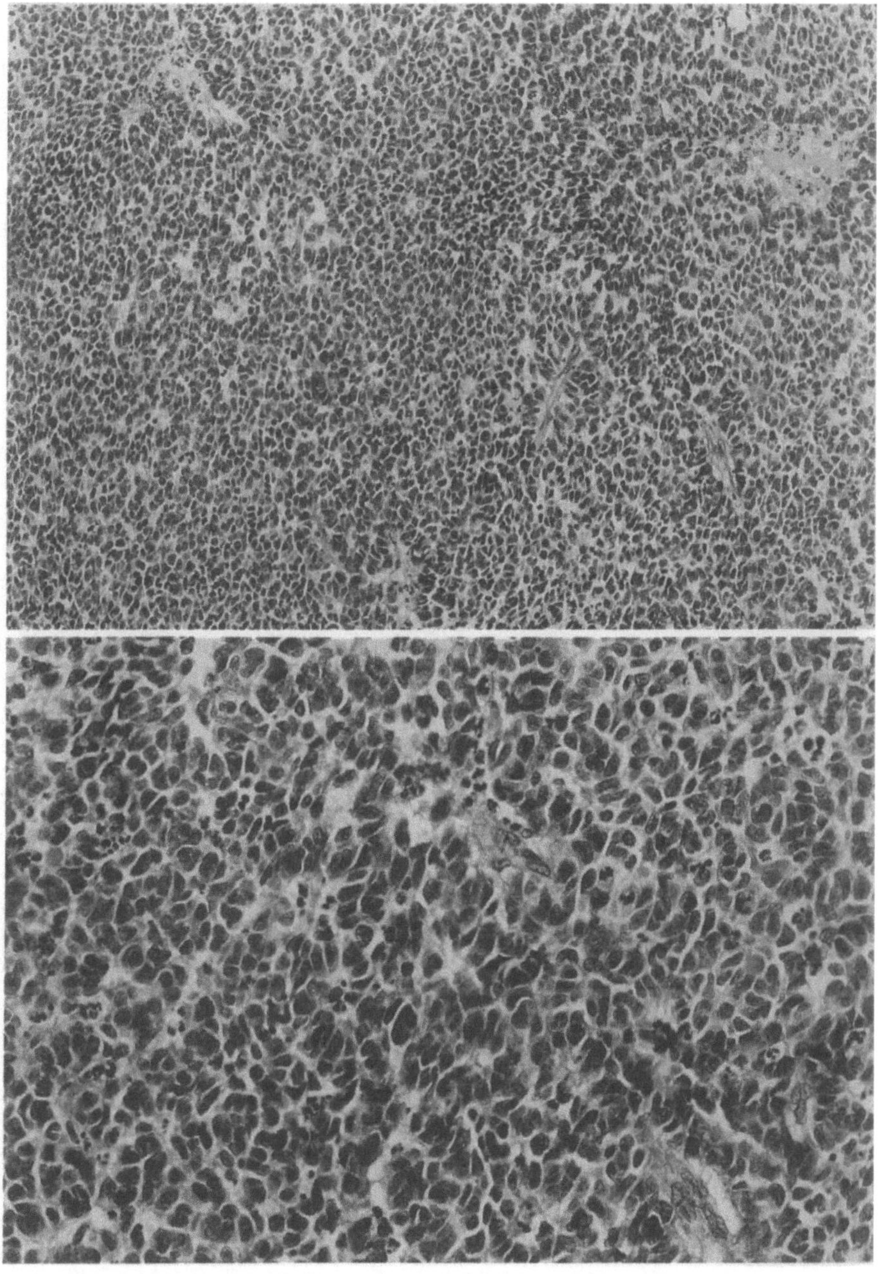

B

Fig. 2A,B. Histologic features of retinoblastoma at two different magnifications – hematoxylin and eosin, ×100 (**A**) and ×250 (**B**). **A** Pseudorosettes and focal necrosis can be observed. **B** Higher magnification shows typical small, round cells with hyperchromatic nuclei, scarce cytoplasm, and stromal tissue

neoplasms still require enucleation. For patients with distant (extraocular) metastasis, chemotherapy has been used with single agents or with combinations of antineoplastic drugs; the overall results, however, are rather poor [7]. Finally, after the operation, affected individuals with unilateral disease should be followed with frequent ophthalmologic examinations for the possible development of Rb in the other eye. This is particularly important for familial cases (i.e., when besides the proband other family members are affected by Rb), but should not be overlooked in apparently sporadic cases either (unilateral, unifocal, and with no family history), owing to the possibility of new germ line mutation of the Rb gene in the proband.

Knudson Model (Two-Hit Hypothesis)

Rb may be hereditary (approximately 40% of all cases) or nonheritable; in 1971 Alfred Knudson proposed a model which could provide a plausible explanation for both types of tumor [1, 2]. The author analyzed retrospectively the clinical data (age of onset, mono- or bilaterality of tumors) of a large series of Rb; he then plotted the logarithm of the proportion of cases not yet diagnosed versus age for both bilateral (all considered hereditary) and unilateral Rb (the large majority presumably sporadic). In the case of bilateral Rb, a straight line was observed, indicating that a single random somatic mutational event was necessary for tumor induction after an initial germ line mutation at the same locus. For unilateral tumors, the curve followed second order kinetics, thus suggesting the occurrence of two somatic mutational events. In addition, by analyzing a group of Rb patients with hereditary disease, the author noticed that the number of tumors per patient followed a Poisson distribution. This pattern suggests that the events leading to cancer development are random and independent.

From these original observations, the two-hit model was postulated and subsequently proposed for other neoplasms, such as neuroblastoma and Wilms' tumor [8]. According to this hypothesis, in hereditary Rb a first mutation exists in the germ line cells and a single (and second) mutation, at the same locus, in any retinal progenitor cell will then produce the tumor. Since there is a high probability of a second genetic event in at least one retinal cell, Rb are transmitted as an autosomal dominant trait. As already discussed, this type of transmission is a paradox, since at a molecular level both copies of the Rb gene should be inactivated for cancer induction, as in the case of recessive diseases. In nonhereditary Rb, there is no germ line mutation, but both mutations occur in the same somatic retinal cell; since the probability of two rare events occurring in the same cell is very low, sporadic cases of Rb are usually monolateral and unifocal.

After the formulation of the two-hit hypothesis and the many validations which accumulated in subsequent years through cytogenetic and biomolecular studies [3–5], the Rb gene is now considered as being representative of a class of genes in which the inactivation of both alleles is critical for tumor development (tumor suppressor genes).

Cytogenetics and Molecular Abnormalities

Evidence favoring the genetic basis of many human cancers has been provided through direct examination of chromosome number and arrangements in tumoral cells. Among the various abnormalities which have been reported, deletions of particular portions of the genome or chromosomal interchanges (translocations) are the most frequent. In Rb, an interstitial deletion of chromosome 13, band q14, was described in the early 1960s [9]. Further studies showed that no more than 5% of all Rb had this deletion [10]; moreover, other chromosomal abnormalities were reported, such as additional copies of 1q, isochromosome 6p, and monosomy 16 [11]. However, 13q14 deletion was particularly useful for localizing the Rb gene, since in the same region of chromosome 13 a gene was mapped which encodes for esterase D, a polymorphic enzyme of unknown physiology but suitable for linkage studies [12]. The activity of esterase D was reduced in patients with deletions 13q14 as compared to family members of normal karyotype; moreover, when large families were assessed, usually a close linkage was found between Rb and esterase D genes [4, 13]. The available evidence indicates that in Rb tumoral cells, a submicroscopic deletion of 13q14 eliminates both esterase D and Rb genes.

Because of its limits, cytogenetic analysis showed deletion of chromosome 13q14 in only a small fraction of Rb cases; the subsequent development of DNA probes and the application of restriction fragment length polymorphism analysis revealed loss of heterozygosity (LOH) for extensive regions of the long arm of chromosome 13 in Rb cancer cells [14]. The frequency of LOH was not different between hereditary and nonhereditary Rb and was in the order of 70% of all cases. Moreover, LOH in Rb tumors was specific for chromosome 13, since the other tested chromosomes maintained their constitutional heterozygosity. For the 30% of Rb tumors which did not show LOH around the Rb locus, more subtle genetic alterations (i.e., point mutations) may be inferred [4].

Retinoblastoma Gene

Cytogenetic studies and restriction fragment length polymorphism strongly suggested that the Rb gene was localized on chromosome 13q14. Definitive isolation of the gene was achieved with a positional cloning strategy by Friend et al. [15, 16], who detected an RNA transcript in an adenovirus-transformed retinal cell line and isolated a complementary DNA clone, which was designated 4.7 R. They noted that this 4.7 R clone was involved in genomic rearrangements in about 30% of Rb tumors and that the 4.7 R message was not expressed in Rb tumors. Taken together, these observations seem to suggest that Rb develops because of the functional inactivation of the 4.7 R fragment (in other words, that this was actually the Rb gene). This contention was further confirmed by the detection of germ line and somatic mutations affecting the putative Rb gene [17, 18].

The Rb gene encompasses 190 kb of DNA mapping to chromosome 13q14. When a mutation of the gene is found in tumoral (Rb) cells, examination of the genomic sequence in the identified exon – in normal lymphocytes or fibroblasts of the affected patient – can indicate whether the mutation was somatic or germ line. It follows: (a) that we are in a position to identify individuals with mutations of Rb gene in their germ line cells who are therefore at high risk of developing RB (or other tumors) and (b) that the precise knowledge of these mutations, within a given family, would be of great help for an accurate genetic counselling.

The Rb gene encodes a 105-kDa phosphoprotein (p105-Rb) which is a substrate of *cdc2* (cell division cycle) kinase [19]. Phosphorylation of Rb fluctuates during the cell cycle; unphosphorylated Rb predominates in resting cells (G-0–G-1), while phosphorylated forms appear as cells enter the S phase and persist during G-2 and M phases [20–23]. p105-Rb has been detected in normal cells of all organs and tissues examined [18, 19]. Thus, the possible involvement of the Rb gene product in cell cycle regulation and its ubiquitous expression in human tissues suggest that p105-Rb plays a central role in some essential cellular activities. This hypothesis has been tested by constructing animals with insertional mutations of the Rb gene [24–26]. While young heterozygous animals (i.e., retaining one normal allele) did not show abnormalities or develop Rb or other tumors, homozygous mutant embryos failed to reach term and died within the first 3 weeks of embryonic life with multiple defects (in particular, massive neuronal cell death and ectopic mitosis in the nervous system and defective hematopoiesis with immature nucleated erythrocytes). These findings clearly show that the Rb gene plays an essential role in the normal mouse development.

Retinoblastoma Gene and Development of Other Tumors

Individuals with the hereditary form of Rb (i.e., those with an inherited mutation of one Rb allele in the germ line cells) who survive after treatment for the disease have an increased risk of developing a second primary cancer, particularly an osteosarcoma [3, 27–29]. In addition, an increased frequency of neoplasms and an excess of cancer-related deaths have been reported among relatives of Rb patients [30, 31]. These clinical observations suggest that the Rb gene might be involved in the development of other neoplasms which do not seem to bear any relation to Rb. Indeed, this is actually not surprising if one considers that the Rb gene is ubiquitously expressed [18, 19].

This contention was further reinforced by several investigations of the Rb gene in solid tumors. Thus, altered expression and various structural alterations of the Rb gene have been reported in some 25%–40% of bone and soft tissue sarcomas, and tumors with markedly reduced expression of the gene tended to be more aggressive than those with normally expressed Rb protein [4, 32, 33]. Similarly, various alterations (mutations, absence of transcripts) of the Rb gene were detected in all major types of lung cancer (small cell, non-small-cell, and adenocarcinoma) [3, 34]. Rearrangements of the Rb gene and alterations of RNA transcripts were found in primary mammary tumors and in breast cancer cell lines [3, 4, 35]; moreover, inactivation of Rb occurs in about one third of bladder carcinomas or their derived cell lines [3, 18, 36]. Finally, the Rb gene has also been implicated in intestinal carcinogenesis; in contrast to all other neoplasms, however, in this case amplification and increased expression of the gene has been reported in approximately 30% of the informative colorectal tumors [37, 38].

The role of Rb gene alterations in the pathogenesis of the above-mentioned malignancies is unclear. Several questions need to be answered before the role of this gene in other, usually more common, neoplasms can properly be assessed [39]: If the gene is expressed in all tissues and if its products play a major role in some essential cellular activity, why do tumors occur predominantly in the retina or in mesenchymal tissue? Moreover, why are lung, breast, and bladder cancer, but not other common carcinomas, associated with consistent genetic changes of Rb? Since in almost all other more frequent malignancies, alterations of other genes (p53, *ras*, *myc*) have invariably been reported, what kind of interaction or interrelation can be imagined between Rb and the other genes presumably involved in tumorigenesis [40–42]? Finally, what is the precise biochemical mechanism by which loss or inactivation of Rb leads to malignancy?

References

1. Knudson AG (1971) Mutation and cancer: statistical study of retinoblastoma. Proc Natl Acad Sci USA 68:820–823
2. Knudson AG (1989) Hereditary cancers disclose a class of cancer genes. Cancer 63:1888–1891
3. Benedict WF, Xu HJ, Takahashi R (1990) Role of retinoblastoma gene in the initiation and progression of human cancer. J Clin Invest 85:988–993
4. Gallie BL, Squire JA, Goddard A et al. (1990) Mechanism of oncogenesis in retinoblastoma. Lab Invest 62:394–408
5. Cavenee WK, Murphree AL, Shull MM et al. (1986) Prediction of familial predisposition to retinoblastoma. N Engl J Med 314:1201–1207
6. Gallie BL, Phillips RA, Ellsworth RM et al. (1982) Significance of retinoma and phthisis bulbi for retinoblastoma. Ophtalmology 89:1393–1397

7. Crist WM, Kun LE (1991) Common solid tumors of childhood. N Engl J Med 324:461–471
8. Knudson AG (1985) Hereditary cancer, oncogenes and antioncogenes. Cancer Res 45:1437–1443
9. Lele K, Penrose L, Stallard HB (1963) Chromosome deletion in a case of retinoblastoma. Ann Hum Gen 27:171–174
10. Balaban G, Gilbert F, Nichols W et al. (1982) Abnormalities of chromosome 13 in retinoblastoma fron individuals with normal constitutional karyotype. Cancer Genet Cytogenet 6:213–221
11. Potluri VR, Helson L, Ellsworth RM et al. (1986) Chromosomal abnormalities of human retinoblastoma. Cancer 58:663–671
12. Sparkes RS, Sparkes MC, Wilson MG et al. (1980) Regional assignement of genes for human esterase D and retinoblastoma to chromosome band 13q14. Science 208:1042–1044
13. Strong LC, Riccardi VM, Ferrell RE et al. (1981) Familial retinoblastoma and chromosome 13 deletion transmitted via an insertional translocation. Science 213:1501–1503
14. Cavenee WK, Dryja TP, Phillips RA et al. (1983) Expression of recessive alleles by chromosomal mechanisms in retinoblastoma. Nature 305:779–784
15. Friend SH, Bernards R, Rogelj S et al. (1986) A human DNA segment with properties of the gene that predisposes to retinoblastoma and osteosarcoma. Nature 323:643–646
16. Friend SH, Horowitz JM, Gerber MR et al. (1987) Deletions of a DNA sequence in retinoblastoma and mesenchimal tumors: organization of the sequence and its encoded protein. Proc Natl Acad Sci USA 84:9059–9063
17. Dunn JM, Phillips RA, Becker AJ et al. (1988) Identification of germline and somatic mutations affecting the retinoblastome gene. Science 241:1797–1800
18. Horowitz JM, Park SH, Bogenmann E et al. (1990) Frequent inactivation of retinoblastoma anti-oncogene is restricted to a subset of human tumor cells. Proc Natl Acad Sci USA 87:2775–2779
19. Weingerg RA (1991) Tumor suppressor genes. Science 254:1138–1146
20. Buchkovich K, Duffy LA, Harlow E (1989) The retinoblastoma protein is phosphorylated during specific phases of the cell cycle. Cell 58:1097–1105
21. DeCaprio JA, Ludlow JW, Lynch D et al. (1989) The product of the retinoblastoma susceptibility gene has properties of a cell cycle regulatory element. Cell 58:1085–1095
22. Hamel PA, Gallie BL, Phillips RA (1992) The retinoblastoma protein and cell cycle regulation. Trend Genet 8:180–185
23. Ludlow JW, Shon J, Pipas JM et al. (1990) The retinoblastoma susceptibility gene product undergoes cell cycle-dependent dephosphorylation and binding to and release from SV40 large T. Cell 60:387–396
24. Clarke AR, Maandag ER, van Roon M et al. (1992) Requirement for a functional Rb-1 gene in murine development. Nature 359:328–3309
25. Lee EY, Chang CY, Hu N et al. (1992) Mice deficient for Rb are nonviable and show defects in neurogenesis and haematopoiesis. Nature 359:288–294
26. Jacks T, Fazeki A, Schmitt EM et al. (1992) Effect of an Rb mutation in the mouse. Nature 359:295–300
27. Weichselbaum RR, Beckett M, Diamond A (1988) Some retinoblastomas, osteosarcomas and soft tissue sarcoma may share a common etiology. Proc Natl Acad Sci USA 85:2106–2109
28. Abramson DH, Ellsworth RM, Kitchin FD et al. (1984) Second monocular tumors in retinoblastoma survivors. Ophtalmology 91:1351–1355
29. Draper GJ, Sanders BM, Kingston JE (1986) Second primary neoplasms in patients with retinoblastoma. Br J Cancer 53:661–665

30. Bonaïti-Pellié C, Briard-Guillemot ML (1980) Excess of cancer death in grandparents of patients with retinoblastoma. J Med Genet 17:95–101
31. Sanders BM, Jay M, Draper GJ et al. (1989) Non-ocular cancer in relatives of retinoblastoma patients. Br J Cancer 60:358–365
32. Cance WC, Brennan MF, Dudas ME et al. (1990) Altered expression of the retinoblastoma gene product in human sarcomas. N Engl J Med 323:1457–1462
33. Wunder JS, Czitrom AA, Kandel R et al. (1991) Analysis of alterations in the retinoblastoma gene and tumor grade in bone and soft-tissue sarcomas. J Natl Cancer Inst 83:194–200
34. Harbour JW, Li SL, Whang-Peng J et al. (1988) Abnormalities in structure and expression of the human retinoblastoma gene in SCLC. Science 241:353–357
35. Lee EY, To H, Shew JY et al. (1988) Inactivation of the retinoblastoma susceptibility gene in human breast cancer. Science 241:218–221
36. Horowitz JM, Yandell DW, Park SH et al. (1989) Point mutational inactivation of the retinoblastoma antioncogene. Science 243:937–940
37. Gope R, Christensen MA, Thorson A et al. (1990) Increased expression of the retinoblastoma gene in human colorectal carcinoma relative to normal colonic mucosa. J Natl Cancer Inst 82:310–315
38. Meling GI, Lothe RA, Borresen AL et al. (1991) Genetic alterations within the retinoblastoma locus in colorectal cancer. Relation to DNA ploidy pattern studied by flow cytometric analysis. Br J Cancer 64:475–480
39. Cowell JK, Hogg A (1992) Genetics and cytogenetics of retinoblastoma. Cancer Genet Cytogenet 64:1–11
40. Hovig E, Andreassen A, Fangan BM et al. (1993) A TP53 mutation detected in cell established from an osteosarcoma, but not in the retinoblastoma of a patient with bilateral retinoblastoma and multiple primary osteosarcoma. Cancer Genet Cytogenet 64:178–182
41. Hortsthemke B (1992) Genetics and cytogenetics of retinoblastoma. Cancer Genet Cytogenet 63:1–7
42. Reuvekamp PTW, Stulp RP, Koops HS et al. (1993) Analysis of a metastasizing testicular mixed gonadal stromal tumor with osteosarcoma components suggests that a malignant tumor with the histology of osteosarcoma may develop without primary involvement of RB1 and TP53. Cancer Res 52:6705–6707

Multiple Endocrine Neoplasia

> *In the MEN syndromes, adenomas predominate in some tissues and carcinomas of varying virulence predominate in others. In some studies, cellular hyperplasia is the abnormality detected, whereas at times hyperplasia precedes tumor formation. What determines the heterogeneity of this pathological response to presumably the same stimuli? Could hyperplasia be the result of the putative germ cell mutation, and tumor formation the consequence of subsequent somatic cell change?*
>
> MARK LESHIN (1985)

Introduction

Multiple endocrine tumors have been recognized from the beginning of this century, when a case of pituitary gland adenoma with concomitant parathyroid hyperplasia was reported [1]. After other reports of individual cases, the familial basis of this clinical entity was documented [2], and this led to the definition of the three main patterns of the disease. Multiple endocrine neoplasia type 1 (MEN-1, or Wermer syndrome) is characterized by a combination of pancreatic islet, pituitary, and parathyroid tumors; in MEN-2A (or Sipple syndrome), there is an association of thyroid (medullary carcinoma, MTC), adrenal medullary, and parathyroid tumors; MEN-2B (also called MEN-3 or multiple mucosal neuroma syndrome), in addition to the features of MEN-2A, shows an unusual phenotype, which includes eye and oral ganglioneuromas, a marfanoid habitus, and facial and skeletal involvement [3]. Finally, some authors described as MEN-4 (MEN of mixed type) the clinical condition featured by some overlap between MEN-1 and MEN-2 [4]. An outline of organs involved, the main type of tumors, and the symptoms occurring in various MEN syndromes are shown in Table 1.

One important feature, common to all types of MEN, is their genetic origin. As initially suggested by Wermer [2], the striking familial aggregation of affected individuals in two or more different generations is compatible with an autosomal dominant type of inheritance; this implies that there are no skipped generations, that men and women are equally affected, and that offspring of an affected patient carry a 50% risk of developing the disease.

Table 1. Multiple endocrine neoplasia (MEN) types 1, 2A, and 2B: organ involvement, type of tumor, main hormones, and symptoms

Organ	Tumor	Hormone	Symptom
MEN-1			
Pituitary	Prolactinoma, somatotropinoma	Prolactin, growth hormone	Galactorrhea, acromegaly
Pancreas (islet)	Gastrinoma, insulinoma, VIPoma	Gastrin, insulin, VIP	Peptic ulcer, hypoglycemia, diarrhea
Parathyroid	Adenoma	Parathyroid hormone	Hypercalcemia, urolithiasis
MEN-2A			
Thyroid	MTC	Calcitonin	Diarrhea
Adrenal medulla	PCC	Catecholamines	Hypertension, palpitations
Parathyroid	Adenoma	Parathormone	Hypercalcemia, urolithiasis
MEN-2B			
Thyroid	MTC	Calcitonin	Diarrhea
Adrenal medulla	PCC	Catecholamines	Hypertension, palpitations
Parathyroid (rare)	Adenoma	Parathormone	Hypercalcemia, urolithiasis
Oral mucosa, conjunctiva, intestinal mucosa	Ganglioneuromas	–	Constipation, diarrhea, vomiting, difficulties in swallowing

VIP, vasoactive intestinal polypeptide; MTC, medulla thyroid carcinoma; PCC, pheochromocytoma.

Penetrance of the responsible gene is usually high, whereas clinical expressivity is extremely variable within and among families. The MEN-1 gene has recently been mapped to chromosome 11 (11q13) [1, 5], and there is evidence that it might act as a tumor suppressor gene, requiring inactivation of both alleles for tumor development; similarly, other investigations have showed that the MEN-2A gene is linked to a locus close to the centromere of chromosome 10 [6].

Two other important aspects of MEN concern the spectrum of pathologic findings and the multiplicity of lesions. Various morphologic patterns can be observed, from hyperplasia to adenoma and carcinoma, in a single patient or in a given family. Moreover, the lesions tend to be multicentric, sometimes with adenomas associated with hyperplasia of the remaining gland. This multiplicity has been observed in the pituitary gland, in more than 70%

of islet cell pancreatic tumors, and in adrenal medullary tissue [3]. It is worth noting that the tendency to develop multiple primaries (in various segments of a single organ, such as colorectum, or in different organs, such as colon and endometrium) is a constant feature of hereditary cancer in general, especially when one or more of these tumors occur at an age which is atypical for that specific neoplasm [7].

A final point of interest, common to all MEN syndromes, concerns the screening of individuals at risk of tumor in affected kindreds. Young members of these families are usually symptom-free for many years, since the various manifastations of the disease usually appear in the second or third decade of life. It is possible therefore to identify persons at risk of MEN before the appearance of symptoms by evaluating specific hormonal levels in basal conditions or after provocative tests. An early diagnosis – as with many other neoplasms – may allow adequate medical and surgical treatment, thus preventing the development of metastatic lesions (particularly frequent in medullary thyroid carcinoma) or the appearance of other complications due to excessive hormonal secretion (i.e., bleeding from peptic ulcer in patients with MEN-1 and gastrin – secreting tumors, severe hypoglycemia due to the excessive secretion of insulin, and others).

Multiple Endocrine Neoplasia Type 1 (Wermer Syndrome)

Clinical Features

The main features of MEN-1 are islet cell pancreatic tumors, adenomas of the anterior pituitary gland, and hyperparathyroidism; carcinoid tumors (especially in bronchi and duodenum) and lipomas also occur with increased frequency in these patients and should therefore be considered as part of the syndrome. The incidence rate of MEN-1 is unknown, but its prevalence is in the order of 0.02–0.2 per 1000 [8].

Clinical manifestations of MEN-1 appear in the third or fourth decade of life and are closely related to the site of tumor and to the type of hormonal secretion. The first symptom of the disease is usually induced by the hyperfunction of a single endocrine gland; as the disease progresses, the involvement of other glands becomes manifest until the complete clinical picture develops. In a large review of the literature, including 122 cases diagnosed between 1963 and 1979, hyperparathyroidism was almost always present at the time of diagnosis, pancreatic neoplasms occurred in 84% and pituitary tumors in 54% [8]. Although only one third of patients showed involvement of all three endocrine glands, autopsy studies suggest that combined pituitary, parathyroid, and pancreatic disease eventually develops in all affected individuals (the "all or none" phenomenon) [9]. A representative pedigree of a MEN-1 family is shown in Fig. 1.

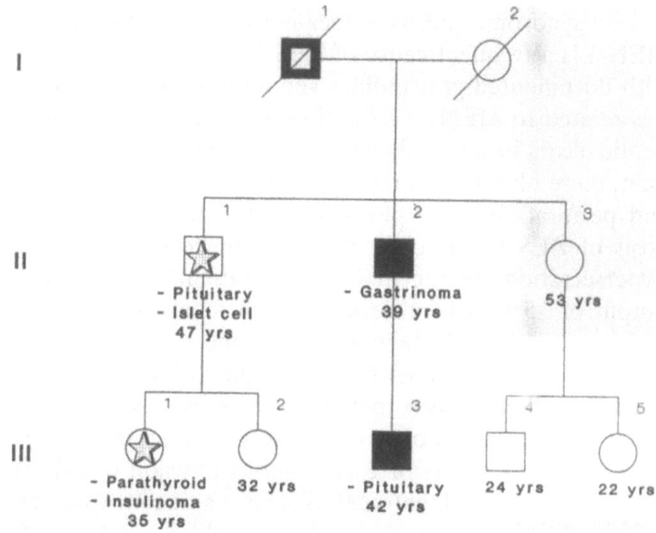

Fig. 1. Representative pedigree of a family with multiple endocrine neoplasia type 1 (MEN-1). Early occurrence of endocrine tumors and multiple primaries are observed in two generations. The clinical history of peptic ulcer of I-1 is fully consistent with the MEN-1 phenotype. *Black squares with white centers*, history of ulcer; *solid black squares*, tumor; *stars*, multiple tumors

Although often asymptomatic, parathyroid disease is the most frequent and presumably the earliest manifestation of MEN-1. Moreover, an underlying MEN-1 or -2 should always be suspected in all forms of primary hyperparathyroidism, since familial cases seem to represent 10%–15% of the total [10]. Hyperplasia of the parathyroid glands and/or adenomas have been reported, though at a morphologic level it is frequently difficult to distinguish between the two. Symptoms related to hyperparathyroidism include decreased bone mineral density (with consequent possible fractures), urolithiasis, cardiac arrhythmias, depression, fatigue, and other complications secondary to hypercalcemia. The diagnosis of hyperplasia of parathyroid glands is based on serum calcium levels (11 mg/dl or higher) and on measurement of plasma concentration of parathyroid hormone. The treatment of choice is subtotal parathyroidectomy with preservation of 30–50 mg of normal tissue [11].

Although most of the pancreatic islet cell tumors secrete gastrin or insulin, many other hormonal substances may be produced, including glucagon, pancreatic polypeptide, vasoactive intestinal polypeptide (VIP), serotonin, adrenocorticotropic hormone (ACTH), and calcitionin; some tumors are nonsecretory and may escape detection. In MEN-1, the clinical condition associated with gastrin-secreting tumors – known as Zollinger-

Ellison syndrome (ZES) – does not differ from sporadic gastrinomas. Since MEN-1 is a frequent cause of ZES (25%–50% of all cases) [12], all patients with documented gastrinomas should also be screened for other abnormalities related to MEN-1. At a clinical level, ZES is characterized by multiple peptic ulcers in the stomach and duodenum; together with severe abdominal pain, these ulcers frequently complicate with active bleeding, piloric stenosis, and perforation of or penetration into the surrounding organs. The diagnosis of ZES is based on the coexistence of hypergastrinemia and gastric hypersecretion. In the majority of patients with ZES, a basal gastric acid output of 15 mEq/h or serum gastrin levels of 1000 pg/ml can be detected and are considered diagnostic. In some cases, however, gastrin levels are within the normal range or only slightly elevated and provocative tests are needed to identify these patients. The most popular of these tests consists in serial measurements of gastrin levels after an intravenous bolus of secretin (2 U/kg body weight) or a continuous infusion of calcium gluconate (4 mg/kg per h) [13, 14]. Treatment of ZES is still controversial and rather unsatisfactory. In the ideal case in which a solitary gastrinoma is identified in the pancreas, surgery alone may be curative. However, despite all recent technologic advances (computed tomography, magnetic resonance imaging, endoscopy, and arteriography) tumors are frequently not identified at laparotomy, and their multicentric origin often render surgery noncurative, thus suggesting a medical approach. Histamine H-2 receptor antagonists or omeprazole are of great value in controlling many of the symptoms related to gastric hypersecretion [3, 15]. In malignant gastrinoma (about 30% of total cases), various combinations of antineoplastic agents or long-acting somatostatin can be used with some benefit [16].

Insulin-secreting tumors (insulinomas) represent about one third of islet cell pancreatic neoplasms in MEN-1. Multiplicity is particularly frequent and some patients may show diffuse beta cell hyperplasia rather then adenomas. Although less frequent than in gastrinoma, malignant changes can be found in approximately one fourth of insulinomas in MEN-1. It has been estimated that MEN-1 accounts for about 4% of all insulinomas [17]. Insulin-secreting tumors induce more or less severe hypoglycemia, with the various clinical manifestations of this metabolic disorder (disturbances of personality, weakness, confusion, convulsions, and eventually coma). The diagnosis is based on the simultaneous occurrence of marked hypoglycemia (45 mg/dl or less) together with a high plasmatic insulin concentration (more than 10 μU/ml); a plasma insulin to glucose ratio (measured in μU/ml and mg/dl, respectively) greater than 0.3 is highly suggestive of an underlying hyperinsulinism. After localization of the tumor with selective arteriography, computed tomography, or magnetic resonance, surgery is the treatment of choice and usually consists in the removal of a large portion of the gland [3].

Glucagon-secreting tumors as well as nonfunctioning A cell adenomas have been reported in MEN-1 patients, usually with concomitant insulinoma and/or gastrinoma [18]; the only symptom is hyperglycemia with glucose intolerance. VIPomas (tumors secreting VIP) have also been documented in MEN-1 [19], though the watery diarrhea, hypokalemia, and achlorhydria syndrome (WDHA or Verner-Morrison syndrome) is rare; however, it is of interest that one of the patients originally described by Verner and Morrison actually had MEN-1 [20]. Hypersecretion of pancreatic polypeptide is frequent in MEN-1 patients, but does not seem to be related to clinical manifestations [1, 3, 19].

The frequency of pituitary tumors in MEN-1 ranges from 60% of clinical studies to more than 90% in autopsy series [1, 3, 9]. Clinical manifestations depend on tumor size and consequent compression (headache, vomiting, abnormalities of the visual field, hypopituitarism) and on hormonal secretions. Prolactinomas account for 50%–70% of all pituitary tumors in MEN-1; hyperprolactinemia may induce amenorrhea and galactorrhea in women and decreased libido in men. Adenomas secreting growth hormone (with consequent acromegaly) are also frequent (20%–30%), whereas basophilic adenomas secreting ACTH, with symptoms of Cushing disease, are relatively rare. Hypopituitarism is found in approximately one fourth of patients with MEN-1 and pituitary tumors. After the detection of an abnormal serum concentration of prolactin, growth hormone, ACTH, or other substances, tumors are identified by computed tomography and/or magnetic resonance imaging. The optimal treatment of these tumors should be individualized; available options include trans-sphenoidal resection of the adenoma, bromocriptine, or simple observation.

Although not as frequently as the parathyroid, pancreas, and pituitary gland, many other organs may be involved in MEN-1. Thus, in approximately one fourth of these patients thyroid lesions can be detected and include adenomas, nonmedullary carcinoma, and Hashimoto thyroiditis [1]. Similarly, adenomas of the adrenal cortex occur in 20%–40% of patients with MEN-1, though an abnormal secretion of corticoid hormones is rare. Carcinoid tumors are undoubtedly more frequent than in the general population and their incidence is in the order of 5%–10% of all patients; these tumors are usually located in the bronchi, duodenum, and thymus and are rarely associated with the typical carcinoid syndrome [21].

Screening of High-Risk Individuals

There are two main categories of individuals at risk of MEN-1. The first includes first-degree relatives of patients in whom the disease has already shown the typical familiarity (aggregation of tumors in various generations). For an autosomal dominant condition, and assuming complete penetrance, the theoretical risk of being affected for these individuals is around 50%. Another risk group is constituted by patients with sporadic gastrinoma, insulinoma, or parathyroid or pituitary gland tumors; if MEN-1 is diagnosed in an apparently sporadic case, then all first-degree relatives of affected individuals are at risk.

Although there is no standardized protocol, a recommended approach is to screen family members at risk every 2 years, starting from the age of 15–20 and continuing up to the age of 60–70 years. Besides physical examination and accurate family history, determination of fasting serum gastrin, calcium, and prolactin levels should be sufficient for an early detection of tumors. Measurement of other hormones, provocative tests, computed tomography, upper endoscopy, and ultrasounds are not advisable for purposes of screening, but should be reserved for individual cases with a strong clinical suspicion of MEN-1.

Multiple Endocrine Neoplasis Type 2A (Sipple Syndrome)

Clinical Features

MEN-2A is featured by the concomitance of MTC (or C cell hyperplasia), pheochromocytoma (PCC), and parathyroid adenoma for hyperplasia. Clinical manifestations usually begin in the third decade with an asynchronous pattern, since symptoms and diagnosis of MTC often antedate those of PCC [3]. After initial reports of the association between thyroid cancer and PCC, further studies clearly defined that the thyroid cancer was actually MTC and that the disorder was transmitted through generations as an autosomal dominant trait [22, 23]. A representative pedigree of a MEN-2A family is shown in Fig. 2.

MTC is a malignant tumor of the calcitonin-producing C cells of the thyroid gland; this rare disease may occur in a sporadic (80% of the total) or in a hereditary (10%–20%) form; however, when MTC is diagnosed, an underlying MEN-2 should always be suspected and abnormal hormonal secretions of other glands accurately evaluated [3]. Calcitonin-producing cells are usually scattered – as single cells or as small groups – among thyroid follicles (they were originally called parafollicular cells). In contrast to follicular cells, which originate from the endoderm, the embryologic origin of C cells is the primitive neural crest. The histogenesis of MTC has been well characterized; the earliest lesion is a focal C cell hyperplasia and replicating cells then penetrate the follicular basement membrane, thus assuming a malignant phenotype. Continuing the proliferation of C cells, follicles gradually disappear and the lesion becomes a neoplastic nodule, which can be locally invasive or can metastatize, especially to mediastinal lymph nodes, lung, liver, soft tissues, and bones. The enzyme histaminase, which is expressed by MTC cells, but not from the precancerous lesions of the gland, can be used for the immunohistochemical evaluation of the transition from hyperplasia to cancer [24].

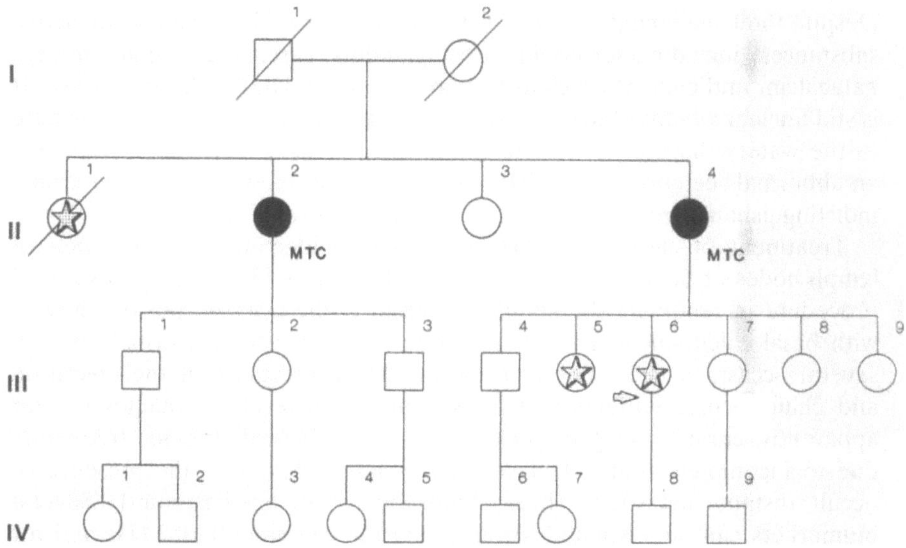

Fig. 2. Representative pedigree of a multiple endocrine neoplasia type 2A (MEN-2A) family. Information on the first generation is very limited. *Black circles*, medullary thyroid carcinoma (MTC) or pheochromocytoma (PCC); *stars*, multiple tumors (MTC and PCC). (Courtesy of Dr. Paola Temperani, Institute of Internal Medicine, University of Modena, Italy)

Being entirely asymptomatic for long periods, MTC may remain undetected and untreated for many years; the main clinical manifestation is often the presence of a small palpable mass in the neck, absolutely indistinguishable from other thyroid nodules. On radioiodine scintiscan the lesions appear as cold nodules. Since thyroid function is normal, affected individuals usually do not develop symptoms of hyper- or hypothyroidism. Another symptom, which develops in approximately 30% of patients with MTC, is secretory diarrhea, which should be related to the increased calcitonin secretion. Calcitonin is an extremely valuable biomarker for diagnosis and management of patients with MTC, as well as for screening programs. Patients with MTC may have elevated serum calcitonin basal levels (normal values up to 200 pg/ml) or show normal baseline values which rise substantially after provocative tests. The most commonly used test consists in a bolus intravenous injection of pentagastrin (0.5 μg/kg body weight) or in a slow infusion of calcium (2 mg/kg for 1 min) immediately followed by the pentagastrin bolus. Blood samples are taken at baseline and then at 1, 2, 3, 5, and 10 min; in the positive cases, a peak value of calcitonin levels, usually at least three to four times the normal range, is observed within 2–5 min [25, 26]. Moreover, the absolute levels of calcitonin observed following a calcium–pentagastrin provocative test seem to be correlated with the extent of the local disease and with its metastatic spread [27].

Despite their malignant nature, MTC secrete many other biologically active substances, including serotonin, prostaglandins, carcinoembryonic antigen, katacalcin, and enzymes such as histaminase and L-DOPA decarboxylase. It is still unclear whether the secretion of serotonin or prostaglandins contribute to the watery diarrhea observed in one third of these patients; in contrast, an abnormal secretion of ACTH may induce a full-blown Cushing syndrome indistinguishable from that seen in pituitary or adrenal tumors [27].

Treatment of choice for MTC is total thyroidectomy and resection of lymph nodes of the central compartment of the neck [3]. Efficacy of surgical procedure in removing the neoplastic mass can be assessed postoperatively with basal calcitonin measurements and provocative tests. Normal tests on several occasions after surgery usually indicate radicality of the operation and clinical cure. Patients with persistently high levels of calcitonin after apparently curative surgery presumably have residual disease, frequently due to incomplete removal of cervical lymph nodes or to the presence of occult distant metastases (liver, lung, bones, or mediastinum). Several biomarkers can be evaluated for assessing the aggressivity of MTC and for prediction fo the clinical outcome; thus, MTC in MEN-2A seem to have a more favorable prognosis when compared to sporadic disease or to MTC in MEN-2B [3]. Age of patients at diagnosis is another prognostic factor: residual tumors are rare in patients operated on during the first decade of life, whereas progressive or metastatic disease is observed in about 30% of patients operated in the second decade and up to 70% in those who undergo surgery in their sixties [3, 28]. Other prognostic factors include: (a) calcitonin immunostaining of the primary tumor (patients with calcitonin-poor tumors seem to have the worse prognosis); (b) DNA content of the tumor (high values of DNA indicate a short survival); and (c) calcitonin concentration doubling time (short doubling time is associated with local recurrence and poor prognosis) [3, 29]. Either chemotherapy (single agent or combination of drugs) or radiotherapy seem to have little role in the management of metastatic MTC, though in individual cases long-term remissions can be observed.

PCC are adrenal tumors characterized by the hypersecretion of catecholamines. These neoplasms may occur in a sporadic (the large majority) or familial (approximately 5%) form. PCC occurs in about 50% of patients with MEN-2 and its incidence increases with advancing age. In MEN-2, PCC is usually bilateral, whereas extra-adrenal disease or malignant PCC are relatively rare. The morphogenesis of PCC is similar to that of MTC, in the sense that there is an initial phase characterized by diffuse hyperplasia of the adrenal medulla and a subsequent development of nodular hyperplasia (nodules larger than 1 cm are designated PCC) [30, 31]. Clinically, PCC can be silent or associated with mild or severe symptoms; these usually develop in attacks of headache, palpitation, tachycardia, pallor, and high blood pressure. The diagnosis of PCC is based on the simultaneous determination of plasmatic and urinary catecholamines and of their main metabolites (vanillylmandelic acid and others); since the secretion of catecholamines is often intermittent, several determinations of the substances should be carried out; moreover, fractionated catecholamines can be of great help for diagnosis. Finally, provocative tests with glucagon or clonidine suppression test may also be of value in patients with normal levels of catecholamines [3]. Besides biochemical tests, computed tomography and [^{131}I]metaiodobenzylguanidine scintiscan are commonly used for the detection of adrenal tumors (of about 1 cm or more) or hyperplasia, respectively [3, 32].

The proper treatment of PCC in MEN-2 is bilateral total adrenalectomy, with an accurate exploration of the paraganglionic areas, removal of paragangliomas, and examination of the liver for metastases. This radical approach has several advantages, though patients require lifelong administration of mineral and glucocorticoid hormones. Despite the fact that symptoms are often mild and that a radical surgical approach can be carried out in many instances, PCC is probably the main cause of mortality in MEN-2; this high mortality rate is due to the possible development of malignant PCC (one fourth of all cases), with consequent metastatic diffusion, and to the severity of vascular changes induced by hormonal secretion.

Parathyroid disease (hyperplasia or adenomas) is present in 30%–60% of patients with MEN-2A. Clinical hyperparathyroidism is, however, minimal or absent in the majority of these families, and involvement of the gland is frequently found only at the time of operation for MTC. When present, symptoms and diagnosis are not different from those discussed for MEN-1. As for management, if symptoms are mild or absent, a conservative approach to parathyroidectomy is usually preferred [3].

Family Screening

As for MEN-1, there are two main groups of individuals at risk of MEN-2A, one represented by first-degree relatives of affected individuals in kindreds with full-blown disease and the other constituted by patients with apparently sporadic MTC or PCC. Since MTC may metastasize early in its natural history, screening should start within the first decade. Baseline and calcium–pentagastrin-induced calcitonin levels should be evaluated in all individuals at risk on an annual basis up to the age of 50–60 years. From the second decade, urinary levels of catecholamines and of their metabolites should also be measured. In the case of clinical suspicion of PCC with negative biochemical tests, fractionated catecholamines excretion can be evaluated after provocative tests, and the frequency of screening should be increased to every 3–6 months. Finally, calcium serum levels should also be assessed as part of the screening protocol.

Multiple Endocrine Neoplasis Type 2B, Mixed-Type Multiple Endocrine Neoplasis, and Familial Medullary Thyroid Carcinoma (Non-Multiple Endocrine Neoplasis)

In MEN-2B (or -3), MTC and PCC are associated with ganglioneuromas and characteristic facial and skeletal abnormalities, whereas parathyroid involvement is rare [33, 34]. Like other MEN syndromes, MEN-2B is a hereditary disease transmitted through generations according to an autosomal dominant model. Single cases (i.e., without family history) are rather frequent (about 50%) and are probably new mutations; it follows that offspring of these single cases are at 50% risk of developing the disease and should be screened accordingly. MTC in MEN-2B tends to be more aggressive than in MEN-2A and to appear earlier in life (anecdotal cases of an affected patient aged 15 months and of metastatic disease at 3 years have been reported) [35]. As far as diagnosis and therapy of MTC and PCC are concerned, there is no relevant difference between MEN-2A and -2B. PCC is equally frequent in both syndromes; however, because of the particular virulence of MTC in MEN-2B, PCC is a less frequent cause of death in the latter.

Mucosal ganglioneuromas (or neuromas) are the hallmark of MEN-2B. These neoformations contain ganglionic cells and thickened (and tortuous) nerve fibers; they are particularly frequent on the lips, tongue, and oral mucosa (though they may affect other epithelia as well, such as laryngeal and conjunctival mucosae). The characteristic facies of these patients is mainly due to pink–yellow nodules, easily observable by the age of 2–3 years, which are responsible for the everted, enlarged, and thickened lips. The marfanoid habitus can be recognized by excessive limb length, loose joints, scoliosis, and chest deformities. Neuromas can also be present in the myenteric plexus of the gastrointestinal tract; involvement of the gut can be associated with symptoms such as constipation, diarrhea, or, less frequently, dysphagia and vomiting [36]. In these patients, barium enema may show megacolon, colonic diverticula, and an abnormal haustral pattern; moreover, segmental esophageal dilatation, gastroesophageal reflux, gastric distension, and delayed gastric emptying have also been described and are presumably related to difficulties in swallowing and to failure to thrive, which may represent an early manifestation of MEN-2B [35]. Finally, the most common neuromuscolar symptoms are regional or diffuse weakness and sensory abnormalities.

There are descriptions of patients with multiple endocrine neoplasms in whom the clinical features of MEN-1 and MEN-2 may overlap. For example, the association of PCC with pancreatic islet cell tumor has been reported in more than one family [37]. Other less common associations reported in the literature include acromegaly, hyperparathyroidism, and PCC or prolactinoma with PCC [38, 39]. Many of these spurious associations might be designated as MEN-4, providing that the main features of the syndrome can be recognized: (a) an autosomal dominant pattern of genetic transmission; (b) multicentricity of tumors; and (c) early age of tumor appearance.

Finally, a new syndrome has recently been identified and designated familial, non-MEN MTC [40, 41]. In this syndrome, MTC is inherited as an autosomal dominant trait, but it is not associated with PCC, hyperparathyroidism, or ganglioneuromas. Moreover, the disease tends to be observed more frequently in older individuals and seems to behave less aggressively than the other types of MTC.

Molecular Biology and Cytogenetics of Multiple Endocrine Neoplasia

MEN-1 gene has recently been mapped to chromosome 11q12–13 by Larsson et al. [42]. By examining three Swedish kindreds, the authors reported a close linkage between the putative MEN-1 gene and the human muscle phosphorylase gene, which had already been assigned to chromosome 11q. Moreover, the authors found evidence of chromosome 11 deletions in insulinomas of two affected brothers in one family. Further linkage studies in larger pedigrees confirmed the location of the MEN-1 gene to chromosome 11q13 [43, 44]; in addition, other investigators showed allelic losses at various loci on chromosome 11q in pancreatic, pituitary, or parathyroid tumors (or hyperplasia) in MEN-1 [45–47]. All these data are suggestive of the possible existence of a tumor suppressor gene on chromosome 11q13 whose loss or inactivation might be related to tumor development in MEN-1. However, the observed findings are not fully consistent with the Knudson model (see above), in which both hereditary and sporadic retinoblastomas are interpreted as due to the successive mutations of two alleles at a single locus. In fact, allelic deletions were found only in tumors of patients with a definite diagnosis of MEN-1, but were invariably absent in sporadic pancreatic islet cell or pituitary tumors [47], thus suggesting that these neoplasms presumably do not develop through alterations of the MEN-1 gene. Interestingly, several other genes with a possible role in tumorigenesis are mapped on chromosome 11q13, including the *sea* gene (an oncogene involved in avian tumors) and *int* and *hst* oncogenes, which encode proteins similar to basic fibroblast growth factor [1]. Although the MEN-1 gene has not yet been cloned, restriction fragment length polymorphism analysis at the 11p12–13 locus may allow the identification of gene carriers in MEN-1 families [42, 44].

Various genetic abnormalities – including chromosome instability and deletions of chromosome 20, band p12.2 – have been reported in MTC [48, 49], but subsequently not confirmed by other investigators [50]; more importantly, the gene for MEN-2A has recently been assigned to chromosome 10. Thus, two research groups reported a linkage between MEN-2A locus and the interstitial retinol-binding protein gene, which is located near the centromere (10p11.2–10q11.2) [51, 52]. The putative MEN-2A gene, however, is approximately 12 cM outside the retinol-binding gene region, and this suggests that the marker is probably not suitable for a precise identification of the affected genotype in families with MEN-2A [52]. However, the results of preliminary studies with this and other probes suggest that restriction fragment length polymorphism analysis is more informative in predicting the disease state than conventional endocrine provocative tests [6]. More recent studies have showed that other genetic changes may contribute to tumor formation in MEN-2A; in particular, LOH at various chromosomal loci, including chromosomes 1, 3, 11, 13, 17, and 22, have been reported [53–55]. On the basis of these findings, it has been proposed that at least seven genes might concur in the development of malignancy in MEN-2A [56]; this includes an initiating event on chromosome 10 and a progressive accumulation of genetic alterations involving several other chromosomes. A similar chain of events has recently been proposed for colorectal and mammary tumorigenesis (see the chapters on "Hereditary and Familial Breast Cancer" and "Hereditary and Familial Colorectal Cancer"). Finally, presymptomatic testing based on DNA polymorphic markers in subjects at risk for MEN-2A showed that a virtual diagnosis could be calculated in 77% and a probable diagnosis in 90% of the individuals at risk [57].

References

1. Brandi ML (1991) Multiple endocrine neoplasia type I: general features and new insights into etiology. J Endocrinol Invest 14:61–72
2. Wermer P (1954) Genetic aspects of adenomatosis of endocrine glands. Am J Med 16:363
3. Becker KL, Bilezikian JP, Loriaux DL et al. (1990) Principle and practice of endocrinology and metabolism. Lippincott, Philadelphia, pp 1393–1400
4. Hansen OP, Hansen M, Hansen HH et al. (1976) Multiple endocrine adenomatosis of mixed type. Acta Med Scand 200:327–331
5. Larsson C, Skogseid B, Oberg K et al. (1988) Multiple endocrine neoplasia type I gene maps to chromosome 11 and is lost in insulinoma. Nature 332:85
6. Sobol H, Narod SA, Nakamura Y et al. (1989) Screening for multiple endocrine neoplasia type 2a with DNA-polymorphism analysis. N Engl J Med 321:996–1001
7. Parry DM, Mulvihill JJ, Miller RW et al. (1987) Strategied for controlling cancer through genetics. Cancer Res 47:6814–6417
8. Eberle F, Grun R (1981) Multiple endocrine neoplasia type I (MEN I). Ergeb Inn Med Kinderheilkd 46:76–149
9. Majewski JT, Wilson SD (1979) The MEA-I-syndrome: an all or none phenomenon? Surgery 86:475–479
10. Jackson CE, Boonstra CE (1967) The relationship of hereditary hyperparathyroidism to endocrine adenomatosis. Am J Med 43:727–734
11. Prinz RA, Gamvros OI, Dinan JJ (1981) Subtotal parathyroidectomy for primary chief cell hyperplasia of MEN-1 syndrome. Ann Surg 193:26–29
12. Lamers CB, Stadil F, van Tongeren JH (1978) Prevalence of endocrine abnormalities in patients with the Zollinger-Ellison syndrome and in their families. Am J Med 64:607–612

13. Lamers CB, Buis JT, van Tongeren J (1977) Secretin-stimulated serum gastrin levels in hyperparathyroid patients from families with multiple endocrine adenomatosis type I. Ann Intern Med 86:719–724
14. Deveney CW, Deveney KS, Way LW (1978) The Zollinger-Ellison syndrome – 23 years later. Ann Surg 188:384–393
15. Jensen RT, Gardner JD, Raufman JP et al. (1983) Zollinger-Ellison syndrome: current concepts and management. Ann Int Med 98:59–75
16. Ellison EC, O'Dorisio TM, Woltering EA et al. (1986) Suppression of gastrin and gastric acid secretion in the Zollinger-Ellison syndrome by long-acting somatostatin (SMS 201-995). Scand J Gastroenterol 21 [Suppl 119]:206
17. Stefanini P, Carboni M, Patrassi N et al. (1974) Beta-islet cell tumors of the pancreas: results of a study on 1067 cases. Surgery 75:597–609
18. Marx SJ, Spiegel AM, Brown EM et al. (1977) Family studies in patients with primary parathyroid hyperplasia. Am J Med 62:698–706
19. Samaan NA, Ouais S, Ordonez NG et al. (1989) Multiple endocrine syndrome type I. Cancer 64:741–752
20. Verner JV, Morrison AB (1958) Islet cell tumor and a syndrome of refractory watery diarrhea and hypokalemia. Am J Med 25:374–380
21. Amano S, Hazama F, Haebara H et al. (1978) Ectopic ACTH-MSH producing carcinoid tumor with multiple endocrine hyperplasia in a child. Acta Path Jpn 28:721–730
22. Williams ED (1965) A review of 17 cases of carcinoma of the thyroid and phaeochromocytoma. J Clin Pathol 18:288–292
23. Schimke RN, Hartmann WH (1965) Familial amyloid-producing medullary thyroid carcinoma and pheochromocytoma: a distinct genetic entity. Ann Intern Med 63:1027–1039
24. Mendelsohn G, Eggleston JC, Weisburger WR et al. (1978) Calcitonin and histaminase in C-cell hyperplasia and medullary thyroid carcinoma: a light microscopic and immunohistochemical study. Am J Pathol 92:35–52
25. Wells SA Jr, Baylin SB, Linehan WM et al. (1978) Provocative agents and the diagnosis of medullary carcinoma of the thyroid gland. Ann Surg 188:139–141
26. Wells SA Jr, Baylin SB, Leight GS et al. (1982) The importance of early diagnosis in patients with hereditary medullary thyroid carcinoma. Ann Surg 195:595–599
27. Keusch G, Binswanger U, Dambacher MA et al. (1977) Ectopic ACTH syndrome and medullary thyroid carcinoma. Acta Endocrinol (Copenh) 86:306–316
28. Sizemore GV, Carney JA, Heath H (1977) Epidemiology of medullary carcinoma of the thyroid gland: a 5-year experience (1971–1976). Surg Clin North Am 57:633–641
29. Miyauchi A, Onishi T, Morimoto S et al. (1984) Relation of doubling time of plasma calcitonin levels to prognosis and recurrence of medullary thyroid carcinoma. Ann Surg 199:461–468
30. Webb TA, Sheps SG, Garney JA (1980) Differences between sporadic pheochromocytoma and pheochromocytoma in multiple endocrine neoplasia type 2. Am J Surg Pathol 4:121–126
31. DeLellis RA, Wofe HJ, Gagel RF et al. (1976) Adrenal medullary hyperplasia. Am J Pathol 83:177–196
32. Valk TF, Frager MS, Gross MD et al. (1981) Spectrum of pheochromocytoma in multiple endocrine neoplasia: a scintigraphic portrayal using ^{131}I-metaiodobenzylguanidine. Ann Intern Med 94:762–767
33. Williams ED, Pollock DJ (1966) Multiple mucosal neuromata with endocrine tumours: a syndrome allied to Von Recklinghausen's disease. J Pathol Bacteriol 91:71–80

34. Khairi MRA, Dexter RN, Burzynski NJ et al. (1975) Musocal neuroma, pheochromocytoma and medullary thyroid carcinoma: multiple endocrine neoplasia type 3. Medicine 54:89–112
35. Jones BA, Sisson JC (1983) Early diagnosis and thyroidectomy in multiple endocrine neoplasia type 2b. J Pediatr 102:219–223
36. Carney JA, Go VLW, Sizemore GW et al. (1976) Alimentary-tract ganglioneuromatosis: a major component of the syndrome of multiple endocrine neoplasia type 2b. N Engl J Med 295:1287–91
37. Carney JA, Go VLW, Gordon H et al. (1980) Familial pheochromocytoma and islet cell tumor of the pancreas. Am J Med 68:515–521
38. Myers JH, Eversman JJ (1981) Acromegaly, hyperparathyroidism, and pheochromocytoma in the same patient: a multiple endocrine disorder. Arch Int Med 141:1521–1522
39. Meyers DH (1982) Association of phaeochromocytoma and prolactinoma. Med J Aust 1:13–14
40. Farndon JR, Leight GS, Dilley WG et al. (1986) Familial medullary thyroid carcinoma withouth associated endocrinopathies: a distinct clinical entity. Br J Surg 73:278–281
41. McHenry CR, Oppenheim DS, Murphy T et al. (1992) Familial nonmultiple endocrine neoplasia medullary thyroid carcinoma: an evolving clinical entity. Surgery 112:728–733
42. Larsson C, Skogseid B, Oberg K et al. (1988) Multiple endocrine neoplasia type 1 gene maps to chromosome 11 and is lost in insulinoma. Nature 323:85–87
43. Bale SJ, Bale A, Stewart K et al. (1989) Linkage analysis of multiple endocrine neoplasia type I with INT2 and other markers on chromosome 11. Genomics 4:320–322
44. Larsson C, Weber G, Kvanta E et al. (1992) Isolation and mapping of polymorphic cosmid clones used for sublocalization of the MEN-1 locus. Hum Genet 89:187–193
45. Yoshimoto K, Iizuka M, Iwahana H et al. (1989) Loss of the same alleles of HRAS1 and D11S151 in two independent pancreatic cancers from a patient with multiple endocrine neoplasia type 1. Cancer Res 49:2716–2721
46. Radford DM, Ashley SW, Wells SA Jr et al. (1990) Loss of heterozygosity of markers on chromosome 11 in tumors from patients with multiple endocrine neoplasia syndrome type 1. Cancer Res 50:6529–6533
47. Bale AE, Norton JA, Wong EL et al. (1991) Allelic loss on chromosome 11 in hereditary and sporadic tumors related to familial multiple endocrine neoplasia type 1. Cancer Res 51:1154–1157
48. Hsu TC, Pathak S, Samaan N et al. (1981) Chromosome instability in patients with medullary carcinoma of thyroid. JAMA 246:2046–2048
49. Babu VR, Van Dyke DL, Jackson CE (1984) Chromosome 20 deletion in human multiple endocrine neoplasia types 2A and 2B: a double-blind study. Proc Natl Acad Sci USA 81:2525–2528
50. Wurster-Hill DH, Noll WW, Bircher LY et al. (1986) A cytogenetic study of familial medullary carcinoma of the thyroid. Cancer Res 46:2134–2138
51. Mathew CGP, Chin KS, Easton DF et al. (1987) A linked genetic marker for multiple endocrine neoplasia type 2A on chromosome 10. Nature 328:527–528
52. Simpson NE, Kidd KK, Goodfellow PJ et al. (1987) Assignment of multiple endocrine neoplasia type 2A to chromosome 10 by linkage. Nature 328:528–529
53. Yang KP, Nguyen CV, Castillo SG et al. (1990) Deletion mapping on the distal third region of chromosome 1p in multiple endocrine neoplasia type II-A. Anticancer Res 10:527–533

54. Khosla S, Patel VM, Hay ID et al. (1991) Loss of heterozygosity suggests multiple genetic alterations in pheochromocytoma and medullary thyroid carcinomas. J Clin Invest 87:1691–1699
55. Moley JF, Brother MG, Fong CT et al. (1992) Consistent association of p1 loss of heterozygosity with pheochromocytomas from patients with multiple endocrine neoplasia type 2 syndrome. Cancer Res 52:770–774
56. Mulligan LM, Gardner E, Smith BA et al. (1993) Genetic events in tumour initiation and progression in multiple endocrine neoplasia type 2. Genes Chromos Cancer 6:166–177
57. Lichter JB, Wu J, Genel M et al. (1992) Presymptomatic testing using DNA markers for individuals at risk for familial multiple endocrine neoplasia 2A. J Clin Endocrinol Metab 74:368–373

Hereditary Tumors of the Nervous System

Given the reliability of the triad of neurofibroma, café au lait spots, and Lisch nodules for the identification of virtually all patients with neurofibromatosis 1 and the reliability of its absence in excluding a sizeable proportion of adults at risk, we have already taken a step towards the future.

V.M. Riccardi (1991)

Introduction

Little is known about the relation between environmental factors and tumors of the nervous system; thus, the most common carcinogens or tumor promoters (tobacco smoking, alcohol, dietary pattern) have never been associated with the development of these neoplasms. In contrast, we know much more about the role of genetic factors on their pathogenesis, since besides the aspecific aggregation of cases in families, several types of tumors of the nervous system recognize a mendelian pattern of inheritance.

Tumors of the nervous system are frequently part of more complex clinical conditions which will be discussed in different sections; thus, hereditary medulloblastoma and glioblastoma, together with breast cancer and sarcoma, define the clinical spectrum of Li-Fraumeni syndrome (see the relevant chapter). Similarly, in Turcot syndrome (see the chapter on "Hereditary Gastrointestinal Polyposis Syndromes"), glioblastomas are associated with colorectal diffuse polyposis. Finally, neuroblastoma has already been discussed in the chapter on "Genetic Factors in Solid Tumors of Childhood" with other hereditary malignancies of childhood.

In this chapter we will focus on meningioma and above all on neurofibromatosis (NF) types 1 and 2. In addition, very rare hereditary syndromes which usually involve the nervous system (tuberous sclerosis, von Hippel-Lindau disease (VHL), and Gorlin syndrome) will also be discussed. Finally, the most recent advances in the molecular biology of brain tumors in general (and not only hereditary) will be reviewed, with particular emphasis on the emerging role of p53 gene mutations.

Familial Meningioma

Meningioma is a relatively rare, usually sporadic tumor of the nervous system; the neoplasm arises from the meninges and accounts for about 10% of all brain tumors. The main symptoms are due to the compression of the brain (headache, vomiting, and other signs of raised intracranial pressure), whereas local invasion is very uncommon, with the exception of the even more rare malignant meningioma (meningiosarcoma). Pressure outwards may cause erosion of the inner table of the skull. Histologically, meningioma may be mainly fibrous (fibroblastic meningioma) or mostly vascular (angioblastic meningioma), the second being more prone to the malignant transformation.

In NF-1, meningioma may occur together with several other types of tumors; however, familial meningioma not associated with other genetic syndromes has also been reported. Thus, meningiomas without NF were reported by Gaist et al. in two members of the same family [1]; similarly, meningiomas were reported in a mother and a daughter [2] and in a pair of identical twins, again without evidence of neurofibromas [3]. Finally, in a large American family meningioma was detected in the father and in three out of eight of his offspring, with clinical onset ranging between 35 and 65 years of age [4]. Although the striking aggregation of meningiomas in some families and the apparent vertical transmission may suggest an autosomal dominant type of inheritance, more observations are needed before the possible genetic basis of this disease can be elucidated. In the abovementioned American family, a constitutional robertsonian translocation - t(14;22)- was found in the three siblings with meningioma and in four of their asymptomatic offspring (probably still too young for assessing the occurrence of tumors); in addition, some of the family members had abnormalities of the *sis* oncogene [4]. The authors hypothesized that in this family a mutant gene on the long arm of chromosome 22 could be involved in the development of meningioma. Subsequent cytogenetic analysis and restriction fragment length polymorphism studies confirmed the frequency of deletions and losses of genes on chromosome 22 [5, 6]. Finally, recent studies showed loss of heterozygosity for loci on chromosome 10, and this suggested a possible model for meningeal tumorigenesis in which an initial genetic event on chromosome 22 is compounded by subsequent allelic deletions at chromosome 10 [7].

Neurofibromatosis-1 (von Recklinghausen Disease)

Clinical Aspects

NF-1 is an autosomal dominant disorder that occurs once in 3000–4000 live births. The syndrome was described in 1849 by Smith and then in 1882 by von Recklinghausen, who gave a detailed description of the various clinical manifestations of the disease [8]. These include:

- Brownish spots of the skin, called café au lait spots, of various sizes and often present at birth; in men, the color intensity of the spots increases up to puberty and then remains stable; in women the spots become darker during pregnancy. The pigmentation is due to an abnormal deposition of melanin in the basal layers of the epidermis.
- Cutaneous and subcutaneous neurofibromas, benign tumors often arising along the course of nerves and ranging in size from a few millimeters to 20 cm. These tumors are usually absent at birth, appear during puberty, and may then increase to number in the thousands. Neurofibromas are characterized by irregular overgrowth of Schwann cells associated with increase of reticulin and collagen.
- Benign melanocytic hamartomas on the iris of the eye (Lisch nodules); these lesions are highly specific for NF-1, appear earlier than neurofibromas, and are particularly helpful for a proper diagnosis in younger individuals [9].

Additional clinical features are freckling in the axillary and inguinal regions, optic gliomas, and various bone lesions (sphenoid dysplasia, thinning of long bone cortex) [10]. NF-1 is usually taken as an example of genetic disease with variable expressivity, since clinical manifestations may range from the simple presence of café au lait spots to disfiguring neurofibromas or to severe deformities. During a recent Consensus Conference it was established that at least two of the above-mentioned clinical manifestations should be present for an appropriate diagnosis of NF-1 [10].

After the initial description of NF-1, evidence accumulated rapidly that it is a hereditary autosomal dominant disorder; however, although there are families in which the disease could be traced in four successive generations [8], single cases are rather frequent and are probably new mutations. The genetic characteristics of the syndrome (autosomal dominant transmission, usually with high penetrance but with an extremely variable clinical expressivity) suggest that all first-degree relatives of affected individuals should be evaluated for the presence of stigmata of NF-1 and then reassessed at regular intervals. This is particularly important for children born to NF-1 patients with no family history of the disease, since in these families the typical pattern of segregation is not yet apparent.

Although for many patients the prognosis is relatively good, severe complications do occur in some individuals, especially when followed up for several years. Osseous deformities develop in about half of these patients, whereas gastrointestinal involvement (multiple neurofibromas in the stomach and small intestine) is less frequent. Neoplasms of the central nervous system (both benign and malignant) occur with increased frequency in NF-1; Sorensen et al. [11] reported a relative risk of 4.0 among probands when compared to the expected numbers, whereas the risk was much smaller for their relatives. Moreover, many non-neurogenic cancer types (gastric, lung, and mammary carcinoma, malignant melanoma, thyroid cancer, sarcomas and leukemias) seem also to occur in excess among these patients [8, 10, 11]. The main clinical manifestations of NF-1 do not need treatment in the majority of affected individuals. Surgical intervention, however, is often necessary for the most common complications; thus, operations can be required for optic gliomas, brain tumors, or neoplasms of other organs. In addition, surgery may be needed for orthopedic problems (kyphoscoliosis, tibial bowing, and other deformities) and for disfigurement. Owing to the large variety of clinical signs and symptoms, and above all to the increased incidence of malignancies, NF-1 patients should have a careful, long-term follow-up, with frequent medical visits and radiologic investigations.

Molecular Biology

The NF-1 gene has been localized on chromosome 17, region 17q11–12. Studying 13 families with typical NF-1 stigmata, Seizinger et al. [12] found a close linkage between NF-1 gene and the locus of the nerve growth factor receptor, which is located on the long arm of chromosome 17 (17q12–22). The gene was subsequently cloned and sequenced through a positional cloning technique [13, 14]; NF-1 gene is 20–30 kb in length and encodes a 2485-amino acid polypeptide (neurofibromin), in which a region shows similarities with the GTPase-activiting proteins [15, 16]. This suggests that the expression product of NF-1 gene may contribute to the control of cell replication by complex interaction with *ras* oncogene products.

The NF-1 gene might act as a tumor suppressor gene (see earlier chapter), requiring the inactivation of both alleles for tumor induction and progression. However, the experimental evidence supporting this contention is still insufficient and, in addition, other genetic alterations could be involved in the pathogenesis of NF-1. Thus, germ line mutations have been found in only a few of the patients so far analyzed [17–19]; similarly, loss of alleles on chromosome 17 was detected in tumors from NF-1 patients, but it was not a constant finding [20, 21] and was observed only in malignant, but not in benign neoplasms [22]. Moreover, in gliosarcoma the common region of deletion was localized on the short arm of chromosome 17 (not on the long arm, where the NF-1 gene was mapped), in the region of p53 gene [21, 22], a tumor suppressor gene frequently mutated in various types of malignancies [23]. By analogy with colorectal tumorigenesis [24], the development of malignant tumors in NF-1 might be the result of a sequence of genetic alterations: the first of these could be the inactivation of one or both alleles of the NF-1 gene, with the consequent formation of neurofibromas; additional genetic changes might lead to loss or mutation of p53 (and/or other tumor suppressor genes) with subsequent transformation of a benign tumor into a malignant neurofibrosarcoma [25, 26]. Finally, recent studies have showed that the NF-1 gene seems to be mutated not only in neurofibromas, but also in several other tumors apparently unrelated to NF-1 [27].

Neurofibromatosis-2 (Bilateral Acoustic Neurofibromatosis or Central Neurofibromatosis)

NF-2 is a rare genetic condition occurring in about one in 50000 individuals and characterized by bilateral neurofibromas of the eighth nerve. The presence of unilateral tumors, but with a first-degree relative affected by typical NF-2 or with the addition of other tumors of the nervous system (cranial and spinal meningiomas, nerve root neurofibromas, or gliomas of the brain stem), is also accepted as evidence of disease [10]. Initial symptoms include hearing loss and vertigo; subsequently, facial paralysis, dysphagia, and hydrocephalus may develop. NF-2 is transmitted as an autosomal dominant trait; thus, offspring of affected individuals bear a 50% risk of developing the disease. First-degree relatives of NF-2 patients should be screened at regular intervals; besides physical examination, audiograms, brain stem auditory evoked potentials, computed tomography (or magnetic resonance), and vestibular tests can be carried out in order to ascertain the presence of NF-2. Surgery is the treatment of choice, and the results have improved dramatically with the new microsurgical techniques [28], so that in a large fraction of cases tumors can be removed with preservation of hearing capacity and of facial nerve function.

The locus of NF-2 gene has recently been assigned to chromosome 22 [29]; thus, despite the similarity of the basic morphologic lesion (neurofibromas), NF-1 and NF-2 are two distinct nosologic entities, either at a clinical level (phenotypically) or genotypically (NF-1 mapped to chromosome 17, NF-2 to chromosome 22). NF-2 was localized on chromosome 22 by linkage studies in a large family spanning six generations and including more than 20 affected individuals [29]; a close linkage was found between NF-2 locus and marker D22S1, which had previously been located in 22q12–22q13. The authors therefore suggested that NF-2 maps in the center of the chromosome 22 long arm, presumably in the region 22q11–22q13. In addition, restriction fragment length polymorphism studies showed that allelic losses on chromosome 22 were frequently detected in both sporadic acoustic neuroma (usually unilateral) and in the bilateral form, which is specific for NF-2 [30]. Rather interestingly, losses of genes on chromosome 22 have also been reported in meningiomas [5, 6], which are frequently associated with NF-2; it is therefore likely that neurofibromas and meningioma share some pathogenetic steps. Moreover, the observation that the same allelic losses were found in sporadic as well as in genetically determined neurofibromas, and the fact that the former is usually unilateral and the latter bilateral, are highly suggestive of a pathogenetic model similar to that proposed by Knudson for retinoblastoma, which represents the paradigm of tumor suppressor genes (see earlier chapters). Thus, we might hypothesize that a couple of alleles at a specific locus on chromosome 22 are strictly involved in the control of Schwann cell replication and differentiation; patients with NF-2 inherit a constitutional mutation of one allele and subsequently undergo a second somatic genetic event, with the consequent inactivation of both alleles. In sporadic acoustic neuromas, both genetic events might occur somatically, which would be a plausible explanation for the much more frequent occurrence of unilateral tumors than bilateral ones. Finally, two independent collaborative studies recently described the identification of the NF-2 gene from the long arm of chromosome 22 [31, 32]; the putative gene encodes for a 587-amino acid protein which shows similarities to proteins at the plasma membrane and cytoskeleton interface, thus suggesting that the NF-2 gene might represent a new class of oncosuppressor genes.

Other Tumors of the Nervous System

Besides the two NF syndromes, tumors of the nervous system may develop more or less frequently in several inherited conditions which usually involve also other organs or apparatus.

VHL (cerebelloretinal hemangioblastomatosis) is characterized by hemangioblastomas of the retina, cerebellum, brain stem, and spinal cord, pancreatic and renal malignancies, pheochromocytomas, and epididymal cysts [33]. VHL is an autosomal dominant disorder, which implies that affected individuals without a well-defined familiality presumably represent new mutations. In some pedigrees, the trait could be recognized for five successive generations. Retinal lesions are present in more than 50% of VHL patients; these lesions can be asymptomatic or, with time, may induce severe complications, such as glaucoma, cataract, and retinal detachment. Treatment of these lesions include cryotherapy and photocoagulation (argon laser). Cerebellar or cerebral involvement develops in some 50%–80% of VHL patients and is associated with symptoms of increased intracranial pressure (headache, vomiting, papilledema), nystagmus, ataxia, and dysmetria. Tumors of the central nervous system show a fine vascular network of endothelial channels and caverns, with no neuronal (or glial) cells; in some cases cysts or pseudocysts may develop. After appropriate diagnosis (computed tomography, magnetic nuclear resonance, and angiography), surgical resection is the treatment of choice. Renal carcinoma is found in approximately 25% of VHL patients and is one of the main causes of death; the diagnosis may not be easy in the presence of multiple renal cysts. Pancreatic cystoadenocarcinomas, pheochromocytomas, and epididymal cysts or tumors may also be found in VHL syndrome, though they are not as frequent as malignant tumors of the kidney.

The molecular basis of VHL disease has recently been investigated in more detail. In nine extended families with VHL syndrome, the VHL gene was found to be linked to the locus of the human homolog of *raf-1* oncogene, which maps to chromosome 3p25 [34], thus suggesting that the gene is located on the short arm of chromosome 3. This might be of relevance, since both cytogenetic studies and restriction fragment length polymorphism analysis showed 3p deletions and loss of heterozygosity in renal cell carcinoma [35, 36] (see the chapter on "Familial Factors in Cancer of the Genitourinary Tract"). It can be speculated, for instance, that VHL syndrome – in which renal cancer is rather frequent – and the apparently sporadic renal cell carcinoma might have some pathogenetic steps in common and that the inactivation of a suppressor gene (mapped to 3p) might play a key role in the development of a series of inherited tumors (i.e., the tumor spectrum of VHL syndrome) and of their sporadic counterpart (i.e., renal cell carcinoma). In a series of elegant investigations, Latif and coworkers [37, 38] recently reported the identification of the VHL gene on the short arm of chromosome 3.

Two other rare inherited conditions in which tumors of the nervous system can be observed are tuberous sclerosis (or Bourneville disease) and basal cell nevus syndrome (or Gorlin disease) [39, 40]. The former is an autosomal dominant condition characterized by the clinical triad of convulsive attacks, mental deficiency, and adenoma sebaceum. The latter are slightly elevated pinkish lesions which show a butterfly distribution over the cheeks and forehead. Brain lesions include gliomas, areas of malformed cortex with extensive astrogliosis, and masses of subependimal glial tissue projecting into the ventricles. Tumors and/or malformations of other organs (liver, pancreas, kidney, and adrenal glands) can also be present.

Gorlin disease is an autosomal dominant disorder with high penetrance and variable clinical expressivity. The main features of the syndrome are multiple basal cell epitheliomas, beginning on average at the age of 15 years and frequently located on exposed areas of the body; their number may vary from a few to many hundreds. Besides cutaneous tumors, additional lesions include soft tissue neoplasms, ocular alterations (cataract, glaucoma, corneal opacities), hypogonadism, osseous abnormalities (spina bifida occulta, kyphoscoliosis, pectus excavatum, oligodactily, or syndactily) oral–facial changes (cleft lip or palate, mandibular prognathism, broad nasal root), and tumors of the nervous system, in particular medulloblastoma, meningioma, and cerebellar astrocytoma.

Genetic alterations have also been studied with increasing interest in many apparently sporadic tumors of the nervous system. Thus, loss of constitutional heterozygosity – indicating chromosomal deletions or rearrangements – was seen for markers of the short arm of chromosome 17 in about 50% of the informative malignant astrocytomas [41]. Although allelic losses were also seen for markers on chromosomes 1 and 10, the authors proposed that chromosome 17 might contain a tumor suppressor gene whose inactivation could be associated with tumorigenesis and suggested that p53 was the most likely candidate. In keeping with these observations, subsequent studies revealed, in addition to chromosomal losses, frequent mutations of p53 in astrocytomas; these changes were clustered in the highly conserved region of the gene (see the chapter on "Oncogenes and Tumor Suppressor Genes"), and at least in some of the studies seemed to be related to tumor progression [42–45]. Moreover, p53 mutations were also reported in nonastrocytic brain tumors (oligodendrogliomas and medulloblastomas), though only in a small fraction of the investigated cases [46]. Finally, preliminary studies indicate that besides p53, other tumor suppressor genes might be involved in the pathogenesis of tumors of the nervous system; thus, a tumor-associated locus on 17p, but distal to p53, seems to be frequently lost in primary neuroectodermal tumors [47], and further studies have reinforced the contention that chromosomes 10 and 22q might contain antioncogenes potentially implicated in the development of these tumors [48, 49].

References

1. Gaist G, Piazza G (1959) Meningiomas in two members of the same family. J Neurosurg 16:110–113
2. Joynt RG, Perrett GE (1961) Meningiomas in a mother and daughter: cases without evidence of neurofibromatosis. Neurology 11:164–165
3. Sedzimir CB, Frazer AK, Roberts JR (1973) Cranial and spinal meningiomas in a pair of identical twin boys. J Neurol Neurosurg Psychiatry 36:368–376
4. Bolger GB, Stamberg J, Kirsch IR et al. (1985) Chromosome translocation t(14;22) and oncogene (c-sis) variant in a pedigree with familial meningioma. N Engl J Med 312:564–567
5. Seizinger BR, de la Monte S, Atkins L et al. (1987) Molecular genetic approach to human meningioma: loss of genes on chromosome 22. Proc Natl Acad Sci USA 84:5419–5423
6. Collins VP, Nordenskjold M, Dumanski JP (1990) The molecular genetics of meningiomas. Brain Pathol 1:19–24
7. Rempel SA, Schwechheimer K, Davis RL et al. (1993) Loss of heterozygosity for loci on chromosome 10 is associated with morphologically malignant meningioma progression. Cancer Res 53:2386–2392
8. Brasfield RD, Das Gupta TK (1972) Von Recklinghausen disease: a clinicopathological study. Ann Surg 175:86–104
9. Lubs MLE, Bauer MS, Formas ME et al. (1991) Lisch nodules in neurofibromatosis type 1. N Engl J Med 324:1264–1266
10. National Institutes of Health Consensus Conference (1988) Neurofibromatosis. Arch Neurol 45:575–578
11. Sorensen SA, Mulvihill JJ, Nielsen A (1986) Long-term follow-up of von Recklinghausen neurofibromatosis. N Engl J Med 314:1010–1015
12. Seizinger BR, Rouleau GA, Ozelius LJ et al. (1987) Genetic linkage of von Recklinghausen neurofibromatosis to the nerve growth factor receptor gene. Cell 49:589–594
13. Viskochil D, Buchberg AM, Xu G et al. (1990) Deletions and translocations interrupt a cloned gene at the neurofibromatosis type 1 locus. Cell 62:187–192
14. Wallace RM, Marchuk DA, Andersen LB et al. (1990) The type 1 neurofibromatosis gene: identification of a large transcript disrupted in 3 NF1 patients. Science 249:181–186

15. Xu G, O'Connell P, Viskochil D et al. (1990) The neurofibromatosis type 1 gene encodes a protein related to GAP. Cell 62:599–608
16. DeClue J, Cohen BD, Lowy DR (1991) Identification and characterization of the neurofibromatosis type 1 protein product. Proc Natl Acad Sci USA 88:9914–9918
17. Riccardi VM (1991) Neurofibromatosis: past, present and future. N Engl J Med 324:1283–1285
18. Xu W, Mulligan LM, Ponder MA et al. (1992) Loss of NF1 alleles in pheochromocytomas from patients with type 1 neurofibromatosis. Genes Chromos Cancer 4:337–342
19. Cawthon RM, Weiss R, Gangfeng X et al. (1990) A major segment of the neurofibromatosis type 1 gene: cDNA, sequence, genomic structure and point mutations. Cell 62:193–201
20. Skuse GR, Kosciolek BA, Rowley PT (1990) Molecular genetic analysis of tumors in von Recklinghausen neurofibromatosis: loss of heterozygosity for chromosome 17. Genes Chromos Cancer 1:36–41
21. Glover TV, Stein CK, Legius E et al. (1991) Molecular and cytogenetic analysis of tumors in von Recklinghausen neurofibromatosis. Genes Chromos Cancer 3:62–70
22. Menon AG, Anderson KM, Riccardi VM et al. (1990) Chromosome 17p deletions and p53 gene mutations associated with the formation of malignant neurofibrosarcoma in von Recklinghausen neurofibromatosis. Proc Natl Acad Sci USA 87:5435–5439
23. Levine AJ, Momand J, Finlay CA (1991) The p53 tumour suppressor gene. Nature 351:453–456
24. Fearon ER, Vogelstein B (1990) A genetic model of colorectal tumorigenesis. Cell 61:759–767
25. Shimizu E, Shinohara T, Mori N et al. (1993) LOH on chromosome arm 17p in small cell lung carcinoma but not in neurofibromas, in a patient with NF-1. Cancer 71:752–758
26. Rey JA, Bello MJ, Kusak ME et al. (1993) Involvement of 22q12 in a neurofibrosarcoma in NF-1. Cancer Genet Cytogenet 66:28–32
27. Seizinger BR (1993) NF-1: a prevalent cause of tumorigenesis in human cancer. Nature Genet 3:97–99
28. Black PML (1991) Brain tumors, part 2. N Engl J Med 324:1555–1564
29. Rouleau GA, Wertelecki W, Haines JL et al. (1987) Genetic linkage of bilateral acoustic neurofibromatosis to a DNA marker in chromosome 22. Nature 329: 246–248
30. Seizinger BR, Martuza RL, Gusella JF (1986) Loss of genes on chromosome 22 in tumorigenesis of human acoustic neuroma (1986) Nature 322:644–647
31. Trofatter JA, MacCollin M, Rutter JL et al. (1993) A novel moesin, ezrin, radixin-like gene is a candidate for the NF-2 tumor suppressor gene. Cell 72: 791–800
32. Rouleau GA, Merel P, Lutchman M et al. (1993) Alteration in a new gene encoding a putative membrane-organizing protein causes NF-2. Nature 363: 515–521
33. Lamiell JM, Salazar FG, Hsia YE (1989) Von Hippel-Lindau disease affecting 43 members of a single kindred. Medicine 68:1–27
34. Seizinger BR, Rouleau GA, Ozelius LJ et al. (1988) Von Hippel-Lindau disease maps to region of chromosome 3 associated with renal cell carcinoma. Nature 332:268–269
35. Kovacs G, Erlandsson R, Boldog F et al. (1988) Consistent chromosome 3p deletion and loss of heterozygosity in renal cell carcinoma. Proc Natl Acad Sci USA 85:1571–1575

36. Morita R, Ishikawa J, Tsutsumi M et al. (1991) Allelotype of renal cell carcinoma. Cancer Res 51:820–823
37. Latif F, Duh FM, Gnarra J et al. (1993) Von Hippel-Lindau syndrome: cloning and identification of the plasma membrane CA^{++}-transporting ATPase isoform gene that resides in the VHL gene region. Cancer Res 53:861–867
38. Latif F, Kalman T, Gnarra J et al. (1993) Identification of the von Hippel-Lindau disease tumor suppressor gene. Science 260:1317–1320
39. Southwick GJ, Schwartz RA (1979) The basal cell nevus syndrome: disasters occurring among a series of 36 patients. Cancer 44:2294–2299
40. Rook A, Wilkinson DS, Ebling FJG et al. (1986) Text of dermatology, 4th edn. Blackwell Scientific, London, pp 122–126
41. El-Azouzi M, Chung RY, Farmer GE et al. (1989) Loss of distinct regions on the short arm of chromosome 17 associated with tumorigenesis of human astrocytoma. Proc Natl Acad Sci USA 86:7186–7190
42. Chung R, Whaley J, Kley N et al. (1991) TP53 gene mutations and 17p deletions in human astrocytomas. Genes Chromos Cancer 3:323–331
43. Frankel RH, Bayona W, Koslow M et al. (1992) p53 mutations in human malignant gliomas. Cancer Res 52:1427–1433
44. Fults D, Brockmeyer D, Tullous MW et al. (1992) p53 mutations and loss of heterozygosity on chromosome 17 and 10 during human astrocytoma progression. Cancer Res 52:674–679
45. Von Deimling A, Eibl RH, Ohgaki H et al. (1992) p53 mutations are associated with 17p allelic loss in grade II and grade III astrocytoma. Cancer Res 52: 2987–2990
46. Ohgaki H, Eibl RH, Wiestler OD et al. (1991) p53 mutations in nonastrocytic human brain tumors. Cancer Res 51:6202–6205
47. Biegel JA, Burk CD, Barr FG et al. (1992) Evidence for a 17p tumor related locus distinct from p53 in pediatric primitive neuroectodermal tumors. Cancer Res 52:3391–3395
48. Biegel JA, Burk CD, Parmiter AH et al. (1992) Molecular analysis of a partial deletion of 22q in a central nervous system rhabdoid tumor. Genes Chromos Cancer 5:104–108
49. Seizinger BR (1992) Antioncogenes and the development of tumors of the human nervous system. Cancer 70:1782–1787

Hereditary Melanoma and Dysplastic Nevus Syndrome

Within the past half century, the population has been exposed to an astronomical number of chemical agents, but more importantly, the recent development of leisure time outdoor sports activities through mass production of inexpensive equipment and apparel has led to a significantly unprecedented large amount of sunlight exposure which starts as early in life as the first decade of life. These exposures are sudden, multiple and excessive. They occur not only in summer but, due to modern transportation, also in the winter. Thus, patients with atypical moles on their trunk are having a hitherto not encountered human experience of sunlight exposure.

R.M. Fusaro and H.T. Lynch (1985)

Introduction

The rapid and continuing increase of incidence of malignant melanoma, especially in developed countries, renders this disease one of the major challenges for oncologists in the future. Melanoma is also of extreme interest in genetic epidemiology; in the introductory chapter, this was defined, in its essence, as the study of the interaction between genes and environmental factors in the etiology and pathogenesis of a given disease. About 10% of all malignant melanomas (MM) have a genetic component; moreover, there is no doubt that environmental factors (sunlight exposure) are also of major importance in their development. We are probably not far from the reality in hypothesizing that a more detailed investigation on the interaction between hereditary predisposition to melanoma (which has now been linked to specific chromosomal loci) and some environmental agents (which can induce highly selective genetic changes) might represent the key passage to the comprehension of this disease.

Hereditary dysplastic nevus (DN) and MM constitute a highly controversial (and in certain aspects confused) area of investigation. A first issue concerns the various denominations which have been proposed for the definition of DN syndrome; thus, hereditary DN syndrome (HDNS), large atypical nevus syndrome, B-K syndrome, familial atypical multiple mole melanoma (FAMMM), and other names have all appeared in the literature, virtually with the same meaning [1]. Second, a similar lack of consensus still exists on the nature of the genetic predisposition to dysplastic nevi and MM; thus, if the prevailing opinion is of a mendelian, autosomal dominant disorder, there are also those who support the multifactorial (i.e., polygenic) model [2]. Finally, molecular biology of MM and HDNS is also controversial: after an initial tentative mapping of the responsible gene on the short arm of chromosome 1 (1p36) [3], subsequent studies in larger series failed to confirm these preliminary observations [4, 5].

Sporadic and Hereditary Melanoma

Clinical and Epidemiologic Features

Data from various cancer registries indicate that the incidence of melanoma continues to increase throughout the world, though more rapidly in developed countries [6, 7], where crude incidence rates of five to ten cases a year per 100000 people (in both sexes) have been reported [8]. In the United States, this increase of incidence is estimated to be in the order of 4% annually, and for 1991 the expected new diagnoses of melanoma range between 27000 and 32000, with approximately one fifth of these patients destined to die of the disease. It is therefore not surprising that the pessimistic hypothesis of a "melanoma epidemic" has been postulated. This bleak outlook is only partially mitigated by the improved overall survival, which is now about 80% at 5 years.

The ultraviolet component (280–320 nm) of sunlight is the most relevent environmental factor involved in the pathogenesis of melanoma [9]. Excessive, multiple, and intermittent exposure to sunlight during leisure time and adolescence increases the risk of melanoma, especially in white, fair-skinned individuals. It follows that the incidence of MM is higher near the equator and tends to be lower in more temperate or cold regions, at least in the white population [9, 10]. Moreover, in accordance with these epidemiological data, we might also expect a further rise of MM incidence rate owing to the recent depletion of the ozone layer of stratosphere and the consequent increase of ultraviolet light reaching the earth [11]. Although not all available literature supports the role of ultraviolet radiation in MM development [12], the particular frequency of MM in patients with xeroderma pigmentosum (see the chapter on "Cancer-Prone Hereditary Diseases Associated with Abnormalities of DNA Repair") deserves some comment. This rare genetic disorder is characterized by a defect of DNA repair after selective DNA damage induced by ultraviolet light [13]; at a clinical level, these patients have an extremely high rate of cutaneous neoplasms, including MM. Moreover, anecdotal reports strongly suggest that the careful control of sunlight exposure to a minimum level (obtained by drastic means, such as avoidance of outdoor activities in certain hours or periods, wearing gloves, and sunscreens in general) can prevent or delay the development of MM [14].

Melanomas can develop anywhere on the cutaneous surface, though they are more worrying in those areas of the body which are not available for direct inspection (i.e., the back). Diagnosis of MM is not always easy, mainly because almost all individuals have pigmented nevi, and these appear to enlarge slowly over the years up to the third fourth decade (and then slowly disappear). Suspicion of MM should always arise when a preexisting mole or a new pigmented lesion undergoes rapid changes in color, size, or shape or when ulceration or bleeding occur. H.K. Koh suggested an "ABCD" rule for the possible diagnosis of melanoma in pigmented lesions of the skin: Asymmetry, Border irregularity, Color (variegation or dark black), and Diameter (more than 0.6 cm) [15]. Despite all these important clinical criteria, there are other skin lesions which are difficult to distinguish from MM unless a skin biopsy is taken; the most frequent are pigmented basal cell carcinoma, juvenile melanoma, blue nevi, and solar keratosis.

Clinical and histologic subtypes of melanoma include: (a) superficial spreading MM (about 70% of all melanomas); (b) lentigo maligna melanoma (i.e., melanoma developing in lentigo maligna, a macular epidermal lesion of slow growth, resulting from the maturation of atypical melanocytes and considered to be a melanoma in situ), which accounts for 5%–10% of all MM; (c) nodular melanoma, developing more rapidly than the other types and usually characterized by dermal invasion by the time of diagnosis; and (d) acral-lentiginous melanoma, which often affects palms and soles and does not seem to be related to sunlight exposure.

Prognosis of MM is correlated with the depth of invasion into the dermis (papillary and reticular) or subcutaneous fat [16]; however, studies have suggested that vertical tumor thickness (in millimeters) could be a better indicator of the clinical outcome [17, 18]. Thus, tumors of less than 0.75 mm show a more favorable prognosis, with prolonged disease-free survival; in contrast, metastasis and short survival are usually observed for lesions thicker than 4 mm. Various staging systems have been proposed for MM [15]; one simple scheme uses three main stages: in stage I, the disease is confined to the local site, and tumors of this category can be divided into five classes depending on their vertical thickness; in stage II tumors, regional lymph nodes are involved, while in stage III, distant metastases are present. The most frequent sites of metastasis include liver, lung, spleen, skin, bones, and central nervous system. New biological indicators of prognosis are under active investigation; among these, cell replication (evaluated with [^{3}H]thymidine or bromodeoxyuridine) and DNA ploidy seem to be the most promising [19, 20].

Morphologic Aspects of Malignant Melanoma and of Precursor Lesions (Dysplastic Nevus)

Melanomas develop from the malignant transformation of melanocytes; these originate from the neural crest during fetal development and then migrate to the skin and to several other organs. This explains why primary melanomas may occur at various other sites besides the skin, especially the gastrointestinal tract, larynx, trachea, and bronchi. In the skin, melanocytes are localized in the basal layer, and their main function is to synthesize melanin, a pigment which protects against ultraviolet radiation.

The common benign nevi are well-circumscribed, cutaneous lesions which are derived from intraepidermal melanocytes. Depending on the type of cell replication, penetration into the dermis, pigmentation, and junctional activity, these lesions can be classified as junctional nevi, compound nevi, intradermal nevi, and other subtypes. Although MM may develop in each of these benign conditions, the rate of transformation is rather low. A more definite precursor lesion is lentigo maligna, which is usually observed in sun-exposed areas; initially, there is a flat pigmented area of the skin – this is the superficial growth phase of the tumor – which expands very slowly over the years. Subsequently, an invasive vertical growth may develop, which is visible as nodules within the lesion.

DN (or atypical nevi) are undoubtedly the most important type of precursor lesion of MM. DN were initially described in familial clusters, but they can also occur sporadically (see later sections in this chapter), although there is still some disagreement about the relative proportion of these two clinical entities [1, 15, 21]. Clinical diagnosis of DN is based on the number of lesions (usually more than 100 melanocytic nevi per patient), their diameter (some of the nevi should be 8 mm or more), color variegation, irregularity of margins, and marked heterogeneity [22]. Histologically, DN are characterized by some architectural and cellular atypia, increased stromal angiogenesis, and the presence of a chronic lymphocytic infiltrate [1, 21, 22]. As recently stated, clinical and histologic characteristics of DN are "qualitatively similar to those seen in melanoma but quantitatively not as extreme" [15]. Panels A, B, and C of Fig. 1 illustrate some of the histologic features more frequently observable in benign melanocytic nevi, DN, and MM.

Familial and Hereditary Aspects of Malignant Melanoma (Not Associated with Dysplastic Nevi)

Although in recent years more emphasis has been given to MM within HDNS, there is evidence that genetically determined melanomas may also occur without a close association with precursor lesions. In 1952, Cawley described a family in which the father and two of the three offspring

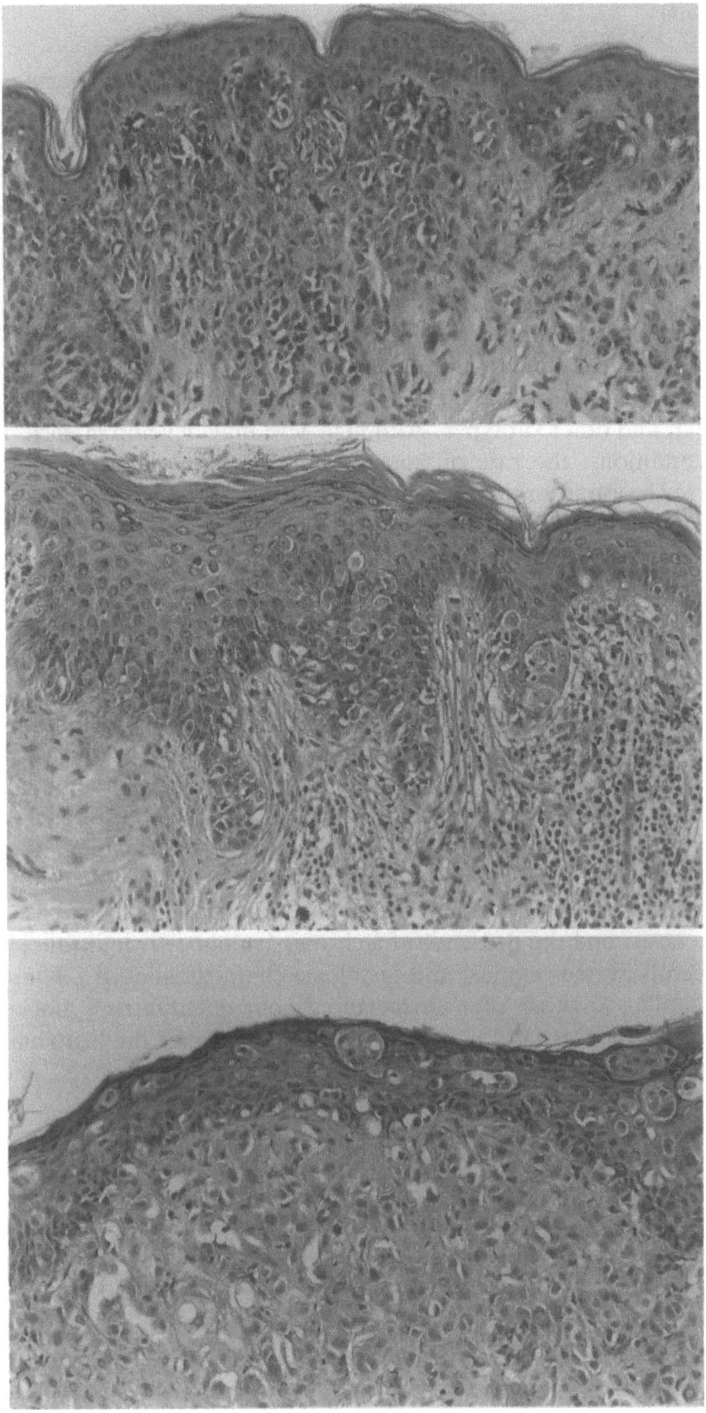

A

B

C

developed cutaneous MM [23]. After subsequent reports of similar familial aggregation of MM [2], two comprehensive studies demonstrated an increased risk of MM among first-degree relatives of affected individuals [24, 25]; in one of these studies (involving 113 families and almost 1000 relatives), the number of observed cutaneous melanomas was almost double the expected value. Even more importantly, the authors noticed that familial melanomas showed some of the clinical features which are typical of hereditary tumors in general, including: (a) early age of onset, often before 40–45 years; (b) frequency of multiple primary neoplasms; and (c) tendency to a more benign overall prognosis. From these observations it was not possible to deduce whether the observed aggregation of tumors in families was compatible with a well-defined model of genetic transmission; the authors, however, suggested that in approximately 10% of their patients the disease could be considered as familial and proposed that polygenic inheritance was the most plausible genetic model.

Classical segregation analyses were carried out by Greene and coworkers [26] in 14 families with cutaneous MM selected on the basis of the presence of at least two pathologically confirmed MM. In these pedigrees, including a total of approximately 400 individuals, single-gene transmission was tested versus alternative (multifactorial) hypotheses. When only the trait "melanoma" was considered, the single-gene dominant hypothesis was not rejected; in contrast, the recessive mode of transmission did not fit the data, and the multifactorial model was only of borderline significance. The authors concluded that in these highly selected kindreds, the distribution of MM was consistent with a mendelian, autosomal dominant type of genetic transmission, with reduced penetrance. In the same study, segregation analysis was also carried out in individuals with either cutaneous MM or DN. Rather surprisingly, both dominant and recessive hypotheses were rejected and, similarly, the multifactorial model did not fit the observed findings. However, the dominant model for MM and DN was actually rejected because there were too many affected patients in the investigated families. The authors suggested that this apparent paradox could be explained by the relative frequency of phenocopies, which can mask the effect of a major gene [26].

Management, Cancer Prevention, and Control

Although there is no doubt that surgery is the primary cure for stage I MM, controversy still exist on the width of surgical excision (wide resections with 4–5 cm margins versus narrow excisions with margins as small as 1 cm) and

Fig. 1. A Histologic features of a benign melanocytic nevus. **B** Typical dysplastic nevus. **C** Morphologic aspects of malignant melanoma

on the usefulness of local lymphadenectomy [15, 27, 28]. Stage II patients require surgery and lymph node dissection, whereas the possible benefit of adjuvant chemotherapy has not been documented [29]. In stage III patients, the aim of treatment is palliative; after the use of dacarbamazine, several combinations of drugs have been given, but the overall results are rather modest and unsatisfactory [15, 30, 31]. Adaptive immunotherapy with interleukin-2, lymphokine-activated killer cells, and/or tumor-infiltrating lymphocytes is a novel approach of great interest in treatment of advanced melanoma, with impressive individual remissions, but with an overall response rate of about 10%–20% [32, 33]. Despite the tendency to a more benign prognosis [2, 25], treatment of hereditary malignant melanoma does not differ from that of the more frequent sporadic counterpart.

After removal of cutaneous MM, the main objectives of follow-up are the prevention and early diagnosis of a second primary melanoma, a fairly frequent event in these patients [34]. Thus, these high-risk individuals should be advised to limit exposure to sunlight and to make regular use of sunscreens or general protection against the sun; in addition, periodic examination of the cutaneous surface by a physician with proper expertise in recognizing melanomas and precursor lesions is also recommended. These measures need to be further detailed in hereditary MM: first of all, an extended genealogical tree should be traced; then, after identification of individuals at risk, these should be followed with accurate dermatologic examinations at intervals of 3–4 months [14]. In addition, patients and their spouses (or close relatives) should be encouraged to perform a continuous inspection of the skin and to refer any new lesion as well as changes in size or color of preexisting nevi. Finally, the striking increase of incidence of cutaneous MM suggests the introduction of preventive measures regarding the whole population, and not only individuals at risk. Besides possible interventions aimed at preserving the ozone layer of stratosphere (decrease in the production of chlorofluorocarbons), a surveillance program for melanoma seems feasible and theoretically appealing, providing that physicians are trained to recognize cutaneous MM and its precursor lesions.

Hereditary Dysplastic Nevus Syndrome

General Features

The first description of HDNS is usually attributed to Norris [35], who reported the occurrence of melanoma in two members (father and son) of the same family; moreover, the attending physician noticed that both affected individuals, as well as other siblings, had many moles on various parts of the body and advanced the hypothesis that the disorder could be hereditary. After more than a century, Lynch and Krush [36] reported two families showing all the clinical components of HDNS, and an even more detailed description of the syndrome was given 10 years later by two different groups [37, 38]. The essential elements of HDNS are multiple DN, MM, and primary cancers of other organs. The main clinical features of the HDNS phenotype can be summarized as follows: (a) the absolute number of nevi (both common and dysplastic) is in the order of 50–100 or more, with lesions of various size and shape; (b) DN are at least 5 mm in diameter, with irregular margins whose color often fades into normal surrounding skin; (c) DN can be variegate or not, with different colors from red to black; (d) DN can be found in all parts of the body, but are more frequent in the trunk and proximal extremities; (e) DN usually appear in the second decade of life, though they have also been described in children; more generally, in these patients nevi that appear normal are recognized in considerable excess from the first decade, and their number continues to increase up to the fourth or fifth decade; both common nevi and DN tend to increase in size and to change their color; and finally (f) MM develop frequently, usually after puberty, and often on preexisting DN [1, 2, 11, 14].

The histologic characteristics of DN have already been discussed and include atypical nuclei with prominent nucleoli, irregular intradermal nests of cells associated with an increased number of isolated melanocytes, inflammatory reaction with a dense lymphocytic infiltrate, angiogenesis, and fibrosis in the papillary dermis [1, 15]. These morphologic features do not seem to be different in hereditary and sporadic DN, although some authors have suggested the possibility of recognizing hereditary lesions by a careful evaluation of particular histologic findings, such as presence of dust-like melanin pigment, irregular nests of melanocytes, and markedly increased junctional activity [39].

DN do not only occur in families with HDNS, but are also frequent in patients with cutaneous MM, and may be present in 2%–10% of the general population [2, 39]. However, the real frequency of sporadic DN is difficult to establish and can reasonably be overestimated; in fact, like virtually all heritable disorders (but in particular those with an autosomal dominant pattern of inheritance, see the chapter on "Genetic Aspects of Disease") HDNS may exhibit reduced penetrance of the gene and variable clinical expressivity. Moreover, family history may be inaccurate, especially for disorders that may be asymptomatic and unobserved for many years; finally, the possibility of new mutation in a patient with apparently sporadic DN should also be considered, which usually requires years of observation before being ruled out.

Genetics of Hereditary Dysplastic Nevus Syndrome

Several lines of evidence indicate that HDNS is inherited as a mendelian, autosomal dominant trait, though with an extremely variable expressivity. Thus, in some families [14] the disorder has been traced for three or four successive generations, usually without skipped generations and often together with other malignancies. Moreover, in HDNS families segregation analyses were carried out by two different groups with almost identical results [40, 41]. Lynch et al. analyzed four kindreds with clinical features of full-blown HDNS (a total of 80 affected or at risk individuals); they reported a segregation ratio of 0.47, which is compatible with an autosomal dominant type of transmission, with a 93% rate of penetrance [40]. Using a different statistical approach, Bale and coworkers reevaluated the same 14 families previously analyzed by Greene et al. [26] (a total of about 400 affected or at risk persons); the estimated lifetime incidence of MM in siblings and offspring of affected patients was 46%, a value which appears fully consistent with a monogenic, autosomal dominant, and highly penetrant type of inheritance [41].

Troupe and colleagues [2, 42] repeatedly questioned the prevailing dogma that HDNS is a monogenic disease and suggested that the multifactorial model was more suitable to explain the aggregation of cutaneous MM in certain families. Their contention is mainly based on three major points. First, they noted that the risk of developing MM in these families was not constant, but depended on the absolute number of precursor lesions (DN); the observation is indicative of a continuous or quantitative trait, and this is more easily interpreted by the multifactorial model. Second, the authors calculated that the frequency of new mutations in HDNS is exceedingly higher than the rate of eliminated mutations; this lack of genetic equilibrium is not consistent with mendelian inheritance and once again suggests a polygenic transmission. The third argument in favor of a multifactorial model was the inability to associate HDNS with the alteration of a single gene; as will be discussed later in this chapter, linkage studies have so far been inconclusive [3, 4], and there is evidence indicating that at least three major genes (probably located on different chromosomes) might be implicated in the pathogenesis of MM and HDNS [2].

Monogenic and multifactorial transmission in MM and HDNS should not be considered mutually exclusive; it is entirely possible that both types of inheritance do exist and are responsible for the aggregation of cancer in some families. The existence of various patterns of transmission – together with truly sporadic cases – has been postulated for many common malignancies and will be discussed in more detail for breast and colorectal neoplasms.

Intraocular Melanoma and Systemic Cancer in Hereditary Dysplastic Nevus Syndrome

Intraocular MM (IMM) is in absolute terms a rare neoplasm, though it is one of the commonest intraocular malignancies in adults of both sexes. The tumor, which usually originates from the choroid, shows various histologic patterns and may have a poor prognosis, with metastases in the liver, lung, and other organs. Although the majority of IMM are sporadic, choroidal melanomas may affect various first-degree relatives in a given family and, more importantly, the disease can be recognized in two or three successive generations [43, 44]. Although the real frequency of these familial (or hereditary) forms is still uncertain, IMM is not rare in kindreds with HDNS. In an informative family spanning four generations and including ten patients affected by MM, the proband had two cutaneous MM with a 1-year interval in between; after 2 years he underwent enucleation of the right eye for choroidal melanoma, and 8 months later a new primary IMM developed in the left eye [46]. Several other reports of IMM in families with defined or suspected HDNS have appeared in the literature [1, 14].

Carcinomas of other organs, in particular the lung, breast, prostate, pancreas, and colorectum, have also been described in HDNS [1, 14, 45]. In four large families, Lynch and coworkers found a fivefold increase of systemic cancer of various anatomic sites [40], including very rare neoplasms (squamous carcinoma of the tonsil in a 28-year-old patient without any apparent risk factor). A similar excess of other neoplasms (besides MM) was observed by Bergmann et al. in three out of nine Dutch families with HDNS [46], with a particularly high incidence of pancreatic cancer. At variance with these observations, Kopf et al. did not observe any excess of systemic cancer in their families with HDNS [47], and similar results were reported by Greene et al. [48] in a prospective study which included the 14 families previously investigated with segregation analysis. In the latter study, however, the follow-up period (5 years) was probably too short for a proper evaluation of cancer occurrence. A representative pedigree of a family with HDNS with the occurrence of cutaneous MM as well as tumors of other organs is shown in Fig. 2.

Molecular Biology of Melanoma

Cytogenetic studies have showed various alterations of chromosome 1 in human melanoma cancer cells, especially deletions and translocation of the short arm [49, 50]. Moreover, Greene et al. [26] reported a "loose linkage" between the putative gene responsible for hereditary MM and the Rh locus, which has been mapped to chromosome 1p. Against this background, Bale et al. carried out linkage studies in six kindreds with hereditary MM and DNS using 26 polymorphic markers for the short arm of chromosome 1 and spanning a region of 185 cM from the distal to the centromeric region of 1p [3]. Significant lod scores were found for two of these markers, D1S47 (an anonymous marker) and the gene locus for pronatrodilatin, indicating their cosegregation with the investigated trait. The authors therefore concluded that the locus for familial cutaneous melanoma–HDNS could be assigned to chromosome 1 (1p36). By combining these observations with the frequently

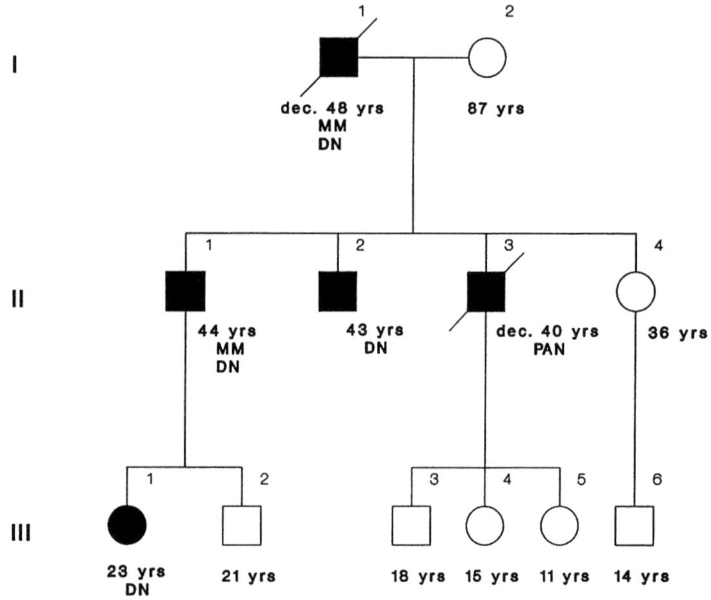

Fig. 2. Representative pedigree of a family with hereditary dysplastic nevus syndrome spanning three generations. Besides melanomas and dysplastic nevi (*DN*), an early-onset pancreatic cancer (*PAN*) can be observed in the second generation. *MM*, malignant melanoma. *dec.*, deceased

reported chromosomal deletions [49, 50] or losses of genetic material from the distal part of chromosome 1p [51], one might hypothesize a sequence of genetic events similar to that described for retinoblastoma and Wilms' tumors (see earlier chapters), in which the sequential inactivation (or loss) of the two alleles in a tumor suppressor gene locus seems to be of critical importance for cancer development.

Two successive investigations, however, failed to confirm these linkage studies. Thus, in six large Dutch families with HDNS, Van Haeringen et al. could not find evidence of linkage between the investigated trait and markers of chromosome 1p [5]. Similarly, in eight Australian families (a total of 118 members, 30 of whom had MM and/or HDNS), Kefford et al. did not find any linkage between the disease and several markers of chromosome 1p (including D1S47 and pronatrodilatin, which had been informative in the study of Bale et al.), thus excluding, at least in these families, the possibility that the putative gene of cutaneous MM–HDNS could be assigned to this chromosomal region [4]. The most likely explanation for these contrasting observations is a basic genetic heterogeneity of cutaneous MM–HDNS, as found (or suggested) for other solid tumors (see relevant chapter). Moreover, as already discussed, Troupe and colleagues consider these contradictory results as one of the main elements in favor of the polygenic model of transmission [2, 42]. In addition, a further element of confusion is the absence of clearly established and accepted minimum criteria for the definition of HDNS, whose phenotypic expression may be extremely variable [1]. Finally, besides deletions and translocation of chromosome 1p, recent cytogenetic analysis of cultured lymphocytes and fibroblasts from HDNS patients showed a certain chromosomal instability, with breakage abnormalities occurring with particular frequency on chromosomes 14, 3, 1, 6, 11, and 22 [1, 11].

Two tumor suppressor genes have recently been investigated in MM. Stretch et al. [52] found mutations of p53 in 85% of 53 melanomas by using the monoclonal antibody Pab 240; moreover, mutations were more frequent in metastatic than in nonmetastatic cancer, thus suggesting a possible role of this gene in the progression of MM and in the development of distal metastases [53]. More recently, high levels of expression of mutant p53 were reported in 12 out of 18 (choroidal) IMM and were associated with point mutations in the evolutionarily conserved regions of the gene; in contrast, p53 was not hyperexpressed in premalignant lesions (choroidal nevi) which can progress to MM [54], again suggesting a possible involvement of p53 in the late stages of tumorigenesis. The nm23 gene represents a new class of tumor-associated genes which might act specifically as suppressors of the metastatic potential. The human nm23 gene has been assigned to chromosome 17 and encodes a protein whose precise biological function is still unknown [55, 56]. Allelic deletions and/or reduced expression of nm23 has been reported in various human neoplasms (breast, colon, lung), more often in the later stages of the disease and in association with distant metastases [57, 58]. Moreover, transfection of murine nm23 cDNA into highly metastatic melanoma cells resulted in a reduced incidence of tumor formation and in a marked inhibition of the metastatic process [55]. In accordance with these observations, Florens et al. reported that the expression of nm23 gene was markedly reduced in human metastatic MM when compared to patients with localized and less aggressive disease and suggested the possible involvement of this gene in the progression of MM [59]. Finally, recent experiments suggest the possible existence of tumor suppressor genes for MM located on chromosomes 6, 11q, and 17q [60–62].

Mutations of the *ras* oncogene have been reported in approximately 20% of melanomas. The majority of these mutations are found in the N-*ras* gene and may occur in primary tumors as well as during the development of metastasis [63]. Interestingly, a correlation was found between occurrence of *ras* mutations and location of tumors at sites (face, back of the hands) which are usually unprotected against sunlight, thus suggesting that ultraviolet light might be involved in the induction of these mutational events [64]. In summary, at least three major aspects regarding the molecular biology of MM should be pointed out. First, despite the efforts of many investigators, the gene (or genes) responsible for hereditary cutaneous MM–HDNS has not yet been identified, although there is some evidence that in certain families a putative gene might be located on the short arm of chromosome 1; genetic heterogeneity seems extremely probable in this syndrome. Second, various alterations of tumor suppressor genes and of dominant oncogenes (*ras*) have been reported; however, in the majority of cases mutations and/or allelic deletions were found in advanced and metastatic disease. These observations, therefore, do not allow the hypothesis of an ordered sequence of mutational events in the pathogenesis of MM, as has recently been suggested for other neoplasms (i.e., colorectum, see later chapters). Third, the available (and limited) experimental evidence does not indicate whether the genetic changes involving oncogenes and tumor suppressor genes are different in sporadic and in hereditary forms of MM.

References

1. Lynch HT, Fusaro RM (1991) Genetic epidemiology and the familial atypical multiple mole melanoma syndrome. In: Lynch HT, Tautu P (eds) Genetic epidemiology of cancer. Springer, Berlin Heidelberg New York
2. Traupe H (1991) Polygenic vs monogenic inheritance of dysplastic nevi and malignant melanoma: yesterday's debate or the answer of tomorrow? In: Lynch TH, Traupe P (eds) Genetic epidemiology of cancer. Springer, Berlin Heidelberg New York
3. Bale SJ, Dracopoli NC, Tucker MA et al. (1989) Mapping the gene for hereditary malignant cutaneous melanoma–dysplastic nevus to chromosome 1p. N Engl J Med 320:1367–1372
4. Kefford RF, Salmon J, Shaw HM et al. (1991) Hereditary melanoma in Australia. Variable association with dysplastic nevi and absence of genetic linkage to chromosome 1p. Cancer Genet Cytogenet 51:45–55
5. Haeringen A, Bergman W, Nelen MR et al. (1989) Exclusion of the dysplastic nevus syndrome (DNS) locus from the short arm of chromosome 1 by linkage studies in Dutch families. Genomics 5:61–64
6. Jensen OM, Bolander AM (1980) Trends in malignant melanoma of the skin. World Health Stat Q 33:2–26
7. Davis DL, Hoel D, Fox J et al. (1990) International trends in cancer mortality in France, West Germany, Italy, Japan, England and Wales, and the USA. Lancet 336:474–481
8. International Agency for Research on Cancer (1987) Cancer incidence in five continents, vol 5. Lyon, France
9. Sober AJ (1987) Solar exposure in the etiology of cutaneous melanoma. Photodermatology 4:23–31
10. Elwood JM, Gallagher RP, Hill GB et al. (1984) Pigmentation and skin reaction to sun as risk factor for cutaneous melanoma: Western Canada Melanoma Study. Br Med J 288:99–102
11. Lynch HT, Fusaro RM (1992) The surgeon, genetics, and malignant melanoma. Arch Surg 127:317–320
12. Koh HK, Kligler BE, Lew RA (1990) Sunlight and cutaneous malignant melanoma: evidence for and against causation. Photochem Photobiol 51:765–779
13. Paterson MC, Gentner NE, Middlestadt MV et al. (1984) Cancer predisposition, carcinogen hypersensitivity, and aberrant DNA metabolism. J Cell Physiol [Suppl] 3:45–62

14. Lynch HT, Fusaro RM, Shannon Danes B et al. (1983) A review of hereditary malignant melanoma including biomarkers in familial atypical multiple mole melanoma syndrome. Cancer Genet Cytogenet 8:325–358
15. Koh HK (1991) Cutaneous melanoma. N Engl J Med 325:171–182
16. Clark WH Jr, From L, Bernardino EA et al. (1969) The histogenesis and biologic behaviour of primary human malignant melanomas of the skin. Cancer Res 29:705–727
17. Breslow A (1970) Thickness, cross-sectional areas and depth of invasion in the prognosis of cutaneous melanoma. Ann Surg 172:902–908
18. Ringborg U, Afzelius LE, Lagerlof B et al. (1993) Cutaneous MM of the head and neck. Cancer 71:751–758
19. Costa A, Silvestrini R, Grignolio E et al. (1987) Cell kinetics as a prognostic tool in patients with metastatic malignant melanoma of the skin. Cancer 60:2797–2800
20. Karlsson M, Boeryd B, Carstensen J et al. (1993) DNA ploidy and S-phase in primary malignant melanoma as prognostic factor. Br J Cancer 67:134–138
21. Elder DE, Goldmann LI, Goldman SC et al. (1980) Dysplastic nevus syndrome: a phenotypic association of sporadic cutaneous melanoma. Cancer 46:1787–1794
22. Rivers JK, Kopf A, Vinokur AF et al. (1990) Clinical characteristics of malignant melanomas developing in persons with dysplastic nevi. Cancer 65:1232–1236
23. Cawley EP (1952) Genetic aspects of malignant melanoma. Arch Dermatol Syph 65:440
24. Anderson DE (1971) Clinical characteristics of the genetic variety of cutaneous melanoma in man. Cancer 28:721–725
25. Wallace DC, Exton LA, McLeod GRC (1971) Genetic factors in malignant melanoma. Cancer 27:1262–1266
26. Greene MH, Goldin LR, Clark WH Jr et al. (1983) Familial cutaneous malignant melanoma: autosomal dominant trait possibly linked to the Rh locus. Proc Natl Acad Sci USA 80:6071–6075
27. Veronesi U, Cascinelli N, Adamus J et al. (1988) Thin stage I cutaneous malignant melanoma: comparison of excision with margins of 1 or 3 cm. N Engl J Med 318:1159–1162
28. Sim FH, Taylor WF, Pritchard DJ et al. (1986) Lymphadenectomy in the management of stage I malignant melanoma: a prospective randomized study. Mayo Clin Proc 61:697–705
29. Koh HK, Sober AJ, Harmon DC et al. (1985) Adjuvant therapy of cutaneous malignant melanoma: a critical review. Med Pediatr Oncol 13:244–260
30. Creagan ET (1989) Regional and systemic strategies for metastatic malignant melanoma. Mayo Clin Proc 64:852–860
31. Cocconi G, Bella M, Calabresi F et al. (1992) Treatment of metastatic malignant melanoma with dacarbazine plus tamoxifen. N Engl J Med 327:516–523
32. Rosenberg SA, Lotze MT, Muul LM et al. (1987) A progress report on the treatment of 157 patients with advanced cancer using lymphokine-activated killer cells and interleukin-2 or high dose interleukin-2 alone. N Engl J Med 316: 889–897
33. Rosenbers SA, Packrad BS, Aebersold et al. (1988) Use of tumor-infiltrating lymphocytes and interleukin-2 in the immunotherapy of patients with metastatic melanoma: a preliminary report. N Engl J Med 319:1676–1680
34. Kang S, Barnhill RL, Mihm MC et al. (1992) Multiple primary cutaneous melanoma. Cancer 70:1911–1916
35. Norris W (1820) A case of fungoid disease. Edin Med Surg J 16:562
36. Lynch HT, Krush AJ (1968) Heredity and malignant melanoma: implications for cancer detection. Can Med Assos J 99:17–21

37. Lynch HT, Frichot BC, Lynch JF (1978) Familial atypical multiple mole melanoma syndrome. J Med Genet 15:352–356
38. Clark WH Jr, Reimer DR, Greene M et al. (1978) Origin of familial malignant melanoma from heritable melanocytic lesions. "The B-K mole syndrome." Arch Dermatol 114:732–738
39. Steijlen PM, Bergman W, Hermans J et al. (1988) The efficacy of histopathological criteria required for diagnosing dysplastic nevi. Histopathology 12: 289–298
40. Lynch HT, Fusaro RM, Kimberling WJ et al. (1983) Familial atypical multiple mole melanoma (FAMMM) syndrome: segregation analysis. J Med Genet 20: 342–344
41. Bale SJ, Chakravarti A, Greene MH (1986) Cutaneous malignant melanoma and familial dysplastic nevi: evidence for autosomal dominance and pleiotropy. AM J Hum Genet 38:188–196
42. Traupe H, Happle R (1990) The dysplastic nevus "syndrome" is not a dichotomic, but a continuous phenotype. Am J Med Genet 35:295–296
43. Bowen SF, Brady H, Jones VL (1964) Malignant melanoma of the eye occurring in two successive generations. Arch Ophtalmol 71:805–806
44. Silcock AQ (1892) Hereditary sarcoma of the eyeball in three generations. Br Med J 1:1079–1082
45. Lynch TH, Fusaro RM, Pester J et al. (1981) Tumour spectrum in the FAMMM syndrome. Br J Cancer 44:553–560
46. Bergman W, Watson P, de Jong J et al. (1990) Systemic cancer and the FAMMM syndrome. Br J Cancer 61:932–936
47. Kopf AW, Hellman LJ, Rogers GS et al. (1986) Familial malignant melanoma. JAMA 256:1915–1919
48. Greene MH, Tucker MA, Clark WH et al. (1987) Hereditary melanoma and the dysplastic nevus syndrome: the risk of cancers other than melanoma. J AM Acad Dermatol 16:792–797
49. Balaban GB, Herlyn M, Clark WH Jr et al. (1986) Karyotypic evolution in human malignant melanoma. Cancer Genet Cytogenet 19:113–122
50. Cowan JM, Halaban R, Francke U (1988) Cytogenetic analysis of melanocytes from premalignant nevi and melanomas. J Natl Cancer Inst 80:1159–1164
51. Dracopoli NC, Harnett P, Bale SJ et al. (1989) Loss of alleles from distal chromosome 1p occurs late in melanoma tumor progression. Proc Natl Acad Sci USA 86:4614–4618
52. Stretch JR, Gatter KC, Ralfkiaer E et al. (1991) Epression of mutant p53 in melanoma. Cancer Res 51:5976–5979
53. Lassam NJ, From L, Khan HJ (1993) Overexpression of p53 is a late event in the development of malignant melanoma. Cancer Res 53:3325–2238
54. Tobal K, Warren W, Cooper CS et al. (1992) Increased expression and mutation of p53 in choroidal melanoma. Br J Cancer 66:900–904
55. Leone A, Flatow U, King CR et al. (1991) Reduced tumor incidence, metastatic potential and cytokine responsiveness of nm23-transfected melanoma cells. Cell 65:25–35
56. Leone A, McBride OW, Weston A et al. (1991) Somatic allele deletion of nm23 in human cancer. Cancer Res 51:2490–2493
57. Steeg PS, Bevilacqua G, Kopper L et al. (1988) Evidence for a novel gene associated with lower tumor metastatic potential. J Natl Cancer Inst 80:200–204
58. Cohn KH, Wang F, DeSoto-LaPaix F et al. (1991) Association of nm23-H1 allelic deletions with distant metastases in colorectal carcinoma. Lancet 338: 722–724

59. Florens VA, Aamdal S, Myklebost O et al. (1992) Levels of nm23 messenger RNA in metastatic malignant melanoma: inverse correlation with disease progression. Cancer Res 52:6088–6091
60. Trent ZM, Stanbridge EZ, McBride HL et al. (1990) Tumorigenicity in human melanoma cell lines controlled by introduction of human chromosome 6. Science 247:568–571
61. Tomlinson IPM, Gammack AJ, Stickland JE et al. (1993) Loss of heterozygosity in MM at loci on chromosome 11 and 17 implicated in the pathogenesis of other cancers. Genes Chromos Cancer 7:169–172
62. Andersen LB, Fountain JW, Gutmann DH et al. (1993) Mutations in the NF-1 gene in sporadic malignant melanoma cell lines. Nature Genet 3:118–121
63. Bos JL (1989) Ras oncogenes in human cancer: a review. Cancer Res 49:4682–4689
64. Van't Veer LJ, Burgering BM, Versteeg R et al. (1989) N-ras mutations in human cutaneous melanoma correlated with sun exposure. Mol Cell Biol 9: 3114–3116

Hereditary and Familial Breast Tumors

Epidemiologists, geneticists, and clinicians need to collaborate on research and discuss the different methodologies used to begin to develop more informative ways of studying complex diseases like breast cancer. Without adequately combining information from all of these disciplines, the etiologies of human breast cancer will remain unfathomable.

A.M. GOLDSTEIN *et al. (1987)*

Introduction

Breast cancer is at the same time a major public health problem in all Western and developed countries, an active field of interdisciplinary collaboration, and an extremely interesting object of genetic and biomolecular investigation. There are several aspects which render this disease of particular interest and importance when compared to other neoplasms. First, breast cancer affects almost exclusively the female sex, where it represents by far the most frequent malignancy and that associated with the highest mortality rates. Second, compared to most other organs the mammary gland is fairly accessible, which explains on the one hand the high number of clinical and experimental investigations (closely dependent on the easiness of sampling) and on the other the theoretical feasibility of screening and surveillance programs. Third, together with colorectal neoplasms, breast cancer is the best example of interaction between environmental and genetic factors in tumor formation. Fourth, at least for certain subtypes of breast cancer (Li-Fraumeni syndrome), subtle biomolecular alterations have been detected which might lead to considerable advances towards the definition of the intimate mechanisms of tumorigenesis.

Despite all these facts, many clinical and biological aspects of breast cancer remain highly controversial, and probably several years of investigation will be required before reaching firm conclusions, for example on the real value of recent prognostic indicators or on the optimal management of node-negative patients. It is virtually impossible to summarize in a few pages the enormous body of investigation which has accumulated on breast cancer, especially in the last decade. Following the main objective of the book, particular emphasis will be given to familial and hereditary aspects of the disease.

Clinical and Epidemiologic Features of Breast Cancer

General Epidemiology

Recent estimates indicate that 10%–12% of women living in Western countries will develop breast cancer during their life, and 3%–4% are destined to die of the disease [1, 2]. With crude incidence rates of 80–100 new cases per 100000 inhabitants per year [3], we should expect more than half a million cases of breast cancer to be diagnosed in Western Europe and USA in 1993. Moreover, data from cancer registries indicate that from 1940 up to the present time there has been a steady increase of incidence of these tumors, which has become even more marked (about 4% per year) in very recent years [4]. An almost similar increase has also been reported in less developed countries, though incidence rates are still much lower than those seen in the most industrialized areas of the world [1]. In contrast to incidence, mortality rates tend to remain stable, which probably reflects both earlier detection and improved overall treatment. Moreover, considering age-specific mortality rates, there is a definite tendency to reduced mortality in younger women and to a slight increase among individuals over the age of 55 [5]. Women living in North America and in Western Europe have the highest incidence rates of breast cancer; women living in Latin America and in some southern European countries can be considered at intermediate risk, whereas individuals living in Africa and Asia show the lowest incidence and mortality rates. However, since the increase of incidence is more or less appreciable in almost all countries, the realistic prediction of a worldwide incidence of more than one million annual cases by the year 2000 has been put forward [2].

Risk Profile

Several risk factors of breast cancer have recently been identified (Table 1). A family history of breast tumors is probably the strongest risk factor and will be discussed later in this chapter. Other well-documented factors associated with an increased risk of mammary tumors include: (a) nulliparity and late age at first birth (the risk for women having their first child after the age of 30 is about the double that of women who have the first child before 20 years) [6] and (b) early menarche and late menopause [7]. Since oral contraceptives and postmenopausal hormonal supplements both seem to induce a slightly increased risk of breast cancer, it is likely that an increased estrogenic stimulation on the mammary gland represents the common

Table 1. Risk profile for breast cancer (see [6–19])

Risk factor	Relative risk	Description
Nulliparity	1.9	Nulliparous women at higher risk of cancer
Age at birth of first child	1.3–1.9	Late age at birth of the first child increases the risk of breast cancer
Age at menarche	1.3	Early age of menarche associated with increased risk
Age at menopause	1.5	Late menopause (after [60]) associated with increased risk
Postmenopausal estrogens	1.2–2.0	Use of estrogens after menopause associated with increased risk
Total calories and dietary fat	1.2–1.5	High caloric intake and dietary fat increase the risk of breast cancer
Obesity	1.2	Increased incidence of breast cancer in postmenopausal women
Alcohol	1.2–2.0	Alcohol consumption (even in moderate amount) increases the risk of breast cancer
Radiation	1.5–3.0	Higher risk of breast cancer among atomic bomb survivors and after repeated fluoroscopies
Benign breast disease	1.5–3.0	Excess risk of breast cancer in women with proliferative disorders of the mammary gland

denominator of several risk factors [8, 9]. The effect of oral contraceptives and of estrogen replacement on mammary carcinogenesis, however, is still controversial [2, 10] and probably dependent on the duration of treatment, age of patients, and specific constituents of contraceptives.

Dietary factors, total calories, and obesity have also been associated with an increased risk of breast cancer [11–14]; among dietary components, total fat and alcohol seem to play a certain role, whereas the possible protective effect of vitamins is still undefined [15].

It is reasonable to expect that high doses of radiation can cause breast tumors as well as many other neoplasms but, with the exception of studies on atomic bomb survivors [16], few clinical studies are available [17] and, in addition, exposure to significant radiation is usually infrequent. The issue, however, is of potential clinical relevance, owing to the widespread diffusion of mammography screening programs for early detection of these tumors.

Benign diseases of the mammary gland might increase the risk of breast cancer; however, the excess risk seems to be limited to women with proliferative lesions, such as atypical hyperplasia, whereas conditions not associated with replicative changes do not seem to bear any substantial risk [18]. Finally, relatively minor risk factors include socioeconomic class, marital status (major risk for those who never marry), place of residence (higher risk for urban areas), race (whites at higher risk than blacks), and physical height (higher risk for taller individuals) [2, 19].

The above-mentioned risk factors deserve some general comments. First, many of these factors (i.e., late age of the first birth, use of contraceptives or postmenopausal hormones, alcohol) are closely related to the modern style of life; although it is theoretically possible to reduce or even abolish the impact of these factors – by changing or modifying our habits – in practical terms this is unfeasible and culturally unacceptable. It follows that modern society will continue to live under the burden of these factors and that the list of them is presumably destined to grow. Second, a crucial question is whether the observed gradual increase of incidence of breast cancer is actually due to the effect of these risk factors or if other unknown etiologic agents are in fact responsible for this trend. Although intuitively one may be led to associate the numerous risk factors to the increased frequency of these neoplasms, it should be noted that for all of them the relative risks are usually low and that rather often the evidence has been contradictory. Finally, whatever their pathogenetic role, the identification of several risk factors is undoubtedly of importance in order to stratify the general population in different "risk categories" for purposes of screening and surveillance.

Clinical Features and Morphology

The large majority of women with breast cancer present to their doctors with a nodule in the breast. In many cases these are benign tumors or cysts; however, as a general rule, all breast lumps should be regarded as potentially malignant, and consequently a morphologic diagnosis is almost always required. Other symptoms, often indicative of a more advanced disease, include bleeding from the nipple, skin infiltration, nipple inversion or retraction, and axillary or supraclavicular lymph nodes enlargements; in less fortunate cases the disease may also begin with symptoms of distant metastasis (frequently in the bones or brain). The diagnosis relies on "fine needle" or excision biopsy and on mammography. Preoperative investigations include, in most centers, liver and bones scintiscans, ultrasounds, and chest X-rays. Preoperative clinical stage is extremely useful for the choice of treatment and for estimation of prognosis. More detailed information is obtained with the pathologic staging; this is usually carried out with the TNM system, which is based on the local extent of the tumor, lymph node involvement, and presence of distant metastasis [20]. Owing to their prognostic relevance, patients are also categorized on the basis of the number of involved axillary lymph nodes into four main classes: (1) no lymph node, (2) one to three, (3) four to nine, (4) ten or more positive lymph nodes.

The majority of breast cancers have invaded into the stroma of the mammary gland by the time of diagnosis and should therefore be regarded as invasive tumors. With the widespread use of screening mammography, however, the frequency of in situ lesions has increased remarkably, opening new problems and controversies about their biologic meaning and the clinical management. In "in situ" carcinoma of the breast, malignant cells proliferate within the duct (ductal carcinoma in situ) or the lobule (lobular carcinoma "in situ"), but there is no invasion or infiltration of the surrounding stromal mammary tissue [21]. The most relevant and still unanswered question concerning these in situ lesions is the likelihood of their progression to invasive carcinoma. In fact, it has been proposed that the natural history of these circumscribed lesions – often discovered in asymptomatic patients during screening mammography – might be different from that of larger, invasive tumors which are detected during physical examination [20]. A recently published autopsy study showed that about 15% of apparently normal breasts of patients who died of unrelated diseases showed carcinomas in situ, thus launching the provocative hypothesis that these tumors may remain clinically silent (and presumably unimportant) for many years [22]. Other studies have suggested that the frequency of these "occult lesions" is probably lower [23], but there is still no satisfactory response to the two basic questions: (1) How many of these in situ carcinoma will progress to invasive cancer? (2) How long does this process take?

Invasive breast tumors are a morphologically heterogeneous group of lesions; the most common are infiltrating ductal carcinomas and infiltrating lobular carcinoma, which account for almost 90% of all invasive cancers. The great variability in histological appearance has led to various attempts to classify these tumors according to their microscopic features. Commonly used descriptive terms include poligonal cell carcinoma, scirrhous (with a marked fibrous stromal component), comedo (with macroscopic appearance suggestive of a small skin papule), and mucinous carcinoma (featured by the abundant accumulation of extracellular mucin around clusters of tumor cells). Moreover, medullary carcinomas are slow-growing tumors with a marked lymphocytic infiltration, a syncytial growth pattern, and overall more favorable prognosis. Finally, in inflammatory carcinoma the subdermal lymphocytes are infiltrated with indifferentiated cancer cells, and at a clinical level there is erythema of the whole gland with tenderness; this histologic subtype of breast cancer seems to be particularly aggressive, with early local invasion and frequent lymph node involvement [20].

At variance with other types of tumors, histologic grading of breast cancer seems to closely reflect the aggressiveness of the neoplastic process. Well-differentiated (low-grade) tumors tend to resemble their cell of origin and to maintain a general architecture; at the other extreme, poorly differentiated (high-grade) tumors do not resemble the original tissue and lose the architectural array entirely. Increase in cell size, degree of pleomorphism, high nuclear to cytoplasmic ratio, loss of nuclear polarity, and cellular pyknosis are all indicators of less-differentiated tumors. The two main problems with grade and grade-related parameters are the frequent lack of agreement among observers (i.e., subjectivity in the interpretation) and the fact that cellular and architectural features may differ in various parts of the tumor, an event which often limits the clinical value of these parameters.

Screening

Besides primary prevention, one of the strategies for reducing mortality rates from breast cancer is early detection. However, the concept of early detection has been questioned, since it was calculated that 15–20 doubling times (in cell growth) are required for producing a 10 mm mass detectable by mammography or palpation; *clinical* earliness, therefore, does not seem to coincide with a *biologically* early lesion [24]. Apart from these considerations, there is a general consensus that an early diagnosis increases the chances of a radical approach, thus improving overall survival [19].

Early detection may be accomplished by mammography or by physical examination of the mammary gland performed by a trained physician, and these are the methods of choice for screening programs. Screening for breast cancer, however, is a controversial issue; several important questions have been raised, especially in very recent years, but the answers are still unsatisfactory. First, detection of precancerous lesions does not necessarily mean reduction of mortality; screening might simply detect in advance malignancies which will be lethal in any case (lead-time bias) or cancers that grow very slowly and are therefore less likely to develop metastasis (length-time bias). Moreover, women participating in a screening program might have different risk factors and may not be representative of the general population (selection bias). Second, the target population of screening has not yet been defined; available evidence indicates that for women in the age-group 50–69, screening may reduce breast cancer mortality by about 25%–40% [25, 26], but preliminary studies showed that no firm conclusion could be reached in women who are 40–50 years old [27, 28]. This is particularly important if we consider that hereditary breast cancer is characterized by early occurrence of tumors, frequently before the age of 40, and that this subgroup of patients should receive high priority in screening programs. Third, cost–benefit ratio should also be considered; Eddy has estimated that for American women in the age-group 40–75 years, annual screening by both mammography and physical examination for 10 years could result in saving 4000 lives per year, but at the annual cost of 1.3 billion dollars [29]. Although the estimates are different from country to country, there is no doubt that every screening program, besides biologic and clinical problems, requires the availability of large funds.

Despite controversies and uncertainties, the American Cancer Society recommends that women older than 40 should have an annual physical examination of their breasts, that screening mammography should begin at the age of 40, and that mammography should be carried out every 1–2 years for women less than 50 and annually for women older than 50 years [19]. An alternative, less expansive but probably more complex approach might consist in designing screening programs after stratification of the population not only by age, but also on the basis of the risk profile (Table 1).

Prognostic Factors and Management

Breast cancer may be a localized or systemic disease; in theory, surgery alone might be sufficient to eradicate local disease, while it should be associated with other forms of treatment (chemiotherapy, antihormones, radiotherapy) when the disease is not confined to the breast. However, the situation is made more complicated by the frequent occurrence of occult metastases, which may become manifest many years after an apparently curative resection. It follows that if the objective is eradication of disease more than local control, surgery should always be associated with some form of systemic treatment. This new, apparently simple paradigm can hardly be accepted for those patients (whose number is rapidly increasing owing to screening mammography) with small (1- to 2-cm) tumors and without axillary lymph nodes metastasis, most of whom (about 70%) are cured by surgery alone, without any adjuvant therapy. However, several biological markers of tumor aggressiveness and clinical outcome have recently been identified; these prognostic indicators might be of help in selecting (not without controversies) those individuals with apparently localized disease, but who presumably require a more "energetic" treatment. A final paradigm, therefore, might be: (a) patients with axillary lymph node metastasis should be treated with surgery and with some form of medical therapy (polychemiotherapy, tamoxifen, or both); (b) axillary node-negative patients are usually cured by surgery alone; however, if various biological markers strongly indicate the presence of a particularly aggressive tumor, antineoplastic drugs or tamoxifen should be recommended; and (c) node-negative patients in whom prognostic biomarkers do not suggest a highly malignant neoplasm can reasonably be considered cured by the operation. Finally, patients with liver, osseous, or brain involvement usually require only palliative treatment.

There is no doubt that the above considerations represent an oversimplification of the problem (for a more detailed discussion see [19, 20, 24, 30–32]); a few other points, however, deserve some general comments.

The standard surgical therapy for breast cancer is total mastectomy and dissection of the axilla (for removal of lymph nodes). Alternative breast-saving treatments include quadrantectomy and lumpectomy (again associated with axillary lymph node removal), which remove the bulk of the tumor surgically and use low doses of radiation to eradicate any residual cancer. Various randomized studies have showed that radical mastectomy and breast-saving approaches are equally effective in controlling the disease, with no difference in overall and disease-free survival [33, 34]. In line with these observations, a panel of experts at the National Cancer Institute agreed that breast conservation treatment is an adequate form of therapy and is preferable to total mastectomy because it "... provides survival equivalent (to mastectomy) ... while preserving the breast" [35]. Despite this apparently conclusive evidence, a recent study reported that in 1986 on average only 12% of American women operated on for breast cancer had breast-conserving surgery (range, 3.5%–21.2% in various States), whereas the large majority (88%) continued to be treated with standard mastectomy [36]. Are tradition and instinct more important than scientific evidence?

A critical evaluation of systemic treatment of early breast cancer by hormonal, cytotoxic, or immune therapy has recently been published [32]; the study included 133 randomized trials, carried out in several countries and a total of 75000 women. The main results of the investigation can be summarized as follows: (a) treatment with either tamoxifen or polychemiotherapy (mostly CMF, i.e., cyclophosphamide, methotrexate, and 5-flurouracil) was associated with a significant reduction of recurrence and of mortality rates; (b) the favorable effect was observed both in node-negative and in node-positive patients, but absolute improvement was more marked in node-positive patients; and (c) tamoxifen was more effective in postmenopausal women and in individuals with estrogen receptor-positive tumors; moreover, tamoxifen therapy reduced serum cholesterol levels, mortality for cardiovascular diseases, and risk of controlateral breast cancer.

The large number of studies on prognostic factors (and not only in breast cancer research) is justified for several reasons. First, these factors or markers may provide further information, besides clinical observation and classical histology, on the behavior and aggressiveness of tumors, so that therapy can be tailored to the biologic features of the neoplasms. This is particularly true for breast cancer, where the majority of node-negative patients can be cured by surgery alone [20], the overall benefit of adjuvant therapy is usually small [32], and the cost of this treatment given indiscriminately to all women with early lesions would be extremely high [31]. Second, even if not directly related to survival, many biological indicators might be of value in identifying subclasses of tumors with a possible different etiology; similarly, biomarkers may select subcategories of neoplasms which are more susceptible to the effect of specific drugs, in breast cancer the most appropriate example being estrogen receptors. Finally, independently of indication on survival, biomarkers contribute to the biological characterization of tumors in general, which simply means that their study increases our knowledge about the basic process of tumor induction and progression. In spite of these (and others) points in favor of biomarker studies, we should also frankly admit that the continuous search for new prognostic indicators has so far produced even more confusion and disillusion (once again, not only in breast cancer research).

Table 2. Prognostic indicators in breast cancer [19, 30, 37–43, 88–118]

Clinical – morphologic indicators
Nodal involvement (yes or not) and number of affected lymph nodes
Tumor size
Estrogen receptors (+ or −)
Tumor grade
Tumor vascularization
Poliferation – ploidy
Labeling index (fraction of DNA synthesizing cells)
Ki-67, PCNA, and AgNor staining
Nuclear ploidy and S-phase fraction (aneuploid vs. diploid tumors)
Oncogenes – antioncogenes
c-*erbB2* (amplification or overexpression)
c-*myc* (amplification or overexpression)
p53 (point mutation)
nm23 (expression)
Others
Cathepsin D
Plasminogen activator
Laminin receptor

PCNA, proliferating cell nuclear antibody; AgNor, nucleolar organizer region.

Traditionally, the most relevant prognostic indicators in breast cancer are axillary nodal status, number of involved lymph nodes, tumor size, histologic grade, and estrogen receptors [30]. A recent study [37] confirmed the primary importance of the nodal status as a predictor of recurrence and survival, while the prognostic information of tumor size and hormone receptors seems to be lower than expected. A second generation of biomarkers is represented by parameters of cell proliferation and nuclear ploidy [31]; in general terms, a high proliferative activity is associated with a higher relapse rate and a decreased overall survival [38–40]. Moreover, patients with aneuploid tumors tend to have a worse prognosis than subjects with diploid neoplasms [41, 42], though other studies failed to confirm these results [43]. A third generation of biomarkers includes oncogenes and tumor suppressor genes (c-*erbB2*, p53, and nm23, in particular), new markers of cell replication (Ki67; proliferating cell nuclear antigen, PCNA) and angiogenesis, and growth factors receptors [31, 44]. For most of these new markers, clinical studies are still preliminary and often controversial. Table 2 summarizes the most important prognostic indicators that have been studied or are under active investigation in breast cancer research.

Familial Breast Cancer

Rather empirically, familial breast cancer can be defined as the aggregation of two or more cases of breast tumor within a family (often two sisters or mother and daughter) [45]. Owing to the frequency of breast cancer in Western countries, this aggregation may be due to chance or can be related to common environmental factors shared by members of a given family; however, it is likely that in many of these cases primary genetic factors are of some relevance. Among various types of genetic transmission, the multifactorial model seems to be the most appropriate for explaining the aspecific aggregation of cancers in these families [45, 46], and the well-documented interaction between many environmental factors and genetic background (see below) lends further support to this interpretation. Evaluation of the real frequency of familial breast cancer is not easy; from a careful follow-up study involving more than 300 consecutive families with probands affected by breast cancer, Lynch and coworkers estimated familial cases to be in the order of 25% of the total [47].

Aggregation of breast cancers in families can also be expressed in terms of risk of developing tumors for members who are first- or second-degree relatives of the proband; this has been the objective of many studies. Macklin obtained detailed information on family history of 295 patients with breast cancer and compared the observed data to the mortality rates of the general population; the results clearly showed that female relatives of cases were more prone to breast cancer development than control relatives [48]. Similarly, Sattin et al. analyzed the clinical data of 4735 cases of breast cancer, diagnosed between 20 and 54 years of age, with those of a matched control group, with the purpose of evaluating whether a family history of breast cancer increased the risk of developing that disease. The authors found that patients with a first-degree relative affected by breast cancer had a 2.3-fold higher risk of developing the disease, whereas the risk was only 1.5-fold higher for second-degree relatives; moreover, among first-degree relatives the risk was similarly elevated (2.1-fold) for both affected mothers and sisters. Finally, for women who had both the mother and a sister with breast cancer, the relative risk (RR) rose to 14 [49]. Several other investigations showed the aggregation of breast cancer in pedigrees and the existence of families with a particular susceptibility to the development of this tumor [50–53]. Of particular interest was the study by Ottman et al. [51], who took into consideration not only family history, but also age of onset of tumors in the proband and mono- or bilaterality of the disease. The RR for sisters of patients with bilateral breast cancer diagnosed within their fourties was equal to 5; sisters of patients with unilateral disease were not at risk when the diagnosis in the proband was reached around the age of 50, but the risk was actually 2.4 when cancer was diagnosed at 40 years (or younger). Finally, a recent study showed that a family history of prostate cancer significantly increased the risk of mammary carcinoma [54].

Hereditary Breast Cancer

In hereditary breast cancer, there is sufficient clinical and biological evidence indicating that primary genetic factors are of major etiologic relevance. Indeed, recent linkage studies suggest that at least in some of these families a putative responsible gene can be located on the long arm of chromosome 17 (see below). However, at present the recognition of hereditary breast cancer requires the careful inspection of an extended family tree, especially if we consider that male individuals are able to transmit the disease to a successive generation, but usually do not express the trait. Several studies indicate that the autosomal dominant type of genetic transmission is fully consistent with the observed aggregation of tumors in breast cancer families [45, 46]; in the most typical cases the main features of monogenic dominant transmission (i.e., verticality, segregation ratio near 0.5, and absence of skipped generations) can be observed. However, the presence of phenocopies (owing to the frequency of breast cancer), the relative late onset of many tumors, and above all the modern tendency to families of small size, all together render the identification of many cases of hereditary breast cancer rather problematic. Besides vertical transmission and familial aggregation, additional features of the disease include early age of onset of tumors (not infrequently in the twenties or thirties), bilateral breast cancer, and multiple primaries. Despite all problems in recognition and identification of families, the most recent estimates of the Creighton group [47] indicate a frequency of hereditary breast cancer of approximately 8% of all breast tumors.

Several studies examined with segregation analysis clusters of familial breast cancer in extended pedigrees [55–59]; in the majority of these investigations, the most likely genetic model was the autosomal dominant type of transmission, with no consistent evidence of residual heritability. Thus, Newman et al. [57] carried out their analysis in a sample of 1579 consecutive nuclear families of breast cancer probands; their main conclusion was that, in this series, an autosomal dominant allele with high penetrance could explain the aggregation of breast tumors; this genetic basis, however, was only evident in 4% of the investigated pedigrees. The authors hypothesized for breast cancer a pathogenetic chain of events similar to that of retinoblastoma and Wilms' tumor. According to this model, families showing genetic transmission might have a germ line mutation of one allele in a tumor suppressor gene locus; a second mutation would then occur at a somatic level (in the same locus), with the consequent inactivation of the gene and development of cancer. In sporadic breast tumors both mutations would occur somatically in the mammary gland. Although attractive, this hypothesis may appear rather simplistic, especially if we consider the apparent genetic heterogeneity of these neoplasms [46]. Similar results were reported by Williams and Anderson [56], who concluded in favor of an autosomal dominant transmission by studying a large series of Dutch families with breast cancer aggregation. However, Goldstein et al. [60] carried out complex segregation analysis in 200 nuclear families in which the proband had bilateral breast cancer; they concluded that monogenic transmission at a single locus was not consistent with the observed distribution of postmenopausal breast tumors and suggested that a mixed model (i.e., a major locus plus other genetic or nongenetic factors) might be more appropriate to explain the distribution of cancer in families. The particular selection of these families (bilateral cancer) and the fact that the analysis was limited to first-degree relatives may partially explain why these findings were at variance with other observations [55, 57].

There are suggestions that some histological subtypes of mammary tumor might be related to hereditary breast cancer [46]; in particular, tubular and medullary carcinomas seem to occur more frequently in the genetic forms of the disease. However, the association was less clear when hereditary and control cases were rigorously matched [61], and more recent studies failed to identify histological markers which could define patients with hereditary breast cancer or individuals who are particularly susceptible to the development of this neoplasm [62].

Hereditary breast cancer is not a homogeneous entity, and several clinical variants have been described. These can be summarized as follows:

1. Site-specific hereditary breast cancer is the most frequent inherited type and is characterized by the absolute predominance of breast cancer in these families (Fig. 1); tumors of other organs are usually absent or, if present, do not show features suggestive of hereditary tumors (i.e., early age of onset, multiple primaries). The recognition can be relatively simple in large kindreds, but extremely difficult in small size families.
2. In hereditary breast/ovarian cancer, neoplasms of these two organs develop in susceptible individuals with a distribution in families which is consistent with dominant inheritance [63, 64]; after initial reports of linkage with the glutamate pyruvate transaminase locus (chromosome 16q) [65], more recent studies suggest that the syndrome might be attributed to a gene located on the long arm of chromosome 17 (see below).
3. Li-Fraumeni syndrome is characterized by early onset breast cancer and by the possible occurrence of several other neoplasms, including soft tissue sarcoma, osteosarcoma, brain tumors, leukemia, and lung, laryngeal, and adrenocortical cancer [66]. Owing to the discovery of p53 mutations in the germ line cells of patients with Li-Fraumeni syndrome, the disease will be treated in more detail in the relevent chapter [67].
4. Cowden disease is a rare type of inherited bilateral breast cancer; besides mammary tumors and cysts, the syndrome is characterized by hamartomatous lesions of the skin, oral fibromas, and benign and malignant thyroid tumors [68]. The disease – which is also known as multiple hamartoma syndrome [69] – seems to be transmitted with an autosomal dominant type of inheritance with high penetrance [46].

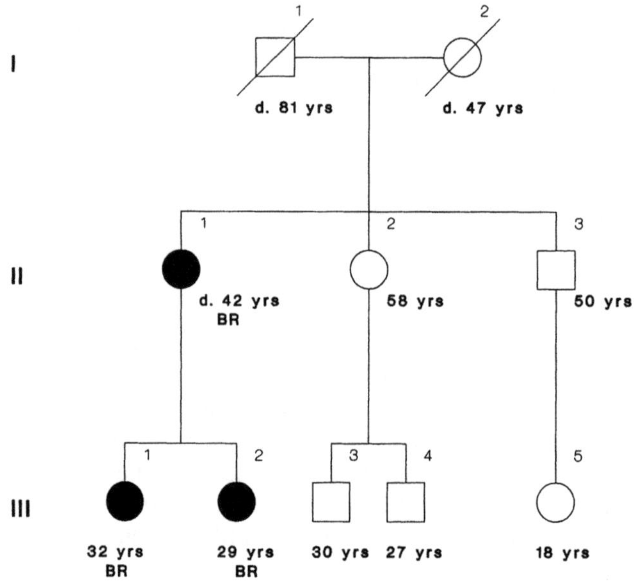

Fig. 1. Pedigree of a family with site-specific hereditary breast cancer. Among the main features of the syndrome, vertical transmission, aggregation, and early age of onset (in all three affected first-degree relatives) are easily observable. *d*, died; *BR*, breast cancer. (Courtesy of Drs. L. Mangone and M. Federico, Division of Oncology, University of Modena, Italy)

5. Finally, several families have been described in which breast cancer was associated with tumors of the digestive organs (especially colorectal carcinoma; Fig. 2) [46, 70].

Interaction Between Environmental and Genetic Factors in Breast Cancer

As already discussed, several environmental factors (mainly hormonal and dietary) are associated with an increased risk of breast cancer; on the other hand, genetic factors also play a major role in the pathogenesis of a large fraction of mammary tumors. We can therefore expect some sort of interaction between environmental factors and genes in breast cancer development. However, this interaction will probably exert a small effect in hereditary tumors, since in this case half of the subjects of affected branches are already at major risk of cancer on a purely genetic basis; in contrast, this interplay should be much more evident in familial tumors, in which a multifactorial model of transmission (i.e., involving the additive affect of both genetic and environmental factors) has been postulated. Experimental carcinogenesis provides some examples of the interaction between environment and genes in breast cancer development. Various strains of mice

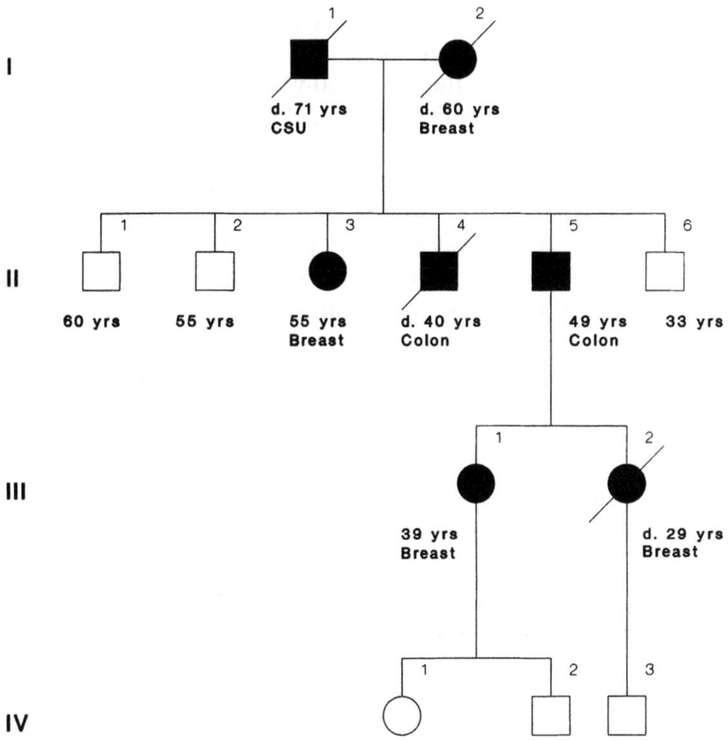

Fig. 2. Genealogical tree of a family showing association of breast cancer (at early onset in the two members of the third generation) with early onset colorectal cancer. The aggregation of cases and the verticality are consistent with an autosomal dominant mode of inheritance. *CSU*, cancer site unknown; *d*, died. (Courtesy of Drs. L. Mangone and M. Federico, Division of Oncology, University of Modena, Italy)

may show different genetic susceptibility to the formation of spontaneous mammary tumors; in less susceptible animals, few neoplasms are seen after estrogen administration, whereas the same dose of estrogens induces the appearance of many tumors in more susceptible animals [71, 72]. In humans, significant differences in urinary estrone and estradiol glucuronides were reported between young women at risk for familial breast tumors and controls [73], thus suggesting that genetically determined neoplasms could be somehow associated with alterations in estrogen conjugation. Moreover, other investigations showed that the promotional effect of oral contraceptives on breast cancer development was much more pronounced among young women (20–40 years of age) with a positive family history for breast cancer, in either paternal or maternal lineage [46]. Anderson et al. evaluated the combined effect of a family history of breast tumors and various reproductive factors on breast cancer risk in sisters of 404 patients affected by mammary cancer [74]. The authors found that early age of menarche and first birth at a late age were both associated with an increased risk of breast cancer, particularly in the 50- to 60-year-old age-group, and suggested that reproductive factors influenced the risk of breast cancer independently (i.e., in an additive way) of the presence of familiality for the disease. Finally, Sellers and coworkers studied the combined effect of family history and various anthropometric (body-mass index, waist to hip ratio) and reproductive factors on breast cancer risk in postmenopausal women [75]. The study, which involved more than 37000 women in the age-range 55–69 years, showed that a high waist to hip ratio was associated to an increased risk of breast tumors almost exclusively in women with a family history of breast cancer; moreover, the increased risk associated with low parity and late age at first pregnancy was much more evident among women with a family history of breast cancer. Besides their potential interest in elucidating the mechanisms underlying mammary tumor development, these observations may be of great value for surveillance, counseling, and follow-up of women with an increased familial risk of breast cancer.

Molecular Biology of Breast Cancer

Search for Genes for Hereditary Breast Cancer

The main objective of linkage studies is to find out the location of genes that determine the susceptibility to a given disease. In hereditary breast cancer, these studies have been inconclusive for many years, and the results are often conflicting, presumably due to the etiologic heterogeneity of the disease. Thus, in 11 breast cancer families showing features of autosomal dominant inheritance, King and colleagues found evidence of possible linkage between the trait (i.e., breast tumor) and the genetic marker GPT [76, 77]; however, in the subsequent years other groups reported no linkage or evidence against linkage of the disease to GPT [78, 79]. Similarly, Skolnick et al., by studying a single large kindred, found evidence of linkage between hereditary breast cancer and the ABO (blood groups) locus, but when the data were combined with those of other breast cancer families, the observed lod scores were no longer consistent with the previous findings [79, 80].

Recent studies, however, suggest that hereditary breast cancer susceptibility is linked, at least in some kindreds, to markers of chromosome 17q [9, 81, 82]. Twenty-three extended pedigrees were evaluated with a total of 146 cases of breast cancer; the families showed clinical features highly suggestive of hereditary disease, i.e., early onset tumors, frequent bilateral disease, and frequent occurrence of cancer among men. Several markers of chromosome 17q21 were used, among them the highly polymorphic marker D17S74. The authors found evidence of linkage (lod score, 5.9) between the trait (breast cancer) and D17S74 only in those families with early onset cancer (average age of breast cancer development less than 48), whereas negative lod scores were seen in families with relatively late onset disease (on average). It was therefore concluded that a gene for early onset breast cancer susceptibility is probably located on chromosome 17q21. Similar results were obtained by Narod et al. in three out of five families with hereditary breast/ovarian cancer [83]. The authors mapped the putative gene to chromosome 17q, but acknowledged that mapping of the cancer susceptibility gene on chromosome 17 was still imprecise and that the distance between D17S74 and breast/ovarian cancer locus may range from 1 to 22 cM, corresponding to bands q12–q23. Finally, further evidence of the possible location of a breast cancer susceptibility gene (BRCA1) on the long arm of chromosome 17 has recently been obtained by other investigators [84–86].

Enthusiasm derived from the above-mentioned studies should be balanced by a note of caution for their interpretation and application. First, positivity for linkage was observed only in part of the investigated families (40% in the study by Hall et al., three out of five kindreds in that by Narod et al.), although clinical evidence of hereditary breast cancer (or breast/ovarian cancer syndrome) was present in all of them; this implies the existence of other genes potentially implicated in the pathogenesis of both syndromes (i.e., genetic heterogeneity). Second, there is already evidence of this heterogeneity if we consider that Li-Fraumeni syndrome, (characterized by early onset breast cancer, sarcomas, and other tumors) is associated with germ line mutations of p53, a tumor suppressor gene mapped to chromosome 17p (see the chapter on "Li-Fraumeni Syndrome"). Finally, since most of the families so far selected and investigated did not show linkage to markers of 17q or 17p, we must conclude that at least one more gene for breast cancer susceptibility exists [87].

Oncogenes, Tumor Suppressor Genes, and Breast Cancer

In the last decade, there has been a veritable explosion of studies on oncogenes and tumor suppressor genes, especially in frequent and accessible neoplasms such as breast cancer; as a result, our knowledge of the biological basis of breast cancer has increased remarkably. It should be stressed, however, that although many molecular alterations were found, "none seems to be unique to breast cancer, and none has been found in all breast cancers" [88]. From the clinical point of view, the main objectives of these studies were: (a) to determine whether specific molecular changes could be associated to a more or less favorable clinical outcome; (b) to explore the possibility that various combinations of genetic events might be of help in the identification of subtypes of tumors with different etiology and pathogenesis; and (c) to find out whether specific genetic alterations, such as mutations, changes of expression, or allelic loss, could be used as targets for possible therapeutical intervention. At present, none of these goals has been reached, and the prevailing attitude among oncologists is towards a certain caution in accepting recent molecular findings as a guide for clinical decisions in addition to the information obtained with acknowledged prognostic indicators (i.e., nodal status, tumor size, and grade) [30]. Nevertheless, several biomolecular alterations appear extremely interesting and deserve some specific comments.

The c-*erbB2* oncogene (also called *neu* or *HER-2*) is a member of the tyrosine kinase oncogene family and encodes for a transmembrane glycoprotein which is structurally similar to the epidermal growth factor receptor. The human gene has been mapped to chromosome 17q21 [88]. In a large series of breast cancer patients, Slamon et al. found that c-*erbB2* amplification (more than five copies) was significantly related to both overall and disease-free survival, in the sense that overamplification was clearly associated with a poor prognosis [89]. Subsequent studies also suggested that c-*erbB2* amplification and expression might be independent prognostic indicators in human breast cancer [88, 90]; moreover, the expression product being a putative growth factor receptor, a possible role of the gene in the pathogenesis of human breast cancer could easily be hypothesized. However, other observations did not confirm these results [91–93], and a recent editorial concluded that at present there is little justification for the introduction of c-*erbB2* gene measurement into clinical practice [94]. Finally, to render the issue even more complicated, it is worth noting that c-*erbB2* amplification has recently been related to a high rate of tumor cell proliferation [95], to an increased mitotic activity [96], and to the presence of tetraploid or near-tetraploid DNA content [97]. Other oncogenes frequently altered in breast cancer include c-*myc* (amplification, in 4%–40% of all cases), and *int-2* (amplification, in 2%–20%), whereas mutations of the *ras* family genes seem rather rare in this neoplasm [88, 98–100]; the biological meaning of all these changes is presently unclear.

Loss of heterozygosity (LOH) on at least nine chromosomes has been reported in breast tumors [88, 98]; since allelic losses are thought to unmask recessive mutations of antioncogenes, it is likely that several tumor suppressor genes are implicated in breast cancer development. LOH is particularly frequent on both arms of chromosome 1 (1p32–p36, 1q21–q43) [101, 102]; on the short arm of chromosome 3 (3p21–25) [98, 103]; on chromosome 7q31 [104], where losses seem to be associated with a significantly shorter disease-free and overall survival; on chromosome 11 (11p14) [105, 106]; on chromosome 13 (13q14), with the frequent loss of the retinoblastoma gene [106, 107]; on chromosome 16q [107, 108]; and on both arms of chromosome 17 (17p13, 17q), with deletions of the two antioncogenes p53 and nm23 [106, 107]. Although less frequently, LOH on other chromosomes (18q and 22q) has also been reported [109, 110].

Point mutations of the p53 gene (see earlier chapter) were found in approximately 40% of breast tumors and are particularly frequent at codons

175, 194, 273, and 280 [111, 112]. In contrast, germ line mutations of the p53 gene are extremely rare and do not seem to play a role in the etiology of hereditary breast cancer [113, 114] (with the exception of Li-Fraumeni syndrome). Rather interestingly, a recent study showed an abnormal expression of wild-type p53 protein in normal epithelial and mesenchymal cells of a young woman from a highly suspected breast cancer family [115]. Expression of the nm23 tumor suppressor/antimetastatic gene (see Table 2 and the chapter on "Hereditary Melanoma and Dysplastic Nevus Syndrome") in human breast cancer tissue seems to be associated with a more favorable prognosis and to lack of lymph node metastasis [116, 117]; these observations are fully consistent with the suggested role of this gene in the suppression of the metastatic phenotype. Moreover, the gene has recently been assigned to chromosome 17q21 [118], a region which is often deleted in breast tumors [106].

Human breast cancer is a heterogeneous and extremely complex neoplasm where many factors may influence the biologic behaviour. Available evidence suggests that several genetic events – activation of oncogenes, altered expression, loss or mutations of tumor suppressor genes – may occur and, in various combinations, are closely linked to tumor development and progression. What we need to know are the genetic events actually responsible for tumor formation (and which of them are only epiphenomena) and the relation (if any) between genetic alterations and environmental factors associated with an increased risk of breast cancer.

References

1. Muir C, Waterhouse J, Mack T et al. (1987) Cancer incidence in five continents, vol 5. Lyon, France (IARC scientific publication, no 88)
2. Kelsey JL, Berkowitz GS (1988) Breast cancer epidemiology. Cancer Res 48:5615–5623
3. Zanetti R, Crosignani P (1992) Cancer in Italy: incidence data from cancer registries 1983–1987. Lega Italiana per la Lotta contro i Tumori, Torini
4. Miller BA, Feuer EJ, Hankey BF (1991) The increasing incidence of breast cancer since 1982: relevance of early detection. Cancer Causes Control 2:67–74
5. Holford TR, Roush GC, McKay LA (1991) Trends in famale breast cancer in Connecticut and the United States. J Clin Epidemiol 44:29–39
6. White E (1987) Projected changes in breast cancer incidence due to trend towards delayed childbearing. Am J Public Health 77:495–497
7. Kampert JB, Whitemore AS, Paffenbarger RS Jr (1988) Combined effect of childbearing, menstrual cycle, and body size on age-specific breast cancer risk. Am J Epidemiol 77:495–497
8. Romieu I, Willet WC, Colditz GA et al. (1989) Prospective studies of oral contraceptives use and the risk of breast cancer in women. J Natl Cancer Inst 81:1313–1321
9. Henderson IC (1993) Risk factors for breast cancer development. Cancer 71[Suppl]:2127–2140
10. Marshall E, Roberts L, Marx J et al. (1993) The politics of breast cancer: search for a killer; zeroing in on a breast cancer gene. Science 259:616–632

11. Graham S, Marshall J, Mettin C et al. (1982) Diet in the epidemiology of breast cancer. Am J Epidemiol 116:68–75
12. Tretli S (1989) Height and weight in relation to breast cancer morbidity and mortality: a prospective study of 570000 women in Norway. Int J Cancer 44:23–30
13. London S, Willet WC (1988) Diet, body size and breast cancer risk. Rev Endocr Relat Cancer 31:19–25
14. Longnecker MP, Berlin JA, Orza MJ (1988) A meta-analysis of alcohol consumption in relation to risk of breast cancer. JAMA 260:652–660
15. Hunter DJ, Manson JA, Colditz GA et al. (1993) A prospective study of the intake of vitamins C, E and A and the risk of breast cancer. N Engl J Med 329:234–240
16. Land CE, Mc Gregor DH (1979) Breast cancer incidence among atomic bomb survivors: implication for radiologic risk at low doses. J Natl Cancer Inst 62:17–21
17. Storm HH, Iversen E, Boice JD et al. (1986) Breast cancer following multiple chest fluoroscopies among tuberculosis patients: a case-control study in Denmark. Acta Radiol Oncol 25:233–238
18. Dupont WD, Page DL (1985) Risk factors for breast cancer in women with proliferative breast disease. N Engl J Med 312:146–151
19. Harris JR, Lippman ME, Veronesi U et al. (1992) Breast cancer, part 1. N Engl J Med 327:319–328
20. Harris JR, Lippman ME, Veronesi U et al. (1992) Breast cancer, part 2. N Engl J Med 327:390–398
21. Stomper PC, Connolly JR, Mayer JE et al. (1989) Clinically occult ductal carcinoma in situ detected with mammography: analysis of 100 cases with radiologic–pathologic correlation. Radiology 172:235–241
22. Andersen J, Nielsen M, Christensen L (1985) New aspects of the natural history of in situ and invasive carcinoma in the female breast: results from autopsy investigations. Verh Dtsch Ges Pathol 69:88–95
23. Barlow SA, Pathak DH, Black WC et al. (1987) Prevalence of benignm atypical, and malignant breast lesions in populations at different risk for breast cancer: a forensic autopsy study. Cancer 2751–2760
24. Plotkin D, Blankenberg F (1991) Breast cancer – biology and malpractice. Am J Clin Oncol 14(3):254–266
25. Shapiro S (1989) Determining the efficacy of breast cancer screening. Cancer 63:1873–1880
26. Wald N, Frost C, Cuckle H (1991) Breast cancer screening: the current position. Br Med J 302:845–846
27. Editorial (1991) Breast cancer screening in women under 50. Lancet 337: 1575–1576
28. Baines CJ, Miller AB, Kopans DB et al. (1990) Canadian national breast screening study: assessment of technical quality by external review. Am J Roentgenol 155:743–749
29. Eddy DM (1989) Screening for breast cancer. Ann Intern Med 111:389–399
30. Bonadonna G (1992) Evolving concepts in the systemic adjuvant treatment of breast cancer. Cancer Res 52:2127–2137
31. McGuire WL, Clark GM (1992) Prognostic factors and treatment decision in axillary node-negative breast cancer. N Engl J Med 326:1756–1761
32. Early Breast Cancer Trialists Collaborative Group (1992) Systemic treatment of early breast cancer by hormonal, cytotoxic or immune therapy. Lancet 339: 1–15, 71–85

33. Veronesi U, Luini A, Del Vecchio M et al. (1993) Radiotherapy after breast-preserving surgery in women with localized cancer of the breast. N Engl J Med 328:1587–1591
34. Fisher B, Costantino J, Redmond C et al. (1993) Lumpectomy compared with lumpectomy and radiation therapy for treatment of breast cancer. N Engl J Med 328:1581–1586
35. Editorial (1991) Treatment of early-stage breast cancer. JAMA 265:391–395
36. Nattinger AB, Gottlieb MS, Veum J et al. (1992) Geographic variation in the use of breast-conserving treatment for breast cancer. N Engl J Med 326: 1102–1107
37. Donegan WL (1992) Prognostic factors: stage and receptor status in breast cancer. Cancer 70:1755–1764
38. Gentili C, Sanfilippo O, Silvestrini R (1981) Cell proliferation and its relationship to clinical features and relapse in breast cancer. Cancer 48:974–979
39. Silvestrini R, Daidone MG, Costa A (1989) Cell kinetics of solid tumors with time and its clinical implication. Tumori 75:367–372
40. Veronese SM, Gambacorta M, Gottardi O et al. (1993) Proliferation index as a prognostic marker in breast cancer. Cancer 71:3926–3931
41. Kallioniemi OP, Blanco G, Alavaikko M et al. (1987) Tumor DNA ploidy as an independent prognostic factor in breast cancer. Br J Cancer 56:637–642
42. Sigurdsson H, Baldetorp B, Borg A et al. (1990) Indicators of prognosis in node-negative breast cancer. N Engl J Med 322:1045–1053
43. Noguchi M, Koyasaki N, Ohta N et al. (1993) Internal mammary nodal status is a more reliable prognostic factor than DNA ploidy. Arch Surg 128:242–246
44. Descotes F, Pavy JJ, Adessi GL (1993) Human breast cancer: correlation study between HER-2 amplification and prognostic factors. Anticancer Res 13: 119–124
45. Lynch HT, Lynch JF (1985) Breast cancer genetics. In: Muller H, Weber W (eds) Familial cancer. Karger, Basel, pp 20–24
46. Lynch HT, Marcus JM, Watson P et al. (1989) Genetic epidemiology of breast cancer. In: Lynch HT, Hirayama T (eds) Genetic epidemiology of cancer. CRC Press, Boca Raton, pp 289–332
47. Lynch HT, Lynch JF (1986) Breast cancer genetics in an oncology clinic: 328 consecutive patients. Cancer Genet Cytogenet 23:369–376
48. Macklin MT (1959) Comparison of the number of breast cancer patients and the number of expected on the basis of mortality rates. J Natl Cancer Inst 22:927–933
49. Sattin RW, Rubin LG, Webster LA et al. (1985) Family history and the risk of breast cancer. JAMA 253:1908–1913
50. Anderson DE, Bodzioch MD (1985) Risk of familial breast cancer. Cancer 56:383–387
51. Ottman R, Pike MC, King MC et al. (1986) Familial breast cancer in a population-based series. Am J Epidemiol 123:15–21
52. Kelsey JL (1979) A review of the epidemiology of human breast cancer. Epidemiol Rev 1:74–109
53. Andrieu N, Clavel F, Demenais F (1989) Familial susceptibility to breast cancer: a complex inheritance. Int J Cancer 44:415–418
54. Anderson DE, Bedzioch MD (1993) Familial breast cancer risk. Cancer 72: 114–119
55. Lynch HT, Albano WA, Heieck JJ (1984) Genetics, biomarkers, and control of breast cancer. Cancer Genet Cytogenet 13:43–92
56. Williams WR, Anderson DE (1984) Genetic epidemiology of breast cancer: segregation analysis of 200 Danish pedigrees. Genet Epidemiol 1:7–20

57. Newman B, Austin MA, Lee M et al. (1988) Inheritance of human breast cancer: evidence for autosomal dominant transmission in high-risk families. Pro Natl Acad Sci USA 85:3044–3048
58. Claus EB, Risch NJ, Thompson WD (1991) Genetic analysis of breast cancer in the cancer and steroid hormone study. Am J Hum Genet 48:232–242
59. Bishop DT, Cannon Albright L, McLellan T et al. (1988) Segregation and linkage analysis of nine Utah breast cancer pedigrees. Genet Epidemiol 5: 151–169
60. Goldstein AM, Haile RWC, Marazita ML et al. (1987) A genetic epidemiologic investigation of breast cancer in families with bilateral breast cancer. J Natl Cancer Inst 78:911–918
61. Marcus JN, Page DL, Watson P et al. (1988) High mitotic grade in hereditary breast cancer. Lab Invest 58:61A
62. Burki N, Buser M, Emmons LR et al. (1990) Malignancies in families of women with medullary, tubular and invasive ductal breast cancer. Eur J Cancer 26:295–303
63. Fraumeni J, Grundy GW, Creagan ET et al. (1975) Six families prone to ovarian cancer. Cancer 36:364–369
64. Lynch HT, Harris RE, Guirgis HA et al. (1978) Familial association of breast/ ovarian carcinoma. Cancer 41:1543–1549
65. King MC, Go RCP, Eltson RC et al. (1980) Allele increasing susceptibility to human breast cancer may be linked to the GPT locus. Science 208:406–408
66. Li FP, Garber JE, Friend FH et al. (1992) Recommendations of predictive testing for germ line p53 mutations among cancer-prone individuals. J Natl Cancer Inst 84:1156–1160
67. Li FP, Fraumeni JF Jr (1969) Rhabdomyosarcoma in children: epidemiologic study and identification of a familial cancer syndrome. J Natl Cancer Inst 43:1365–1373
68. Browstein MH, Wolf M, Bikowski JB (1978) Cowden's disease: a cutaneous marker of breast cancer. Cancer 41:2393–2398
69. Starink TM, van der Veen JPW, Arwent F et al. (1986) The Cowden syndrome: a clinical and genetic study in 21 patients. Clin Genet 29:222–233
70. Lynch HT, Krush AJ, Lemon HM et al. (1972) Tumor variation in families with breast cancer. JAMA 222:1631–1634
71. Gardner WU (1939) Estrogens in carcinogenesis. Arch Pathol 127:138–143
72. Loeb L (1940) The significance of hormones in the origin of cancer. J Natl Cancer Inst 1:169–171
73. Fishman J, Fukushima DK, O'Connor J et al. (1979) Low urinary estrogen glucuronides in women at risk for familial breast cancer. Science 204:1089–1091
74. Anderson DE, Badzioch MD (1989) Combined effect of family history and reproductive factors on breast cancer risk. Cancer 63:349–353
75. Sellers TA, Kushi LH, Potter JD et al. (1992) Effect of family history, body-fat distribution, and reproductive factors on the risk of postmenopausal breast cancer. N Engl J Med 326:1323–1329
76. Goldstein AM, Haile RW, Spence MA et al. (1989) A genetic epidemiological investigation of breast cancer in families with bilateral breast cancer. Clin Genet 36:100–106
77. King MC, Go RCP, Lynch HT et al. (1983) Genetic epidemiology of breast cancer and associated cancers in high-risk families. J Natl Cancer Inst 71: 463–467
78. Anderson DE, Ferreu RE, Williams RW (1985) A linkage study of human breast cancer. Cytogen Cell Genet 40:568–569
79. Human gene conference 9 (1987) Cytogenet Cell Genet 46:1–101

80. Skolnick MH, Thompson EA, Bishop DT et al. (1984) Possible linkage of a breast cancer susceptibility locus to the ABO locus: sensitivity of lod scores to a single new recombinant observation. Genet Epidemiol 1:363–373
81. Hall JM, Lee MK, Newman B et al. (1990) Linkage of early-onset familial breast cancer to chromosome 17q21. Science 250:1684–1689
82. Hall JM, Friedman L, Guenther C et al. (1992) Closing in on a breast cancer gene on chromosome 17q. Am J Hum Gen 50:1235–1242
83. Narod SA, Feunteun J, Lynch HT et al. (1991) Familial breast/ovarian cancer locus on chromosome 17q12–q23. Lancet 338:82–83
84. Skolnick MH, Cannon-Albright L, Goldgar DE et al. (1990) Inheritance of proliferative breast disease in breast cancer kindreds. Science 250:1715–1720
85. Haile RW, Cortessis VK, Millikan R et al. (1993) A linkage analysis of D17S74 in 35 families with premenopausal bilateral breast cancer. Cancer Res 53: 212–214
86. Arason A, Barkardottir RB, Egilsson V et al. (1993) Linkage analysis of chromosome 17q markers and breast–ovarian cancer in Iceland families. Am J Human Genet 52:711–717
87. Skolnick MH, Cannon-Albright LA (1992) Genetic predisposition to breast cancer. Cancer 70:1747–1754
88. Wolman SR, Pauley RJ, Mohamed AN et al. (1992) Genetic markers as prognostic indicators in breast cancer. Cancer 70:1765–1774
89. Slamon DJ, Clark GM, Wong SG et al. (1987) Human breast cancer: correlation of relapse and survival with amplification of the HER-2/neu oncogene. Science 235:177–181
90. Wright C, Angus B, Nicholson S et al. (1989) Expression of c-erbB-2 oncoprotein: a prognostic indicator in human breast cancer. Cancer Res 49:2087–2090
91. Parkes HC, Lillycrop K, Howell A et al. (1990) C-erbB-2 mRNA expression in human breast tumours. Br J Cancer 61:39–45
92. Borg A, Tandon AK, Sigurdsson H et al. (1990) HER-2/neu amplification predicts poor survival in node positive breast cancer. Cancer Res 50:4332–4337
93. Clark GM, McGuire WL (1991) Follow-up study of HER-2/neu amplification in primary breast cancer. Cancer Res 51:944–948
94. Levine MN, Andriulis I (1992) The HER-2/neu oncogene in breast cancer: so what is new? J Clin Oncol 10:1034–1036
95. Borg A, Baldetorp B, Ferno M et al. (1991) ERBB2 amplification in breast cancer with a high rate of proliferation. Oncogene 6:137–143
96. Heintz NH, Leslie KO, Rogers LA et al. (1990) Amplification of the c-erb-B-2 oncogene and prognosis of breast adenocarcinoma. Arch Pathol Lab Med 114:160–163
97. Bacus SS, Bacus JW, Slamon DJ et al. (1990) HER-2/neu oncogene expression and DNA ploidy analysis in breast cancer. Arch Pathol Lab Med 114:164–169
98. Callahan R, Campbell G (1989) Mutations in human breast cancer. J Natl Cancer Inst 81:1780–1786
99. Locker AP, Dowle CS, Ellis IO et al. (1989) c-myc oncogene product expression and prognosis in operable breast cancer. Br J Cancer 49:357–360
100. Richiltz FC, Scott GK, Dodson JM et al. (1989) Incidence of activating ras oncogene mutations associated with pripary and metastatic human breast cancer. Cancer Res 49:357–360
101. Chen LC, Dollbaum C, Smith HS (1989) Loss of heterozygosity on chromosome 1p in human breast cancer. Proc Natl Acad Sci USA 86:7204–7207
102. Bieche I, Champeme MH, Matifas F et al. (1993) Two distinct regions involved in 1p deletion in human primary breast cancer. Cancer Res 53:1990–1994

103. Ali IU, Lidereau R, Callahan R (1989) Presence of two members of c-erbA receptor gene family in smallest region of somatic homozygosity on chromosome 3p21–p25 in human breast carcinoma. J Natl Cancer Inst 81:1815–1820
104. Bieche I, Champeme MH, Matifas F et al. (1992) Loss of heterozygosity on chromosome 7q and aggressive primary breast cancer. Lancet 339:139–143
105. Mackay J, Elder PA, Porteous DJ et al. (1988) Partial deletion of chromosome 11p in breast cancer correlates with size of primary tumours and oestrogen receptor level. Br J Cancer 58:710–714
106. Ander sen TI, Gaustad A, Ottestad L et al. (1992) Genetic alterations of the tumours suppressor gene regions 3p, 11p, 13q, 17p, and 17Q in human breast carcinoma. Genes Chromos Cancer 4:113–121
107. Sato T, Tanigami A, Yamakawa K et al. (1990) Allelotype of breast cancer: cumulative allele losses promote tumor progression in primary breast cancer. Cancer Res 50:7184–7189
108. Lindblom A, Rotstein S, Skoog L et al. (1993) Deletions on chromosome 16 in primary familial breast carcinoma are associated with distant metastases. Cancer Res 53:3707–3711
109. Devilee P, van der Broek M, Mannens M et al. (1991) Differences in patterns of allelic loss between two common types of adult cancer, breast and colon carcinoma and Wilms' tumor of childhood. Int J Cancer 47:817–821
110. Thompson AM, Morris RG, Wallace M et al. (1993) Allele loss from 5q21 and 18q21, and DCC mRNA expression in breast carcinoma. Br J Cancer 68:64–68
111. Coles C, Condie A, Chetty U et al. (1992) p53 mutations in breast cancer. Cancer Res 52:5291–5298
112. Prosser J, Thompson AM, Cranston G et al. (1990) Evidence that p53 behaves as a tumour suppressor gene in sporadic breast tumours. Oncogene 5:1573–1579
113. Prosser J, Elder PA, Condie A et al. (1991) Mutations of p53 do not account for heritable breast cancer: a study in 5 affected families. Br J Cancer 63: 181–184
114. Thorlacius S, Borresen AL, Eyfjord JE (1993) Somatic p53 mutations in human breast carcinomas in an icelandic population. Cancer Res 53:1637–1641
115. Barnes DM, Hanby AM, Gillett CE et al. (1992) Abnormal expression of wild type p53 protein in normal cells of a cancer family patient. Lancet 340:259–263
116. Hennessy C, Henry JA, May FEB et al. (1991) Expression of the antimetastatic gene nm23 in human breast cancer: an association with good prognosis. J Natl Cancer Inst 83:281–285
117. Slamon DJ (1991) Expression of the nm23 gene and breast cancer prognosis. J Natl cancer Inst 84:229–231
118. Varesco L, Caligo MA, Simi P et al. (1992) The nm23 gene maps to human chromosome band 17q22 and shows a restriction fragment length polymorphism with Bg/II. Genes Chromos Cancer 4:84–88

Hereditary and Familial Ovarian Cancer

As far as we can determine, there is no one at greater risk for ovarian cancer than a patient who is in the direct genetic lineage of a hereditary ovarian cancer syndrome kindred and whose mother, sister, and/or daughter is affected with this disease and/or an integrally related syndrome cancer.

H.T. LYNCH et al. (1991)

Introduction

Ovarian cancer is a common and frequently lethal condition, especially in well-developed and industrialized countries. The disease shows several analogies with breast carcinoma, and both neoplasms represent examples of probable, or possible, interaction between environmental and genetic factors in tumor promotion and progression. Thus, hormonal and reproductive factors are thought to be of some pathogenetic relevance in breast as well as in ovarian carcinoma, and a "risk profile" can tentatively be traced for both neoplasms. Many of these factors are closely related to modern habits and lifestyle; interestingly, some of these factors (i.e., oral contraceptives) might actually be protective against ovarian cancer development.

Analogies with breast tumors also concern familial and hereditary aspects; inherited ovarian cancer is a well-defined clinical condition which can be associated with breast tumors (breast/ovarian cancer syndrome), can consist in ovarian cancer only (site-specific ovarian cancer), or may be part of a syndrome with a broader neoplastic spectrum (Lynch syndrome II; see later chapter). Moreover, familial cases have also been reported and are characterized by the frequent occurrence of ovarian cancer among first- and second-degree relatives of probands, but without evidence of a mendelian type of transmission. Finally, biomolecular studies indicate that the same genetic events (p53 mutations, c-*erbB2*, and c-*myc* amplification or overexpression) may underlie the development of a certain proportion of either ovarian or breast carcinoma.

General Features of Ovarian Cancer

Clinical and Epidemiologic Features

Ovarian cancer occurs frequently in Western and northern Europe, in USA, and, more generally, in all industrialized countries, with adjusted incidence rates in the order of ten to 20 new cases per 100 000 inhabitants a year [1, 2]. At the other extreme, these neoplasms are rare in China, Japan, and Middle Eastern countries, but in Japanese women who have emigrated to USA, after one generation, incidence rates approach those of white American women, which strongly suggests the pathogenetic role of environmental factors. Finally, mortality rates for ovarian cancer have remained relatively stable over the last 30 years [3].

Among dietary components, meat and animal fat consumption has been linked to the incidence of ovarian cancer, whereas alcohol and smoking do not seem to bear any relationship to the disease [4]. Cramer and coworkers put forward the attractive hypothesis that milk consumption (typically high in northern countries) could be associated with an enhanced risk of ovarian cancer [5]; although these observations were confirmed by subsequent studies [6], it is still unclear whether this high risk has to be attributed to galactose or to other components of the milk (i.e., fat). Some studies indicate that the use of cosmetics might increase the risk of ovarian carcinoma, presumably owing to their content of asbestos [7]; the evidence, however, is rather weak (relative risk less than 2.0), and other authors have not confirmed this association [8]. Moreover, in a case–control study, Mori et al. found a significantly lower use of cosmetics in patients with ovarian cancer than in matched controls [9].

Among reproductive and endocrine factors, there is evidence indicating that multiparity and use of oral contraceptives show a protective effect against ovarian cancer formation [10, 11], though in other studies this protection was less clear [12]. Rather interestingly, according to some authors a reduced risk of the disease can be observed for several years after discontinuing the use of contraceptives [13]. In 1971, Fathala suggested that the protective effect of pregnancy and oral contraceptives might be reconciled to the hypothesis of an "incessant ovulation" [14]; according to this theory, cyclic ovulation induces damage to the ovarian epithelium, and these repeated traumas may ultimately lead to malignant changes. Moreover, ovulation exposes the ovarian surface epithelium to estrogen-rich follicular fluid. Pregnancy, as well as contraceptive use, suppresses ovulation and protects the epithelium from these continuous insults, thus preventing ovarian cancer formation; in contrast, the risk of the disease should be related to the number of times a woman ovulates in her life. However, in addition to the incessant ovulation, various other theories and hypotheses have been postulated in order to explain this protective effect [15, 16]. Finally, in line with this reasoning, early age of menarche, late menopause, and low parity have been found to be associated with an increased ovarian cancer risk [9, 15, 17].

The large majority of ovarian tumors arise from the ovarian surface epithelium; this consists of cuboidal–columnar cells separated from the ovarian cortex by a layer of connective tissue. Ovarian surface epithelial cells are cytologically similar to mesothelial peritoneal cells, with which they share a common embryologic origin. The main histologic types of epithelial cancer include serous cystoadenocarcinoma and mucinous, endometrioid, clear cell, and undifferentiated carcinoma. Ovarian tumors may show various degrees of differentiation, though the importance of histologic grade as a prognostic indicator is still unclear [18, 19].

As for most carcinomas, staging is of considerable prognostic importance in ovarian cancer. The International Federation of Gynecology and Obstetrics (FIGO) proposed a staging system which is mainly based on the extent of spread at laparotomy [20]. In stage I tumors, the neoformation is limited to the ovary (this class can be subdivided into three subclasses), whereas in stage II lesions the neoplastic growth extends outside the ovary to gynecological adnexae or other pelvic tissues, but it remains limited to the pelvis. Stage III tumors invade the abdominal cavity, including peritoneal surface and omentum (the undersurface of the diaphragm represents a common site of intra-abdominal dissemination and, thus, a particularly important area for inspection at surgery); moreover, metastasis in retroperitoneal or inguinal lymph nodes can be detected. Finally, in stage IV distant metastases are observed, especially to the liver and lung. Staging, however, is not a simple task in ovarian carcinoma, and it is not unusual to find patients with the same FIGO stage, but with striking differences in survival. Young and coworkers reevaluated patients with an initial diagnosis of stage I or II ovarian carcinoma [21]; with a supplement of clinical investigation (including laparotomy), a change of stage occurred in approximately one third of the patients, with stage II subjects being frequently reclassified as stage III. Sites of disease which were unrecognized at the first investigation included pelvic and para-aortic lymph nodes, peritoneal folds, omentum, and subdiaphragmatic areas.

Clinical manifestations of ovarian carcinoma usually present late, and only one third of these tumors are localized lesions at diagnosis. Early ovarian cancer is quite often asymptomatic; when symptoms develop, they tend to be mild or vague and can be overlooked by the patient as well as by the doctor. Anorexia, fatigue, and lower abdominal pain are among these common symptoms, which are usually not so specific as to raise suspicion of tumor or to suggest further investigations. Late symptoms, indicative of advanced disease, include ascites and a palpable abdominal mass. Definite diagnosis of ovarian carcinoma is based on ultrasounds and/or computed tomography, laparoscopy, and cytology of peritoneal washing.

Prognosis and Treatment

It is worth noting that one of the main biological features of ovarian cancer is its variable behavior, which ranges from relatively benign borderline tumors to rapidly progressive disease.

Despite its limits, staging at laparotomy remains the main determinant factor of the clinical outcome. Thus, stage I and II patients may show 50%–90% survival at 5 years, whereas prognosis is much more severe for stage III and IV individuals, with only 5%–15% of them surviving at 5 years from diagnosis [22]. Histologic type and degree of differentiation are of limited prognostic significance [18, 19], while more recent observations suggest that nuclear ploidy and cell kinetics might be valuable indicators of prognosis. Thus, several studies showed that aneuploid tumors tend to be associated with a shorter survival, whereas diploid tumors usually have a more favorable overall prognosis and may require less intensive chemotherapy [22–25]. Similarly, some studies suggest that a high proliferative activity (expressed as [^{3}H]thymidine labeling index or as S-phase fraction) seems to be indicative of a worse clinical outcome [26, 27]. However, the independent prognostic significance of these relatively new biomarkers is still uncertain, and further observations are needed. Finally, for stage II and III neoplasms, tumor residuum (i.e., the remaining neoplastic mass after debulking surgery) is an important prognostic factor; rather intuitively, a large residuum will be correlated with a poor prognosis [25, 28].

Treatment of ovarian carcinoma is not simple and requires close collaboration between surgeons and oncologists. For stage I tumors, surgery alone may be the treatment of choice and usually consists of hysterectomy and bilateral salpingo-oophorectomy; careful inspection of the whole abdominal cavity and, in particular, of diaphragmatic surfaces and paracolic gutters is an essential aspect of the initial surgical procedure, since it may reveal an unsuspected dissemination of the disease. For stage II and IV disease, the traditional approach includes extensive surgical ablation (for the purpose of removing as much tumor as possible), followed by mono- or polychemiotherapy, clinical reevaluation (by ultrasounds, computed tomography, or magnetic resonance imaging), and "second look" operation, with the specific objective of restaging the disease (and thus assessing whether postoperative treatment has succeeded in eradicating residual tumor) and of removing, if technically possible, any remaining tumor [29]. More recent approaches take into account the striking clinical benefit of associating cisplatin (or carboplatin) to an alkylating agent, with objective response, symptom relief, and prolonged survival in approximately 80% of the patients [30]. According to this view, treatment for ovarian carcinoma can now be limited to the initial surgical cytoreduction followed by an appropriate polychemiotherapy, whereas second look procedures do not seem to provide any further survival benefit [31]. Finally, follow-up of patients operated on for ovarian carcinoma is mainly based on serial measurements of the cancer-associated antigen CA-125 [29, 30, 32]; in patients with raised CA-125 (about 75% of the total), response to therapy (i.e., tumor regression) is associated with a significant reduction of serum marker levels, and, as long as no further rise is detected, progression of the disease can reasonably be excluded.

Familial Aspects of Ovarian Carcinoma

In the introductory chapter, familial cancer was defined as an aspecific aggregation of neoplasms in families, which is often reconciled to the multifactorial mode of inheritance; in contrast, in hereditary tumors there is sufficient evidence to believe that primary genetic factors are of major etiologic importance, and in the large majority of cases this implies an autosomal dominant type of transmission. As far as ovarian cancer is concerned, both conditions seem to exist, although their contribution to the overall burden of ovarian tumors is still unclear.

A large case–control population-based investigation was carried out by Schildkraut and Thompson with the objective of assessing the degree of aggregation of ovarian carcinoma in families [33]. The study included 493 patients with histologically verified ovarian tumor in the age-range 20–54 years and a group of 2465 controls selected by random digit dialing from the same geographic area during the same period (1980–1982). The authors reported a significant excess of ovarian cancer among case families, with odds ratios of 3.6 for first-degree relatives and of 2.9 for second-degree relatives. Moreover, the relative risk for mothers was almost three times greater than for sisters of cases and controls, and this was more in favor of a possible dominant type of inheritance. The statistical approach of the study (i.e., case–control investigation, not segregation analysis), however, did not allow various models of genetic transmission to be differentiated. Finally, the data suggested that this susceptibility to ovarian cancer development could pass through both the maternal and paternal lineages. A noticeable excess (7 versus 0) of ovarian cancer among case relatives was found by Casagrande et al. [15] in a study including 150 patient–control pairs; interestingly, the affected relatives were mothers ($n = 4$), aunts ($n = 2$), or grandmother ($n = 1$) of the proband, while no affected sister was reported. Similarly, in another case–control investigation (215 patient–control pairs; average age, 53 years for both), Cramer and colleagues referred a family history of ovarian tumors only among case relatives (4 versus 0) and estimated (by empirical logic) an 11-fold increase in the risk of the disease for women with a positive history of ovarian carcinoma [34]. Cancer of the lung, colorectum, prostate, head, and neck also occurred significantly more often among case relatives. Moreover, patients with ovarian carcinoma of serous, endometrial, and clear-cell histologic type reported a greater frequency of consanguinity in their ancestry; as discussed in the chapter on "Genetic Aspects of Disease," this suggests the possible involvement of recessive factors in the genetic transmission of the disease, though the hypothesis is rather at variance with the apparent "verticality" observed in other studies [15, 33]. A significant increase in the risk of ovarian cancer (odds ratio, 18.2) was reported by Hildreth et al. for first-degree relatives of affected patients in a hospital-based case–control study [35]. In a large Italian case–control study involving 755 cases of ovarian carcinoma and 2023 control women residing in the same area, Parazzini et al. found that a family history of ovarian neoplasms was significantly more frequent among case families (odds ratio, 1.9) than in controls, though the fraction of cases with aggregation of ovarian carcinoma was rather small, representing less than 1% of total cases [36]. Finally, it is worth noting that other case–control studies did not show any excess or clustering of ovarian cancers among case relatives, although these negative findings might partially be attributed to the relatively small size of some investigated series [9, 12, 37].

In 1950, A.F. Lieber described a remarkable family in which ovarian cancer developed in the mother and in five of her daughters [38]. In the following years, clustering of either site-specific ovarian tumors or breast/ovarian cancers in extended pedigrees were reported by several other investigators. Thus, Li et al. described another family with a marked aggregation of ovarian tumors [39]; after this initial report, the same authors described six more families with multiple cases of ovarian cancer [40]. Three of these families had concomitant clustering of breast tumors, whereas no aggregation of other neoplasms was observed. The authors suggested that the familial occurrence of cancer could be consistent with an autosomal dominant type of genetic transmission, and this led to prophylactic oophorectomy in 14 asymptomatic women from four families. At histology, three of these apparently normal ovaries showed abnormalities of the ovarian surface cells consisting in hyperplastic foci of epithelial and mesothelial tissues of possible preneoplastic significance. However, despite prophylactic surgery, three patients at risk for ovarian neoplasms developed disseminated intra-abdominal cancer resembling ovarian carcinoma, thus suggesting that in these cancer-prone kindreds the tissue susceptibility to neoplastic changes is not limited to the ovary, but might include other derivatives of the coelomic epithelium [41].

Several families with various aggregations of breast/ovarian carcinoma were repeatedly described by Lynch and coworkers [42–47]. The authors pointed out that both tumors tended to occur earlier than in sporadic cases, a feature which is constantly observed in almost all hereditary forms of cancer. Cumulative risk of breast/ovarian cancer, in the age-span 20–80 years, was estimated to be in the order of almost 46%, which is fully consistent with dominant inheritance; moreover, in one of these families ovarian carcinoma developed in two identical twins and in their progeny. Evidence was also provided indicating that the trait (i.e., ovarian or breast tumor) could be passed from one generation to another through both maternal and paternal lineages, thus reinforcing the contention of an autosomal dominant type of transmission. Finally, reevaluation of an extended pedigree 10 years after the initial ascertainment revealed a significant increase of breast and ovarian cancer occurrence in high-risk individuals during this decade when compared to the values expected on the basis of age- and sex-specific incidence rates from the Connecticut Cancer Registry (for the period 1979–1989).

In 1981, after the description of a family with a striking aggregation of ovarian cancer [48], Piver and coworkers instituted a Familial Ovarian Cancer Registry, with the specific purpose of genetic counseling and appropriate management of high-risk individuals. During the first 4 years of activity, a total of 201 cases of ovarian carcinoma in 94 families were reported [49], and by December 1990 the number of registered patients reached 1336 cases in 587 families [17]. A careful analysis of this large series confirmed the main features of the syndrome: (a) hereditary ovarian cancer seems to be inherited as an autosomal dominant trait; this implies a theoretical 50% risk of the disease for members of affected branches, which should be compared with the 1.4% average risk in the general population; it follows that prophylactic oophorectomy around the age of 35 is recommended for high-risk individuals; (b) two major clinical subtypes of hereditary ovarian cancer can be observed; in one of these the neoplastic spectrum is limited to ovarian tumors (site-specific ovarian cancer) in the other, breast and ovarian carcinomas aggregate in extended families (breast/ovarian cancer syndrome). In addition, significant ovarian cancer excess has been observed in hereditary nonpolyposis colorectal cancer (or Lynch syndrome II, see relevant chapter) [45, 46], whereas nonepithelial ovarian tumors seem to occur with increased frequency in Peutz-Jeghers syndrome (see the chapter on "Hereditary Gastrointestinal Polyposis Syndromes") and in basal cell nevus disease [17, 50]. A representative pedigree of a family with breast/ovarian cancer syndrome is illustrated in Fig. 1.

Molecular Biology of Ovarian Carcinoma

Putative Gene for Hereditary Ovarian/Breast Cancer

As already discussed in the previous chapter, recent experimental evidence suggests that a gene for hereditary ovarian/breast cancer syndrome can be assigned to chromosome 17q [51]. Narod et al. carried out linkage studies in five large families with full-blown disease using a polymorphic marker of chromosome 17q21. Lod scores indicative of linkage were observed in three out of five families, thus suggesting that a high proportion of hereditary breast/ovarian cancers map to chromosome 17q21–23. The authors, however, stressed that mapping of the gene on chromosome 17 was still imprecise and estimated that the genetic distance between the polymorphic marker (D17S74) and the putative locus of ovarian/breast cancer was in the order of

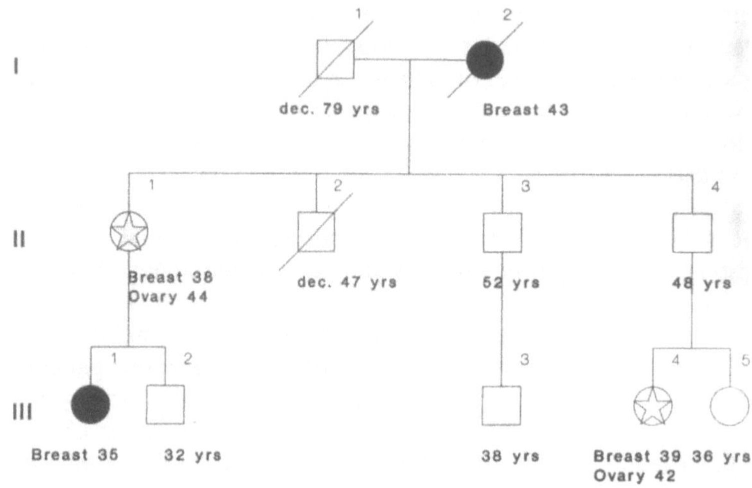

Fig. 1. Representative genealogical tree of a large family with breast/ovarian cancer syndrome spanning three generations. *Solid black symbols*, verified cancer; *stars*, multiple tumors; *dec.*, deceased

10–20 cM. Finally, no linkage was found between the trait and 60 additional polymorphic DNA markers distributed among various chromosomes [51]. As fas as we know, neither linkage study nor attempts at gene mapping have been reported for hereditary site-specific ovarian cancer; in contrast, it has recently been reported that hereditary nonpolyposis colorectal cancer (which may frequently include cases of ovarian carcinoma, see the chapter on "Hereditary and Familial Colorectal Cancer") does not seem to be linked to specific DNA markers of chromosomes 5q21 and 18q [52, 53].

Oncogenes, Antioncogenes, and Ovarian Carcinoma

Several lines of evidence support the contention that molecular events controlling tumorigenesis probably involve abnormal cell proliferation induced by altered expression of oncogenes and/or inactivation of tumor suppressor genes. This suggests that for many human tumors the accumulation of genetic changes is the most likely mechanism of tumor development and progression through a multistage process [54]. The complex genetic abnormalities observed in ovarian cancer are fully consistent with this pathogenetic sequence. In fact, several cytogenetic and biomolecular changes have been reported in these tumors. Some of these alterations might be early events, presumably associated with the initial steps of carcinogenesis, whereas others seem to act in the later stages of cancer progression. Our limited knowledge, however, does not allow a clear definition of the role of each of these changes in the development of ovarian cancer. Moreover, there is no abnormality of oncogenes or tumor suppressor genes which has specifically been related to familial or hereditary ovarian carcinoma; in addition, no genetic change has been found in all ovarian cancers or only in ovarian cancer.

Overexpression and/or amplification of the c-*myc* gene has been detected in approximately 10% of ovarian carcinomas [55]; similarly, activation (by point mutation) of the *ras* genes (N and K) was reported in an even smaller fraction of cases (3%–5%) and does not seem to be related to the clinical outcome [56]. Interestingly, ovarian mucinous tumors show K-*ras* mutations in a much larger fraction of cases (75% of total) than the other histologic types [57]. The biological relevance of *myc* and *ras* changes in ovarian tumors is at present still undefined. Several studies indicate that c-*erbB2* (or *HER-2/neu*) oncogene is amplified and overexpressed in 5%–20% of ovarian cancers; moreover, gene amplification seems to be associated with a poor prognosis, which suggests that the gene might play an important role in ovarian tumorigenesis [55, 58, 59]. More recent studies, however, did not show a close association between c-*erbB2* and prognosis in serous ovarian neoplasms [60].

Cytogenetic studies showed various reproducible and specific structural changes in invasive ovarian carcinoma, such as frequent abnormalities of chromosome 1, short arm deletion of chromosome 3, and long arm deletion of chromosome 6 [61, 62]. The frequent loss of genetic material on various chromosomes was confirmed by Southern blot analysis with probes that recognize restriction fragment length polymorphisms. Thus, genetic losses involving chromosomal segments 3p, 6q 11p, 13q, and 17p were observed at nonrandom frequency in ovarian cancer, suggesting the possible pathogenetic role of tumor suppressor genes located on these chromosomes [63, 64]. Similar results were reported by Zheng et al. in 30 human ovarian carcinomas; the authors suggested that allelic losses on chromosome 6 could be involved in the initial stages of ovarian carcinogenesis (together with c-*erbB2* amplification or overexpression), whereas loss of heterozygosity on chromosomes 3 and 11 seems to be associated with later steps of this process [65]. More recently, allele losses on chromosomes 17q, 18q, and Xp have been described in approximately 60% of ovarian carcinomas, especially in the more advanced stages [66–69].

Finally, p53 and Rb (retinoblastoma) genes might also been involved in ovarian tumorigenesis, which is of particular biological interest owing to their well-documented tumor suppressor activity (see relevant chapter). Allele loss from the short arm of chromosome 17 (where the human p53 has been located) have frequently been reported in ovarian carcinoma [70, 71]; moreover, overexpression of nuclear p53 protein and of p53 mRNA was detected in 50%–70% of these tumors [72, 73]. In addition, high-level expression was closely correlated with the presence of p53 point mutations, almost invariably in the highly conserved regions of the gene [72, 74–76]. Point mutations and altered expression of the p53 gene have also been found in several human ovarian carcinoma cell lines [77]. Taken together, these findings suggest a two-step inactivation of the normal p53 gene, which is in accordance with the general paradigm of tumor suppressor genes (see the chapters on "Oncogenes and Tumor Suppressor Genes" and "Retinoblastoma"): mutation of one copy of the gene followed by deletion of the remaining wild-type allele. However, the role of p53 inactivation in the promotion and progression of epithelial ovarian cancer is still unclear, and it is likely that the gene acts in concert with other oncogenes/antioncogenes [76, 78].

Two recent studies suggest the possible involvement of the Rb gene in ovarian cancer development. Sasano et al. [79] found evidence for homozygous deletion of the Rb gene in one out of 24 specimens of human ovarian tumors. Subsequently, Li et al. examined the DNA from 23 human ovarian carcinomas using a series of polymorphic markers of various chromosomes [80]; a high frequency (22%–44%) of allele deletion on chromosome 13q12–q32 (the Rb gene has been mapped to 13q14, see the chapter on "Retinoblastoma") was found with four of these probes. On the basis of these findings, the authors speculated that Rb gene might play a certain role in ovarian cancer development, although they could not exclude the possibility that other unidentified genes on chromosome 13, close to the Rb locus, may also be involved in ovarian tumorigenesis.

References

1. Whelan SL, Parkin DM, Masuyer E (1990) Pattern of cancer in five continents. IARC Sci Publ 102:1–168
2. Zanetti R, Crosignani P (1992) Cancer in Italy: incidence data from cancer registries 1983–1987. Lega Italiana per la Lotta contro i Tumori, Torino
3. Davesa SS, Silverman DT, Young JL et al. (1987) Cancer incidence and mortality trends among whites in USA, 1947–1984. JNCI 79:710–770
4. Cramer DW, Welch WR, Hutchison GB et al. (1984) Dietary animal fat in relation to ovarian cancer risk. Obstet Gynecol 63:833–837
5. Cramer DW, Willet WC, Bell DA et al. (1989) Galactose consumption and metabolism in relation to the risk of ovarian cancer. Lancet II:66–68
6. Piver MS, Mettlin CA (1990) A case-control study of milk drinking and ovary cancer risk. Am J Epidemiol 132:871–876
7. Cramer DW, Welch WR, Scully RE et al. (1982) Ovarian cancer and talc: a case-control study. Cancer 50:372–377
8. Whittemore AS, Wu ML, Paffenbarger RS et al. (1988) Personal and environmental characteristics related to epithelial ovarian cancer II. Exposure to talcum powder, tobacco, alcohol and coffee. Am J Epidemiol 128:1228–1234
9. Mori M, Kiyosawa H, Hirotsugu M (1984) Case-control study of ovarian cancer in Japan. Cancer 53:2746–2752
10. The cancer and steroid hormone study of the centers for Disease Control and the National Institute of Child Health and Human Development (1987) The reduction in risk of ovarian cancer associated with oral contraceptive use. N Engl J Med 316:650–655
11. Kvale G, Heuch I, Nilssen S et al. (1989) Reproductive factors and risk of ovarian cancer. Int J Cancer 42:246–251

12. Shu XO, Brinton LA, Gao YT et al. (1989) Population-based case-control study of ovarian cancer in Shanghai. Cancer Res 49:3670–3674
13. Cramer DW, Hutchison GB, Welch WR et al. (1982) Factors affecting the association of oral contraceptives and ovarian cancer. N Engl J Med 307:1047–1051
14. Fathala MR (1971) Incessant ovulation. A factor in ovarian neoplasia. Lancet II:163–164
15. Casagrande JT, Louie EW, Pike MC et al. (1979) Incessant ovulation and ovarian cancer. Lancet II:170–172
16. Godwin AK, Testa JR, Hamilton TC (1993) The biology of ovarian cancer development. Cancer 71:530–536
17. Piver SM, Baker TR, Piedmonte M et al. (1991) Epidemiology and etiology of ovarian cancer. Semin Oncol 18:177–185
18. Sorbe B, Frankendal BO, Veress B (1982) Importance of histologic grading in the prognosis of epithelial ovarian carcinoma. Obstet Gynecol 59:576–582
19. Jacobs AJ, Deligdisch L, Deppe G et al. (1982) Histologic correlations of virulence in ovarian adenocarcinoma. Am J Obstet Gynecol 143:574–580
20. Petterson F, Kolstad P, Ludwig H et al. (1988) Annual report of the results of treatment in gynecological cancer. Int Fed Gynecol Obstet 20
21. Young RC, Decker DG, Wharton JT et al. (1983) Staging laparotomy in early ovarian cancer. JAMA 250:3072–3076
22. Friedlander ML, Dembo AJ (1991) Prognostic factors in ovarian cancer. Semin Oncol 18:205–212
23. Hedley DW, Friedlander ML, Taylor IN (1985) Application of DNA flow cytometry to paraffin-embedded archival material for the study of aneuploidy and its clinical significance. Cytometry 6:327–333
24. Brescia RJ, Barakat RA, Beller U et al. (1990) The prognostic significance of nuclear DNA content in malignant epithelial tumors of the ovary. Cancer 65:141–147
25. Khoo SK, Battistutta D, Hurst T et al. (1993) The prognostic value of clinical, pathological, and biological parameters in ovarian cancer. Cancer 72:531–537
26. Kallioniemi OP, Punnonen R, Mallila J et al. (1988) Prognostic significance of DNA index, multiploidy and S-phase fraction in ovarian cancer. Cancer 61:334–339
27. Conte PF, Alama A, Rubagotte A et al. (1989) Cell kinetics in ovarian cancer. Relationship to clinico-pathologic features, responsiveness to chemotherapy and survival. Cancer 64:1188–1191
28. Delgado G, Oram DH, Petrelli EG (1984) Stage III epithelial ovarian cancer: the role of maximal surgical reduction. Gynecol Oncol 18:290–297
29. Griffiths CT (1975) Surgical resection of tumour bulk in the primary treatment of ovarian carcinoma. Natl Cancer Inst Monogr 42:101–104
30. Neijt JP (1991) Ovarian cancer treatment: time for some hard thinking. Eur J Cancer 27:680–681
31. Van der Burg MEL, Hoff AM, van Lent M et al. (1991) Carboplatin and cyclophosphamide salvage therapy for ovarian cancer patients relapsing after cisplatin combination chemotherapy. Eur J Cancer 27:248–250
32. Bast RC, Klug TL, St John E et al. (1983) A radioimmunoassay using a monoclonal antibody to monitor the course of epithelial ovarian cancer. N Engl J Med 309:883–887
33. Schildkraut JM, Thompson WD (1988) Familial ovarian cancer: a population-based case-control study. Am J Epidemiol 128:456–466
34. Cramer DW, Hutchison GB, Welch WR et al. (1983) Determinants of ovarian cancer risk. I. Reproductive experiences and family history. JNCI 71:711–716

35. Hildreth NG, Kelsey JL, LiVolsi VA et al. (1981) An epidemiologic study of epithelial carcinoma of the ovary. Am J Epidemiol 114:398–405
36. Parazzini F, La Vecchia C, Restelli C et al. (1992) Family history of reproductive cancers and ovarian cancer risk: an Italian case-control study. Am J Epidemiol 135:35–40
37. Grover S, Quinn MA, Weideman P (1993) Pattern of inheritance of ovarian cancer. Cancer 72:526–530
38. Lieber AF (1950) Ovarian cancer in mother and five daughters. Arch Pathol 49:280–290
39. Li FP, Rapoport AH, Fraumeni JF et al. (1970) Familial ovarian carcinoma. JAMA 214:1559–1561
40. Fraumeni JF, Grundy GW, Creagan ET et al. (1975) Six families prone to ovarian carcer. Cancer 36:364–369
41. Tobacman JK, Greene MH, Tucker MA et al. (1982) Intra-abdominal carcinomatosis after prophylactic oophorectomy in ovarian-cancer-prone families. Lancet II:795–797
42. Lynch HT, Krush AJ (1971) Carcinoma of the breast and ovary in three families. Surg Gynecol Obstet 133:644–648
43. Lynch HT, Harris RE, Guirgis HA et al. (1978) Familial association of breast/ovarian carcinoma. Cancer 41:1543–1549
44. Lynch HT, Watson P, Bewtra C et al. (1991) Hereditary ovarian cancer: heterogeneity in age at diagnosis. Cancer 67:1460–1466
45. Lynch HT, Conway T, Lynch J (1991) Hereditary ovarian cancer: pedigree studies, part II. Cancer Genet Cytogenet 52:161–183
46. Lynch HT, Watson P, Lynch JF et al. (1993) Hereditary ovarian cancer: heterogeneity in age at onset. Cancer 71:573–581
47. Amos CI, Strueving JP (1993) Genetic epidemiology of epithelial ovarian cancer. Cancer 71:566–572
48. Lurain JR, Piver MS (1979) Familial ovarian cancer. Gynecol Oncol 8:185–192
49. Piver MS, Mettlin CJ, Tsukada Y et al. (1984) Familial ovarian cancer registry. Obstet Gynecol 64:195–199
50. Gorlin RJ (1987) Nevoid basal-cell carcinoma syndrome. Medicine 66:98–113
51. Narod SA, Feunteun J, Lymch HT et al. (1991) Familial breast-ovarian cancer locus on chromosome 17q12–q23. Lancet 338:82–83
52. Peltomaki P, Sistonen P, Mecklin JP et al. (1991) Evidence supporting exclusion of DCC gene and a portion of chromosome 18q as the locus for susceptibility to hereditary non-polyposis colorectal carcinoma in five kindreds. Cancer Res 51:4135–4140
53. Peltomaki P, Sistonen P, Mecklin JP et al. (1992) Evidence that the MCC-APC gene region in 5q21 is not the site for susceptibility to hereditary non-polyposis colorectal carcinoma. Cancer Res 52:4530–4533
54. Vogelstein B, Fearon ER, Hamilton SR et al. (1988) Genetic alterations during colorectal-tumor development. N Engl J Med 319:525–532
55. Perez RP, Godwin AK, Hamilton TC et al. (1991) Ovarian cancer biology. Semin Oncol 18:186–204
56. Rodenburg C, Koelma I, Nap M et al. (1988) Immunohistochemical detection of the ras oncogene product p21 in advanced ovarian cancer: lack of correlation with clinical outcome. Arch Pathol Lab Med 112:151–154
57. Enomoto T, Weghorst CM, Inoue M et al. (1991) K-ras activation occurs frequently in mucinous adenocarcinomas and rarely in other common epithelial tumors of the human ovary. Am J Pathol 139:775–785
58. Slamon D, Godolphin W, Jones L et al. (1989) Study of the Her-2/neu protooncogene in human breast and ovarian cancer. Science 244:707–712

59. Berchuck A, Kamel A, Whitaker R et al. (1990) Overexpression of Her-2/neu is associated with poor survival in advanced epithelial ovarian cancer. Cancer Res 50:4087–4091
60. Seidman JD, Frisman DM, Norris HJ (1992) Expression of the HER-2/neu proto-oncogene in serous ovarian neoplasms. Cancer 70:2857–2860
61. Bello M, Rey J (1990) Chromosome aberration in metastatic ovarian cancer. Int J Cancer 45:50–54
62. Trent J, Kaneko Y, Mitelman F (1989) Report of the committee on structural chromosome changes in neoplasia. Cytogenet Cell Genet 51:533–562
63. Ehlen T, Dubeau L (1990) Loss of heterozygosity on chromosomal segments 3p, 6q and 11p in human ovarian carcinoma. Oncogene 5:219–223
64. Cliby W, Ritland S, Hartmann L et al. (1993) Human epithelial ovarian cancer allelotype. Cancer Res 53:2393–2398
65. Zheng J, Robinson WR, Elhen T et al. (1991) Distinction of low grade and high grade human ovarian carcinomas on the basis of losses of heterozygosity on chromosomes 3, 6 and 11 and HER-2/neu gene amplification. Cancer Res 51:4045–4051
66. Eccles DM, Russell SEH, Haites NE et al. (1992) Early loss of heterozygosity on 17q in ovarian cancer. Oncogene 7:2069–2072
67. Chenevix-Trench G, Larry J, Kerr J et al. (1992) Frequent loss of heterozygosity on chromosome 18 in ovarian adenocarcinoma which does not always include the DCC locus. Oncogene 7:1059–1065
68. Yang-Feng T, Li S, Han H et al. (1992) Frequent loss of heterozygosity on chromosome Xp and 13q in human ovarian cancer. Int J Cancer 52:575–580
69. Jacobs IJ, Smith SA, Wiseman RW et al. (1993) A deletion on chromosome 17q in epithelial ovarian tumors distal to the familial breast/ovarian cancer locus. Cancer Res 53:1218–1221
70. Eccles DM, Cranston G, Steel CM et al. (1990) Allele losses on chromosome 17 in human epithelial ovarian carcinoma. Oncogene 5:1599–1601
71. Black DM, Solomon E (1993) The search for the familial breast/ovarian cancer gene. Trends Genet 9:22–26
72. Marks JR, Davidoff AM, Kerns BJ et al. (1991) Overexpression and mutation of p53 in epithelial ovarian cancer. Cancer Res 51:2979–2984
73. Eccles DM, Brett L, Lessells A et al. (1992) Overexpression of the p53 protein and allele loss at 17p13 in ovarian carcinoma. Br J Cancer 65:40–44
74. Okamoto A, Sameshima Y, Yokoyama S et al. (1991) Frequent allelic losses and mutations of the p53 gene in human ovarian cancer. Cancer Res 51:5171–5176
75. Milner BJ, Allan LA, Eccles DM et al. (1993) p53 mutation is a common genetic event in ovarian cancer. Cancer Res 53:2128–2132
76. Teneriello MG, Ebina M, Linnoila RI et al. (1993) p53 and Ki-ras gene mutations in epithelial ovarian neoplasms. Cancer Res 53:3103–3108
77. Yaginuma Y, Westphal H (1992) Abnormal structure and expression of the p53 gene in human ovarian carcinoma cell line. Cancer Res 52:4196–4199
78. Mok SCH, Bell DA, Knapp RC et al. (1993) Mutation of K-ras protooncogene in human ovarian epithelial tumors of borderline malignancy. Cancer Res 53:1489–1492
79. Sasano H, Comerford J, Silverberg SG et al. (1990) An analysis of abnormalities of the retinoblastoma gene in human ovarian and endometrial carcinoma. Cancer 66:2150–2154
80. Li S, Schwartz PE, Lee WH et al. (1991) Allele loss at the retinoblastoma locus in human ovarian cancer. JNCI 83:637–640

Genetic Factors in Lung Cancer

The sharp and continuing rise in death from lung cancer, nearly all from cigarette smoking, is now widely recognized as a medical, social and political scandal.

J.C. BAILAR and E.M. SMITH (1986)

Introduction

Lung cancer is the commonest malignancy in the male sex and a major public health problem in the world. These tumors provide the most appropriate example of what is usually associated with the concept of neoplasia: pain, suffering, distress, and rapid death. This dismal outlook should not obscure the progress achieved in the basic knowledge of lung tumor biology and the consequent hope of a gradual improvement in prevention and clinical management.

Biologically, the interest of these tumors stems from several observations. First, lung cancer is one of the few examples in which a single etiologic factor (i.e., cigarette smoking) which outweights all other possible causes of the neoplasms has been identified. Second, several lines of evidence indicate the presence, in many patients, of a genetic predisposition to the disease; thus, despite the undoubted primary role of an exogenous agent, the development of these tumors should be viewed as consequent to a complex interaction between environmental and genetic factors. As already discussed in the introductory chapter, this might explain why not all heavy smokers, but only one in three or four, develop the disease. Third, various studies showed genetically determined differences between individuals in the metabolism of specific carcinogens found in tobacco smoke (such as polycyclic aromatic hydrocarbons), thus suggesting that susceptibility to lung cancer might be related to inherited alterations of a few enzymatic activities. Finally, recent studies indicated that various oncogenes and especially tumor suppressor genes are presumably involved in different phases of pulmonary tumorigenesis; these observations open new fields of application, which might be particularly rewarding in a disease where the advancements of knowledge have so far been frustrated by an almost constant increase in incidence and mortality rates.

General Features of Lung Cancer

Epidemiology

Almost all reports from cancer registries indicate a continuing increase in lung cancer incidence and mortality. In USA, age-adjusted incidence rate rose, among men, from 27 new cases per 100000 in the late 1940s to almost 90 per 10000 in 1981–1982, an increase of more than 200%, or 3% per year [1]. Although the rates are appreciably lower in women, the proportional increase has been even higher (from just under seven to 35 per 100000 in 1983–1984, an overall increase of more than 400 or almost 6% per year) [1]. During the same years, mortality rates showed parallel increases, with a mortality to incidence ratio close to 1. Similar figures were reported from several other sources [2–4], although there is some evidence that incidence rates reached a plateau in the late 1970s and early 1980s, at least in white American men [5]. In 1987, the number of deaths from lung cancer recorded in United Kingdom was 40137, whereas 142000 deaths were estimated in the United States for 1989 [4, 6].

After the classic observations of Doll and colleagues [7, 8], there is no longer any doubt that cigarette smoking is the major etiologic factor in lung cancer. The existence of an incontravertible link between these tumors and smoking has opened a political debate in almost all Western countries, the main arguments for discussion being on the one hand health education and reduction of productivity (due to illness) and on the other freedom of choice of adult individuals. The debate became even fiercer after the discovery that "passive smoking" (i.e., living in a smoky atmosphere, as in the case of spouses of heavy smokers) may increase the risk of these tumors. The deleterious effect of smoking, however, seems to be reversible, and there is evidence indicating that after 10–12 years of complete abstinence from cigarettes, the risk of lung cancer (and of other smoking-related diseases) tends to become as low as in nonsmokers [9, 10].

The strong causative role of smoking, its ample diffusion, and the possible effect of passive smoke in lung cancer development rendered extremely difficult the identification of other, well-grounded etiologic factors. Despite these problems, various authors estimated that some 10%–15% of all lung tumors should be attributed to occupation more than to cigarette smoking [12–14]. In particular, elevated relative risks (RR) were found for uranium and underground miners (RR, 1.9–2.1), painters (RR, 2.7), and especially for welders (RR, 3.2) [13]. Welding involves exposure to asbestos and to toxic gases that may affect the lung, while underground miners can be exposed to radon daughters, diesel exhaust, and silica. In addition, examples of non-tobacco-related carcinogens include several other agents, such as chromium, nickel, isopropyl alcohol, various radioisotopes, haloethers, and polycyclic aromatic hydrocarbons [15].

Evidence has been accumulated indicating that nutritional factors might be somehow related to lung cancer; thus, Carroll and Khor found a correlation between fat consumption and lung cancer mortality for 40 countries [16]. Moreover, in a case–control study, Hinds et al. [17] suggested that dietary cholesterol intake could be related to the risk of developing lung cancer, and more recent observations showed a highly significant correlation between calories from dietary fat and lung cancer mortality (after controlling for the possible confounding effect of many other variables) [18]. There are studies indicating that a high-fat diet may affect either the induction or the progression of lung cancer [18]; these findings are consistent with the well-known effect of dietary fat on experimental carcinogenesis [19, 20]. Finally, several studies support the existence of an association between low plasma levels of vitamins A and E selenium and the risk of lung carcinoma, though other authors did not confirm these observations [21, 22].

Clinical Features and Morphology

Unfortunately, early manifestations of lung cancer are infrequent, and the development of symptoms (cough, hemoptysis, and chest pain are the most common) usually indicates local or lymphatic spread of the disease. Moreover, the patient may be used to these symptoms because of chronic obstructive lung disease (which is frequent in heavy smokers), which may lead to a further delay in diagnosis. Other late manifestations of the disease include hoarseness of the voice or dysphonia (due to tumor invasion of the left recurrent laryngeal nerve), dysphagia (caused by enlarged mediastinal lymph nodes compressing the esophagus), dyspnea (by airways obstruction), severe pain of the shoulder and arm, owing to infiltration of the brachial plexux, and signs of vena cava obstruction. Paraneoplastic syndromes are common in lung cancer and may appear as the presenting finding or the first sign of recurrence [23, 24].

Lung carcinomas are highly malignant neoplasms, with a marked tendency to both local and metastatic diffusion. Thus, the tumor may spread into the mediastinum or through the bronchial wall and lung parenchima, reaching the pleura and ribs and infiltrating various nerves or plexi. Lymphatic spread primarily involves hilar, mediastinal, and tracheobronchial lymph nodes, although involvement of more distant lymphonodal areas (i.e., supraclavicular, cervical, axillary, and para-aortic) is not infrequent. Finally, the most common sites of distant metastasis include the bones (especially vertebrae and pelvis), brain, liver, and adrenal glands. TNM staging applies only to non-small cell carcinoma (in small cell cancer, staging is virtually of no help) and is a rather complex procedure, taking into consideration four main anatomical subsites and 14 different lymphonodal regions [25].

Despite the current definition of lung cancer, the tumor often originates in large and medium-sized bronchi. Histologic types are numerous, but four of these account for more than 90% of all cases with morphologic verification [3]. Squamous cell (or epidermoid) carcinoma is the most frequent histologic type found in males (30%–50% of total) and is characterized by the presence of keratinization; the large majority of these tumors arise in large–medium bronchi, where it is likely that their development is preceeded by squamous metaplasia. Adenocarcinomas (20%–30% of total) show a typical glandular array, with formation of acini, papillae, and mucin; this histologic type is particularly frequent in females and does not seem to be strictly related to cigarette smoking; various studies indicate that the frequency of adenocarcinoma has increased significantly since 1974 [26]. Large cell carcinomas (10%–20%) tend to present as peripheral nodules with well-defined borders; these tumors are often poorly differentiated and may show a variety of appearences, usually large cells with little tendency to keratinization and acinous formation. Small cell carcinomas (20%–30% of total) have spread beyond the bounds of curative surgery at time of presentation, and in many cases these tumors are diagnosed by biopsy of palpable cervical or supraclavicular lymph nodes; it follows that management of small cell cancer often does not involve surgery, but is limited to chemotherapy (with or without radiotherapy). Histologically, the tumor is characterized by a diffuse growth of small cells with hyperchromatic nuclei, indistinct nucleoli, and scant cytoplasm; electron microscopy shows the presence of dense neurosecretory granules, representing the morphologic basis of the various hormonal secretions (adrenocorticotropic hormone calcitonin; antidiuretic hormone); typical of these tumors [23, 24]. The main clinical properties of the four major histologic subtypes are summarized in Table 1; however, the fundamental decisions on management of these patients are taken on the basis of the classification of tumors as small cell or non-small cell carcinomas (the latter including squamous carcinoma, adenocarcinoma, and large cell tumor).

When symptoms and signs suggest the presence of lung cancer, the main objectives are to reach a firm morphologic diagnosis and to establish whether

Table 1. Clinical features of the major lung cancer histologic types

	Frequency (% of total)	Morphologic appearance	Five-year survival (% of resectable cases)
Non-small-cell carcinoma			
Squamous	30–50	Presence of keratinization	30–40
Adenocarcinoma	20–30	Typical glandular array	20–30
Large cell	10–20	Undifferentiated cells with various appearances	20–30
Small cell carcinoma	20–30	Small cells with hyperchromatic nuclei	0–5

the tumor is surgically resectable or whether it is preferable to treat the patient with chemotherapy and/or radiotherapy. In a large proportion of patients with lung tumors, malignant cells can be found in the sputum, especially when several samples are examined. Tumor tissue, or tumor cells in lavage fluid, can also be obtained with fiberoptic bronchoscopy, whereas other ways of obtaining neoplastic specimens include mediastinoscopy, subcutaneous lymph node biopsy, examination of pleural fluid or transthoracic fine-needle aspiration biopsy. Chest X-ray, bone scintiscan, computed tomography, and nuclear magnetic imaging – together with bronchoscopy and mediastinoscopy – are extremely valuable techniques for clinical staging of non-small-cell lung cancer. Presence of distant metastases or mediastinal involvement are definite contraindications to surgery. Small cell lung carcinomas are characterized by early hematogenous and lymphatic metastases, which render surgical intervention unsuitable in the majority of cases; clinical staging, therefore, is of limited value, and these tumors are simply classified as limited stage or extensive stage disease.

Prognostic Factors and Management

In patients with non-small-cell lung cancer, TNM staging (which reflects size of the primary neoplasm, involvement of lymph nodes, and presence of distant metastases) is the most important prognostic factor [27]. Thus, 5-year survival of all patients resected for cure is approximately 30%; however, for stage I patients with squamous carcinoma, survival is in the order of 50%, while it is reduced to 10%–15% for stage III tumors. Similarly, 5-year survival of stage III patients with adenocarcinoma or large cell carcinoma is about 5%–10%. Finally, in patients with small cell cancer, prognosis remains extremely poor, with 5-year survival of 2%–8% for limited disease and of 0%–1% for extensive disease [28].

In recent years several biomarkers of potential prognostic significance have been assessed. Among these, DNA ploidy remains one of the most actively investigated, owing to the availability of archive material. The results of several observations are fairly concordant and suggest that patients with diploid lung tumors tend to survive significantly longer than patients with aneuploid neoplasms; moreover, in some of these studies DNA ploidy appears to be a stage-independent prognostic factor [29–31]. Thymidine labeling index has also been assessed as a prognostic indicator; thus, Alama et al. [32] reported a much better survival in patients with a low replicative activity than in patients with a high proliferative rate; in addition, labeling index maintained its independent significance in multivariate analysis. Recent studies suggest that in non-small-cell carcinomas angiogenesis might be related to the metastatic potential of these neoplasms. Macchiarini et al. [33] evaluated microvessel density (by immunohistochemistry, using anti-factor VIII antibodies) in a large series of resectable lung cancers; only six out of

65 tumors (9.2%) with a relatively low microvessel count per microscopic field showed postoperative metastasis; in contrast, all patients with highly vascularized neoplasms manifested metastatic disease during follow-up. It was concluded that intensity of neovascularization, in resectable stage I lung tumors, correlates independently with the development of metastasis and might be a useful parameter in order to identify those patients who may benefit from adjuvant therapy. Finally, Miyake and colleagues [34] found that the expression of a carbohydrate antigen related to blood group H was an indicator of the clinical outcome of patients with non-small-cell carcinomas. The interest of these observations lies mainly in the fact that cell surface carbohydrates may have a role in the interaction between cells and extracellular matrix and thus in tumor progression and development of the metastatic phenotype [35].

Unfortunately, the majority of patients with lung cancer present with extensive and inoperable disease, i.e., tumors infiltrating the chest wall, diaphragm, or mediastinal structures or presence of distant metastasis. For these patients, prognosis remains extremely poor despite modern chemotherapy; moreover, radiotherapy is only an acceptable palliative treatment for symptoms such as pain, airway or vena cava obstruction, and dysphagia. For patients with non-small-cell carcinoma, surgery remains the only possibility of cure, although only a fraction of such patients can be operated on; despite some encouraging results, chemotherapy is usually ineffective in these patients [28, 36]. In contrast, small cell lung carcinoma can rarely be cured by surgery, since tumor dissemination is almost always present at diagnosis; in these patients, single agent or combination chemotherapy can prolong survival and may offer some prospect of cure in a small fraction of cases [37–39].

Familial Lung Cancer

Because of its strong association with cigarette smoking and certain occupations, lung cancer is usually considered as a neoplasm almost exclusively determined by environmental factors. Indeed, the pathogenetic relevance of smoking is so great that it can obscure the role of a possible genetic predisposition to the disease; the issue became even more complex after the recognition that passive smoking (which cannot be easily controlled as a confounding factor in epidemiologic studies) is associated with an increased risk of lung cancer [11]. On the other hand, it is also true that the presence of these well-grounded exogenous agents makes lung tumors particularly interesting for studying the possible interaction between environmental and genetic factors in tumor development. It is therefore not surprising that several investigators since the late 1950s have raised the possibility and accumulated evidence that genetic factors might play a definite role in the etiology of lung cancer [40].

Several authors described the aggregation of lung cancer and other tumors in isolated families. Thus, Brisman et al. reported a family in which lung carcinoma of the same histologic type developed in four siblings [41], while Joishi et al. [42] reported the occurrence of alveolar cell carcinoma in two identical twins; similarly, Goffman and colleagues described two families with lung and other respiratory tract carcinomas [43]. Takuhata and Lilienfeld [44] provided the first epidemiologic evidence of a possible role of genetic factors in lung cancer development; in a case–control study, the authors evaluated the frequency of respiratory tumors among relatives of lung cancer patients; a significantly increased risk for lung tumors among first-degree relatives was found, suggesting the presence of a susceptibility gene to these neoplasms. Similar results were reported by Ooi et al. [45] in a series of 2720 first-degree relatives of 336 patients who had of lung cancer; 70 case families with one relative affected by lung cancer and 14 families with two affected individuals were found, as compared to 25 and five control families, respectively (RR, 3.0). Rather interestingly, female relatives of patients over the age of 40 years showed a ninefold higher risk of lung cancer than female control relatives of the same age, and an excess risk was found even among relatives who did not smoke or report excessive exposure to hazardous occupations. Moreover, cancers of several other sites occurred more frequently among relatives of the proband than in control relatives (RR, 1.3–4.6). The authors concluded: (a) that an increased risk for lung cancer was present in their case families even after controlling for the confounding effect of smoking, occupation, and several other variables; (b) that the risk for the disease among relatives was a function of age; and (c) that the results could lend support to the existence of a susceptibility gene to lung carcinoma. In a further analysis of the same series [46], the authors confirmed a significantly greater overall risk of tumors of the respiratory tract among case relatives. In addition, the analysis showed that the increased risk was confined to neoplasms of three main sites: (1) trachea, bronchus, and lung; (2) nasal cavity and larynx; (3) female reproductive organs (RR, 1.9–4.4). Once again, the observed findings supported the hypothesis of a genetic predisposition to cancer of various organs in families with lung cancer. Clustering of cancer in relatives of patients with lung carcinoma was reported by McDuffie [47] in a large Canadian series of 359 case families and 234 matched control families. Besides lung tumors, several other neoplasms occurred significantly in excess among case relatives (i.e., cancer of the vocal cord, esophagus, colorectum, and pancreas); moreover, aggregation of tumors was more pronounced among siblings than in parents. The authors concluded that a family history of lung cancer can be considered an additional risk factor which interacts with environmental exposure in tumor development and progression.

Lynch and coworkers [48] evaluated cancer family histories in 254 lung cancer probands and 231 patients with other smoking-related tumors. At variance with other investigations, the authors did not find any increased familial risk of lung cancer per se when only this tumor was considered; however, a significant risk was observed for cancer of all sites among relatives of lung cancer probands; in addition, most of these neoplasms were not associated with cigarette smoking and were not greatly influenced by secular trends. The authors were led to the conclusion that the observed findings were consistent with the hypothesis of an underlying genetic susceptibility to cancer development, though the data were insufficient to analyze the possible types of genetic transmission.

Recent studies have provided evidence for mendelian inheritance in lung cancer. Thus, Sellers et al. [49] applied segregation analyses to 337 families of lung cancer probands – in which information on complete three-generation pedigrees was available – with the specific objective of determining whether the aggregation of tumors was consistent with the hypothesis of monogenic inheritance. Using the maximum likelihood method [50], the authors tested five hypotheses of genetic transmission: (1) the autosomal dominant allele; (2) the Mendelian inheritance of a single recessive gene; (3) the monogenic inheritance of a susceptibility allele with no dominance restriction ("codominant" inheritance); (4) Random environmental factors; (5) no major type of genetic transmission. While all other hypotheses were rejected or were close to the critical value for rejection, the mendelian codominant hypothesis was not rejected and showed a good fit to the data, suggesting that this type of inheritance of a rare autosomal gene might play a certain role in the etiology of lung cancer. Finally, in a recent investigation Sellers and colleagues [51] evaluated whether there were differences in clustering of lung cancers according to tumor histologic type. The results showed that a family history of lung tumor tended to be more frequent in patients with small cell compared with non-small-cell lung carcinoma, although the difference was not statistically significant (odds ratio, 1.9; confidence intervals, 0.9–4.1). Other authors, however, reported a more frequent familial aggregation of cancer in patients with squamous cell lung carcinoma [52].

In conclusion, aggregation of cancers is a frequent event in families of patients with lung carcinoma, which suggests that genetic factors might play an etiologic role in this common and frequently lethal malignancy. However, clustering of lung tumors is rarely as marked as that observed in other hereditary cancer syndromes (i.e., hereditary breast/ovarian cancer or hereditary nonpolyposis colorectal cancer); in addition, other stigmata of hereditary tumors, such as early age of onset and multiple primaries, are not observed with any particular frequency. It follows that the lack of these distinctive features, together with the presence of a strong confounding factor, such as cigarette smoking, may render extremely difficult the identification of these families. Representative pedigrees with a more or less marked aggregation of lung tumors are illustrated in Fig. 1 (see also Fig. 1 in the introductory chapter).

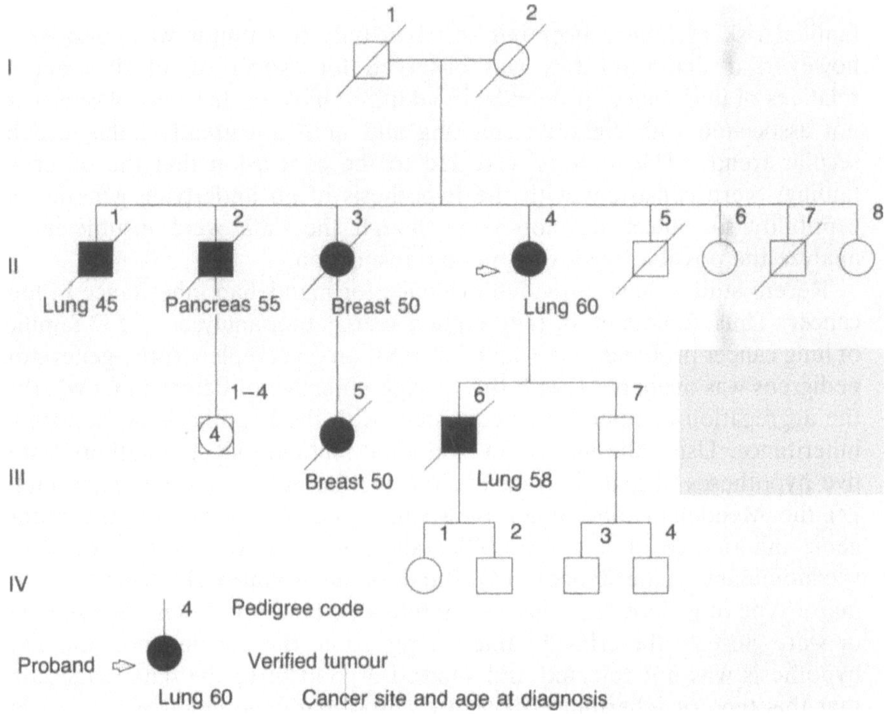

Fig. 1. Pedigree of a large family with an excess of lung and breast carcinomas in two different generations. Note the relative early onset (ages shown) of almost all neoplasms developed among family members (*solid black symbols*, affected subjects)

Metabolic Markers of Increased Susceptibility to Lung Cancer

If one considers the undoubted importance of cigarette smoking in lung cancer development and, on the other hand, the existence of a familial basis for many of these tumors, it is tempting to speculate that a genetically determined variation in the metabolism of carcinogens contained in tobacco smoke might be related to lung cancer predisposition. These basic concepts led to the search for and the investigation of various metabolic markers of lung cancer risk, despite the fact that it is not yet clear which are the constituents of tobacco smoke that actually cause lung cancer in humans [53, 54].

The enzymatic activity aryl-hydrocarbon-hydroxylase (AHH) can provide an estimate of the metabolism of benzopyrene and other polycyclic aromatic hydrocarbons found in tobacco smoking. AHH activity has been measured in bronchial mucosa, in alveolar macraphages, and in peripheral blood lymphocytes of patients with lung cancer; although some studies revealed a higher enzymatic activity in affected subjects than in normal controls, other investigations failed to show significant differences, so that the possible role of AHH as a metabolic marker of an increased susceptibility to lung neoplasms remains undetermined [55–57].

Antipyrine metabolism has also been assessed in lung tumor patients; this drug might be a suitable marker of lung cancer risk, since it is metabolized through the cytochrome P-450 pathway (as many smoke-related carcinogens) and, in addition, its half-life correlates with benzopyrene hydroxylation. Various authors investigated antipyrine clearance from blood or saliva of lung cancer patients and of normal individuals, but once again conflicting results have been reported [58, 59].

Studies on debrisoquin metabolism as a possible marker of genetic predisposition to lung cancer have been so far the most rewarding. Debrisoquine is an anti-hypertensive agent which can be excreted unchanged or after hydroxylation to 4-hydroxydebrisoquine [60]. Debrisoquin metabolism is determined by a single gene which has recently been mapped to chromosome 22; it follows that the ratio of debrisoquin to 4-dehydroxy-debrisoquin in biological fluids is largely under genetic control and that extensive and poor hydroxylation are two distinct phenotypes [61, 62]. Since the metabolism of several drugs and chemical compounds correlates with that of debrisoquin, it is possible that a similar relation exists with the metabolism of some carcinogens present in tobacco smoking, although direct proof of this is lacking. Following this line of reasoning, several authors investigated debrisoquin metabolism in lung cancer patients; the results of these studies showed that there is an increased risk of lung cancer among individuals who metabolize debrisoquin extensively as compared to poor metabolizers, with odds ratio ranging between 1.7 and 5.9 and confidence intervals of borderline significance [63–65]. It is likely therefore that lung cancer patients show a preponderance of the homozygous dominant "extensive metabolizer" phenotype as compared to controls and that the gene controlling debrisoquin hydroxylation may be a host genetic determinant of susceptibility to lung tumors. Further studies might lead to a better definition of metabolic groups characterized by a different extent of debrisoquin hydroxylation and to the screening of high-risk individuals (i.e., heavy smokers, workers exposed to carcinogens, members of families with clustering of lung cancers) with this or others metabolic markers.

Oncogenes, Antioncogenes, and Lung Cancer

Several lines of evidence suggest that the occurrence of malignant tumors is closely associated with the selection of multiple somatic mutations which may deregulate normal tissue development or provide selective growth advantage to the tumor cell. In general terms, these mutations affect two classes of genes: cellular proto-oncogenes and tumor suppressor genes. Accumulating evidence indicates that lung cancers develop due to multiple genetic changes involving both oncogenes and tumor suppressor genes.

Among the genes implicated in the pathogenesis of lung tumors, *ras* and p53 have been the most extensively investigated, especially owing to their possible relation to tobacco smoking [66].

Reynolds et al. [67] used the NIH 3T3 focus assay and the NIH 3T3 cotransfection–nude mouse tumorigenicity assay in order to analyze ras oncogene activation in a series of non-small-cell lung cancers from smokers. Eighty-six percent of the investigated tumors contained activated oncogenes, an incidence which is almost as high as that reported in pancreatic cancer [68]; rather interestingly, the two tumor types showing the highest frequency of *ras* mutation recognize cigarette smoking as a common risk factor. A further link between oncogene activation and tobacco smoking was established by studying the mutation profile of the activated *ras* gene; in fact, G to T transversions were the most frequently detected mutations in lung tumor, and the same type of mutation of the *ras* gene is usually detected in the benzopyrene-induced mouse lung tumor. The authors suggested that carcinogens in tobacco smoking which give rise to aromatic or bulky hydrophobic DNA adducts can be responsible for activation of the *ras* genes in human lung cancer; as a matter of fact, several studies showed the existence of this kind of DNA adduct in the lung tissue of smokers and their persistence for several years after cessation of smoking [67, 69]. Although eight out of ten metastatic lung tumors contained activated *ras* genes, mutational activation was also frequent in nonmetastatic cancer; thus, on the basis of these findings it is unclear whether *ras* oncogene activation is an early or late event in lung cancer development. Finally, altered expression of the N-*myc*, c-*raf*, *jun*, and *bcl-2* genes and of numerous growth factors (and/or their receptors) has also been reported in primary lung tumors [66, 70–72].

Although the existence of specific chromosomal changes in lung tumors is rather controversial, cytogenetic studies showed a high frequency of chromosome 3p and chromosome 13 deletions, especially in small cell cancer [73, 74]. Subsequently, restriction fragment length polymorphism analysis confirmed these preliminary observations and revealed loss of heterozygosity for loci on three different chromosomes in almost 100% of patients with small cell lung cancer [75, 76]. Since allele losses were detected in various cases of stage I tumors, it is likely that these genetic changes occur relatively early in the development of these carcinoma rather than being secondary events that take place during tumor progression. Moreover, common regions of allele loss were 3p14, 13q12, and 17p13; it is noteworthy that these regions contain the retinoblastoma locus (13q) and the p53 locus (17p), both tumor suppressor genes which are frequently lost or altered in several human neoplasms (see earlier chapters).

In line with these observations, there is evidence implicating p53 inactivation (usually by point mutation) in lung cancer pathogenesis. Thus, several studies showed point mutations changing the p53 coding sequence in 40%–60% of lung tumors of all histologic types, whereas no structural abnormalities of the p53 gene was found in the corresponding normal tissue [77–81]. In non-small-cell cancer, p53 mutations were distributed between codons 132 and 283 – with a hot spot at codon 273 – and included tumors with or without loss of heterozygosity at 17p [79]. Suzuki et al. [82] detected point mutations changing the coding sequence of p53 in 14 out of 30 (47%) non-small-cell lung cancers, especially G:C to T:A transversion. The authors could not find any association between the presence of these mutations and various clinical and morphologic variables; in contrast, a close relation was observed between lifelong cigarette consumption and p53 mutations, thus suggesting that the gene may be a suitable target for studying the interaction between environmental and genetic factors in tumor development. Two recent studies showed loss of allele at 17p and p53 mutations in dysplastic bronchial epithelium adjacent lung tumors [83, 84], raising the possibility that changes in the gene may take place at an early stage of lung tumorigenesis; this is of particular importance, since in several other neoplasms p53 mutations are considered a late event, usually associated with the appearance of metastatic phenotype [85, 86]. Similarly, Sameshima et al. [87] recently suggested that alterations in the p53 gene are common, early events also in the development of small cell lung cancer. Finally, Takahashi et al. [88] further documented the strong tumor suppressor activity of the normal p53 gene. The authors introduced a wild-type p53 complementary DNA into lung cancer cell lines containing a homozygous deletion or a point mutation of p53; a marked inhibition of cell proliferation was observed, whereas no significant effect was seen by transfecting with the mutated gene. Moreover, in accordance with these observations, Lavigueur et al. [89] found that transgenic mice carrying the mutant gene tend to develop lung tumors.

Finally, alterations of the retinoblastoma gene have also been reported in lung cancer [90–93], though the precise role of the abnormal expression of this gene in lung tumorigenesis remains unclear.

References

1. Davesa SS, Silverman DT, Young JL et al. (1987) Cancer incidence and mortality trends among white in the USA, 1947–1984. JNCI 79:701–770
2. Levi F, Te VC, La Vecchia C (1990) Changes in cancer incidence in the Swiss canton of Vaud 1978–87. Ann Oncol 1:293–297
3. Zanetti R, Crosignani P (1992) Cancer in Italy: incidence data from cancer registries 1983–87. Lega Italiana per la Lotta contro i Tumori, Torino
4. Silverberg M, Lubera JL (1989) Cancer statistics, 1989. CA 39:3–21
5. Horm JW, Kessler LG (1986) Falling rates of lung cancer in men in USA. Lancet I:425–426
6. Bleehen NM (1989) Lung cancer – still a long road ahead. Br J Cancer 61: 493–494
7. Doll R, Hill AB (1964) Mortality in relation to smoking: ten years' observation on British doctors. Br Med J 1:1399–1410, 1460–1467

8. Doll R, Peto R (1986) Mortality in relation to smoking: 20 year's observation on male British doctors. Br Med J II:1525–1531
9. Boyle P (1993) The hazard of passive – and active – smoking. N Engl J Med 328:1708–1709
10. Halpern MT, Gillespie BW, Warner KE (1993) Pattern of absolute risk of lung cancer mortality in former smokers. J Natl Cancer Inst 85:457–464
11. Dalager NA, Pickle LW, Mason TJ et al. (1986) The relation of passive smoking to lung cancer. Cancer Res 46:4808–4811
12. Doll R, Peto R (1981) The causes of cancer: quantitative estimates of avoidable risk of cancer in the USA today. JNCI 66:1191–1308.
13. Lerchen ML, Wiggins CL, Samet JM (1987) Lung cancer and occupation in New Mexico. JNCI 79:639–645
14. Tomasek L, Darby S, Swerdlow AJ et al. (1993) Radon exposure and cancers other than lung cancer among uranium miners in West Bohemia. Lancet 341: 919–923
15. Blot WJ, Fraumeni JF (1976) Geographic patterns of lung cancers: industrial correlations. Am J Epidemiol 103:539–547
16. Carroll KK, Khor HT (1975) Dietary fat in relation to tumorigenesis. Prog Biochem Pharmacol 10:308–353
17. Hinds MW, Kolonel LN, Lee J et al. (1983) Dietary cholesterol and lung cancer risk among men in Hawaii. Am J Clin Nutr 37:192–193
18. Wynder EL, Hebert JR, Kabat GC (1987) Association of dietary fat and lung cancer. JNCI 79:631–637
19. Tannenbaum A (1942) The genesis and growth of tumors. III. Effect of a high fat diet. Cancer Res 2:468–475
20. Beems RB, van Beek L (1984) Modifying effect of dietary fat on benzopyrene-induced respiratory tract tumors in hamsters. Carcinogenesis 5:413–417
21. Stahelin HB, Buess E, Brubacher G (1984) Cancer, vitamins and plasma lipids: prospective Basel study. JNCI 73:1463–1468
22. Menkes MS, Comstock GW, Vuilleumier JP et al. (1986) Serum beta-carotene, vitamins A and E, Selenium, and the risk of lung cancer. N Engl J Med 315:1250–1254
23. Baylin S, Mendelsohn G (1980) Ectopic hormone production by tumors. Endocr Rev 1:45–77
24. Korman LY, Carney DN, Citron ML et al. (1986) Secretin/VIP stimulated secretion of bombesin/gastrin releasing peptide from human small cell carcinoma of the lung. Cancer Res 46:1214–1218
25. Spiessl B, Beahrs OH, Hermanek P et al. (1990) TNM atlas. Springer, Berlin Heidelberg New York, pp 134–144
26. Dodds L, Davis S, Polissar L (1986) A population-based study of lung cancer incidence trends by histologic types, 1974–81. JNCI 76:21–29
27. Naruke T, Goya T, Tsuchiya R et al. (1989) Prognosis and survival in resected lung carcinoma based on the new international staging system. J Thorac Cardiovasc Surg 97:350
28. Idhe DC (1992) Chemotherapy of lung cancer. N Engl J Med 327:1434–1441
29. Volm M, Hahn EW, Mattern J et al. (1988) Five-year follow-up study of independent clinical and flow cytometric prognostic factors for the survival of patients with non-small cell lung carcinoma. Cancer Res 48:2923–2928
30. Sahin AA, Ro JY, El-Naggar AK et al. (1990) Flow cytometric analysis of the DNA content of non-small cell lung cancer. Cancer 65:530–537
31. Miyamoto H, Harada M, Isobe H et al. (1991) Prognostic value of nuclear DNA content and expression of the ras oncogene product in lung cancer. Cancer Res 51:6346–6350

32. Alama A, Costantini M, Repetto L et al. (1990) Thymidine labelling index as prognostic factor in resected non-small cell lung cancer. Eur J Cancer 26: 622–625
33. Macchiarini P, Fontanini G, Hardin MH et al. (1992) Relation of neovascularization to metastasis of non-small-cell lung cancer. Lancet 340:145–146
34. Miyake M, Taki T, Hitomi S et al. (1992) Correlation of expression of H/Le/Le antigens with survival in patients with carcinoma of the lung. N Engl J Med 327:14–18
35. Hakamori S (1989) Aberrant glycosylation in tumors and tumor-associated carbohydrate antigens. Adv Cancer Res 52:257–331
36. Ihde DC, Minna JD (1991) Non-small cell lung cancer II treatment. Curr Probl Cancer 15:105–154
37. Lowenbraun S, Birch R, Buchanan R et al. (1984) Combination chemotherapy in small cell lung carcinoma: a randomized study of two intensive regimens. Cancer 54:2344–2350
38. Jackson DV Jr, Case LD, Zekan PJ et al. (1988) Improvement of long-term survival in extensive small-cell lung cancer. J Clin Oncol 6:1161–1169
39. Fukuoka M, Furuse K, Saijo N et al. (1991) Randomized trial of cyclophosphamide, doxorubicin, and vincristine versus cisplatin and etoposide versus alternation of these regimens in small-cell lung cancer. JNCI 83:855–861
40. Lynch HT, Lynch JF (1989) Genetic epidemiology of lung cancer. In: Lynch HT, Hirayama T (eds) Genetic epidemiology of cancer. CRC Press, Boca Raton, pp 279–288
41. Brismam R, Baker RR, Elkins R et al. (1967) Carcinoma of lung in 4 siblings. Cancer 20:2048–2053
42. Joishi SK, Cooper RA, Bowley PT (1977) Alveolar cell carcinoma in identical twins. Ann Intern Med 87:447–450
43. Goffman TE, Hassinger DD, Mulvihill JJ (1982) Familial respiratory tract cancer. JAMA 247:1020–1023
44. Tokuhata GK, Lilienfeld AM (1963) Familial aggregation of lung cancer in humans. JNCI 30:289–312
45. Ooi WL, Elston RC, Chen VW et al. (1986) Increased familial risk for lung cancer. JNCI 76:217–222
46. Sellers TE, Ooi WL, Elston RC et al. (1987) Increased familial risk for non-lung cancer among relatives of lung cancer patients. Am J Epidemiol 126:237–246
47. McDuffie HH (1991) Clustering of cancer in families of patients with primary lung cancer. J Clin Epidemiol 44:69–76
48. Lynch HT, Kimberling WJ, Markvicka SE et al. (1986) Genetics and smoking-associated cancers. Cancer 57:1640–1646
49. Sellers TA, Bailey-Wilson JE, Elston RC et al. (1990) Evidence for mendelian inheritance in the pathogenesis of lung cancer. JNCI 82:1272–1279
50. Elston RC, George VT (1989) Age of onset, age of examination, and other covariates in the analysis of family data. Genet Epidemiol 6:217–220
51. Sellers TA, Elston RC, Atwood LD et al. (1992) Lung cancer histologic type and family history of cancer. Cancer 69:86–91
52. Ambrosone CB, Rao J, Michalex AM et al. (1993) Lung cancer histologic types and family history of cancer. Cancer 72:1192–1198
53. Law MR (1990) Genetic predisposition to lung cancer. Br J Cancer 61:195–206
54. Nazart-Stewart V, Motulsky AG, Eaton DL et al. (1993) The glutathione S-transferase polymorphism as a marker for susceptibility to lung carcinoma. Cancer Res 53:2313–2318
55. Oesch F, Schmassmann H, Ohnhaus E et al. (1980) Mono-oxygenase, epoxide hydrolase, and glutathione-S transferase activities in human lung. Carcinogenesis 1:827–832

56. Harris CC, Autrup H, Connor R et al. (1976) Interindividual variation in binding of benzopyrene to DNA. Science 194:1067–1069
57. Kouri RE, McKinney CE, Slomiany DR et al. (1982) Positive correlation between high aryl hydrocarbon hydroxylase activity and primary lung cancer as analysed in cryopreserved lymphocytes. Cancer Res 42:5030–5035
58. Ambre J, Graeff D, Bures F et al. (1977) Antipyrine metabolism and bronchogenic carcinoma. J Med 8:57–64
59. Danhof M (1980) Antipyrine metabolite profile as a tool in the assessment of the activity of different drug oxidising enzymes in man. Doctoral thesis, University of Leiden, The Netherlands
60. Idle JR, Mahgoub A, Angelo MM et al. (1979) The metabolism of debrisoquine in man. Br J Clin Pharmacol 7:257–263
61. Eichelbaum M, Baur MP, Dengler HJ et al. (1987) Chromosomal assignment of human P-450 (debrisoquine/spartein type) to chromosome 22. Br J Clin Pharmacol 23:455–459
62. Steiner E, Iselius L, Alvan G et al. (1985) A family study of genetic and environmental factors determining polymorphic hydroxylation of debrisoquine. Clin Pharmacol Ther 38:394–399
63. Ayesh R, Idle JR, Ritchie JC et al. (1984) Metabolic oxidation phenotypes as markers for susceptibility to lung cancer. Nature 312:169–171
64. Caporaso N, Hoover R, Aisner S et al. (1988) Debrisoquine metabolic phenotype and the risk of lung cancer. Proc Am Soc Clin Oncol 8:336–338
65. Roots I, Drakoulis N, Ploch M et al. (1988) Debrisoquine hydroxylation phenotype, acetylation phenotype and ABO blood groups as genetic host factors of lung cancer risk. Klin Wochenschr 66[Suppl XI]:87–92
66. Richardson GE, Johnson BE (1993) The biology of lung cancer. Semin Oncol 20:105–127
67. Reynolds SH, Anna CK, Brown KC et al. (1991) Activated protooncogenes in human lung tumors from smokers. Proc Natl Acad Sci USA 88:1085–1089
68. Motoijma K, Urano T, Nagata Y et al. (1991) Mutations in the K-ras oncogene are common but lack correlation with prognosis and tumor stage in human pancreatic carcinoma. Am J Gastroenterol 86:1784–1788
69. Pursiaines KH, Hackman P, Ridanpaa M et al. (1993) K-ras mutations in human adenocarcinoma of the lung. Int J Cancer 53:250–256
70. Saksela K, Makela TP, Alitao K (1989) Oncogene expression in small-cell lung cancer cell lines and a testicular germ-cell tumor. Int J Cancer 44:182–185
71. Veale D, Kerr N, Gibson GJ et al. (1989) Characterization of epidermal growth factor receptor in primary human non-small cell lung cancer. Cancer Res 49: 1313–1317
72. Pezzella F, Turley H, Kuzu I et al. (1993) bcl-2 protein in non-small-cell lung carcinoma. N Engl J Med 329:690–694
73. Whang-Peng J, Kao-Shan CS, Lee CS et al. (1982) Specific chromosome defect associated with human small-cell lung cancer. Science 215:181–182
74. Morstyn G, Brown J, Novak U et al. (1987) Heterogeneous cytogenetic abnormalities in small cell lung cancer cell lines. Cancer Res 47:3322–3327
75. Yokota J, Wada M, Shimosato Y et al. (1987) Loss of heterozygosity on chromosomes 3, 13, and 17 in small-cell carcinoma and on chromosome 3 in adenocarcinoma of the lung. Proc Natl Acad Sci USA 84:9252–9256
76. Mori N, Yokota J, Oshimura M et al. (1989) Concordant deletions of chromosome 3p and loss of heterozygosity for chromosome 13 and 17 in small cell lung carcinoma. Cancer Res 49:5130–5135
77. Horio Y, Takahashi T, Kuroishi T et al. (1993) Prognostic significance of p53 mutations and 3p deletion in primary resected non-small cell lung cancer. Cancer Res 53:1–4

78. Iggo R, Gatter K, Bartek J et al. (1990) Increased expression of mutant forms of p53 oncogene in primary lung cancer. Lancet 335:675–679
79. Chiba I, Takahashi T, Nau MM et al. (1990) Mutations of p53 are frequent in primary, resected non-small cell lung cancer. Oncogene 5:1603–1610
80. Marchetti A, Buttitta F, Merlo G et al. (1993) p53 alterations in non-small cell lung cancers correlate with metastatic involvement of hilar and mediastinal lymph nodes. Cancer Res 53:2846–2851
81. Morkve O, Halvorsen OJ, Skjaevern R et al. (1993) Prognostic significance of p53 protein expression and DNA ploidy in surgically treated non-small cell lung carcinomas. Anticancer Res 13:571–578
82. Suzuki H, Takahashi T, Kuroishi T et al. (1992) p53 mutations in non-small cell lung cancer in Japan: association between mutations and smoking. Cancer Res 52:734–736
83. Sozzi G, Miozzo M, Donghi R et al. (1992) Deletions of 17p and p53 mutations in preneoplastic lesions of the lung. Cancer Res 52:6079–6082
84. Sundaresan V, Ganly P, Hasleton P et al. (1992) p53 and chromosome 3 abnormalities, characteristics of malignant lung tumors, are detectable in preinvasive lesions of the bronchus. Oncogene 7:1989–1997
85. Vogelstein B, Fearon ER, Hamilton SR et al. (1988) Genetic alterations during colorectal tumor development. N Engl J Med 319:525–532
86. Mazars R, Pujol P, Maudelonde T et al. (1991) p53 mutations in ovarian cancer: a late event? Oncogene 6:1685–1690
87. Sameshima Y, Matsuno Y, Hirohashi S et al. (1992) Alterations of the p53 gene are common and critical events for the maintenance of the malignant phenotypes in small-cell lung carcinoma. Oncogene 7:451–457
88. Takahashi T, Carbone D, Takahashi To et al. (1992) Wild-type but not mutant p53 suppresses the growth of human lung cancer cells bearing multiple genetic lesions. Cancer Res 52:2340–2343
89. Laviguer A, Maltby V, Mock D et al. (1989) High incidence of lung, bone and lymphoid tumors in transgenic mice overexpressing mutant alleles of the p53 oncogene. Mol Cell Biol 9:3982–3991
90. Harbour JW, Lai SL, Wang-Peng J et al. (1988) Abnormalities in structure and expression of the human retinoblastoma gene in SCLC. Science 241:353–357
91. Hensel CH, Hsieh CL, Gazdar Af et al. (1990) Altered structure and expression of the human Rb susceptibility gene in small cell lung cancer. Cancer Res 50:3067–3072
92. Murakami Y, Katahira M, Makino R et al. (1991) Inactivation of the retinoblastoma gene in a human lung carcinoma cell line. Oncogene 6:37–42
93. Reissmann PY, Koga H, Takahashi R et al. (1993) Inactivation of the Rb susceptibility gene in non-small cell lung cancer. Oncogene 8:1913–1919

Genetic Factors in Precancerous Lesions and Cancer of the Esophagus

One of the most intriguing features of esophageal cancer is its considerable geographic variation. Data worldwide present a mosaic of changing incidence rates and sex ratios. In most countries, incidence rates of esophageal cancer per 100 000 are approximately 2.5–5.0 for males and 1.5–2.5 for females. However, in certain areas the incidence rates are remarkably high, varying up to 500-fold from one area to another, from one country to another, and between ethnic groups within the same country.

(F. Change et al. 1992)

Introduction

Esophageal carcinoma is a highly malignant disease in which the various therapeutic approaches so far have been discouraging. It follows that prognosis remains extremely poor, with 5-year overall survival in the order of 5% or less.

Perhaps the most surprising and still largely unexplained characteristic of this neoplasm is the marked geographic variation of its frequency, with a few well-defined areas and populations showing very high incidence rates, which fall off sharply in neighboring areas. Precursor lesions of esophageal cancer have also been identified (especially in high-risk populations), and this led to the definition of a hypothetical pathogenetic sequence of morphologic changes, from chronic esophagitis with various degrees of dysplasia to the fully malignant phenotype.

Until a few years ago, genetic factors were virtually unknown in esophageal cancer, and the disease was usually considered as an example of a neoplasm strongly related to environmental factors only. More recent data revealed a possible role of heritable factors in determining susceptibility to the disease, at least in certain high-risk ethnic groups. Because of the relative rarity of esophageal tumors in most Western countries, familial aspects have not been extensively investigated in these populations. Finally, there is no doubt that its epidemiologic features and the underlying genetic predisposition render esophageal cancer an interesting model for studying the interaction between environmental factors and genetic background in the induction and progression of neoplasia.

General Aspects

Descriptive Epidemiology and Etiologic Factors

In most Western countries the incidence of esophageal cancer ranges between 1 and 5 new cases/100 000 inhabitants per year, with a male : female ratio of about 2 : 1 [1, 2]. However, several investigators have identified some high-risk countries in which incidence rates appreciably higher are usually observed; these include China, Iran, States of the former Soviet Union, South Africa, Brazil, and France [3–5]. Among these countries, the highest incidence and mortality rates for esophageal cancer are observed in three well-defined areas: the Caspian littoral of northern Iran, the Henan and Shanxi provinces of China, and the Transkei region of South Africa [6–8]. In these particular areas, age-standardized incidence rates of 150–300 new cases/100 000 per year have been reported for both sexes, and deaths due to esophageal carcinoma account for approximately 15% of total mortality, and for more than 60% of cancer-related deaths [9–11]. Rather interestingly, these markedly elevated rates are highly specific of certain provinces and populations (Turkoman in Iran, Linxian in China, and Xhosa in South Africa), but tend to drop sharply even a short distance into neighboring areas (Fig. 1).

The etiologic factors implicated in esophageal cancer development differ either between low-risk and high-risk areas, or among countries with a greatly elevated frequency of the disease. In Western countries, alcohol and tobacco appear to be the most relevant risk factors for esophageal carcinoma, with relative risks (RR) up to 10–15 for heavy smokers who also drink more than 70–80 g ethanol per day [12–14]. Suspected risk factors include nutritional deficiencies (i.e., poor intake of fresh fruit and raw vegetables), excessive intake of certain foods (i.e., fried bacon and ham), chronic esophagitis and columnar (Barrett's) esophagus (which are frequently associated with gastroesophageal reflux), Plummer-Vinson syndrome, and long-lasting achalasia [12–16].

The high risk of esophageal carcinoma among the Turkoman of the Caspian littoral has been attributed to many factors. The large majority of the adult population are used to drinking tea at a temperature of over 65°C, which is remarkably high compared with other populations at low risk for the disease; besides chronic thermal irritation, hot tea might facilitate the passage of putative carcinogens through the esophageal mucosa [6, 9, 11]. In addition, tea might exert a direct mutagenic effect – owing to its content of tannins, phenols, and other cancer-promoting substances [6, 9]. Opium presumably represents another risk factor; in fact, in this high-risk population, a large fraction of individuals of both sexes are used to smoking or eating opium (which is a mutagenic compound) [17]. Moreover, because of the dry environment and the nomadic lifestyle, the consumption of fresh fruits and vegetables among the Turkoman tribes is very low, and this may result

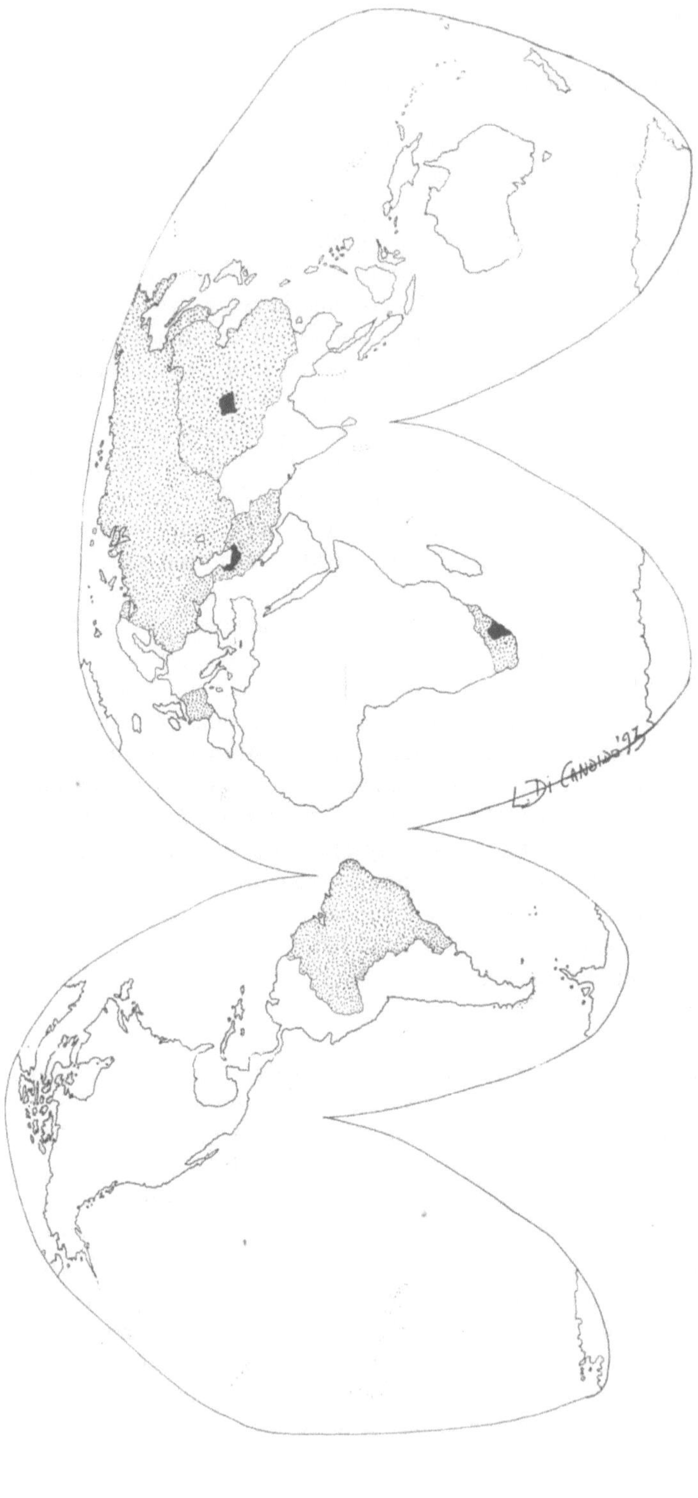

Fig. 1. Geographic variation of esophageal cancer incidence. *Hatched areas* represent countries with incidence rates higher than average (i.e., France, China, Russia, Iran, and some South American regions). *In black* are shown the three geographic zones with the highest prevalence of esophageal tumors (northern Iran, Linxian provinces, and Transkei)

in chronic vitamin deficiency, especially riboflavin, retinol, and ascorbic acid [18]. Finally, at variance with Western countries, cigarette smoking and alcohol do not seem to play a significant role in esophageal cancer development in this population [9].

In the People's Republic of China, esophageal carcinoma is particularly common in Linxian county [19]. Traditionally, this population is used to collecting and storing water in "dry wells"; this water is often contaminated with microorganisms of human and animal waste, so that high concentrations of *N*-nitroso compounds (nitrosamines and their precursors nitrate and nitrite, well-known inducers of tumors in many organs) are usually found in the drinking water [20]. Moreover, in Linxian, maize, millet, and other foods are frequently contaminated with fungi (*Aspergillus*, *Penicillium*, and many others) which are able to reduce nitrate to nitrite and to decompose proteins, thus increasing the amount of amines in these foods and favoring the production of nitrosamines [21]. The consumption of pickled and fermented vegetables is also common in this region; once again, several species of fungi usually contaminate these foodstuffs, and it is therefore not surprising that extracts of pickled vegetables are highly mutagenic in the Ames test [22]. Finally, both fungal and bacterial esophagitis are common in several regions of China; consequently, high concentrations of *N*-nitroso compounds have been detected in gastric juice, saliva, and urine in the Linxian population [11, 20, 23, 24].

Despite the considerable geographic distance, some of the risk factors considered for Linxian inhabitants seem to play an etiologic role also in the Xhosa tribes of Transkei, South Africa. In these regions, food is often contaminated with fungi of various species, and this process is further facilitated by the zinc and molybdenum deficiency of the soil, which increases the susceptibility of maize to *Fusarium*, *Aspergillus*, and other fungi capable of producing mutagenic metabolites [25]. Moreover, maize is fermented to make a traditional Xhosa beer, which contains an elevated concentration of nitrosamines [26]. In this population, both males and females are heavy smokers from a young age; in addition, the pipe stem juice – which contains a high concentration of nitrosamines – is usually chewed and swallowed while still hot [27]. The poor nutritional status of Xhosa and the consequent vitamin deficiency are additional factors which may contribute to cancer development in this population [10].

Finally, there is accumulating evidence that certain viruses – such as herpes simplex, human papillomavirus, and cytomegalovirus, which have been implicated in the pathogenesis of various human cancers – may infect the esophageal epithelium, and should therefore be considered potential etiologic factors in tumors of the esophagus [11, 28–30]. The main factors implicated in the pathogenesis of esophageal carcinoma are summarized in Table 1.

Table 1. Risk variables for esophageal carcinoma in different populations [12–29]

Population and/or geographic area	Associated risk factors
A. Western countries	Alcohol consumption and cigarette smoking Low intake of fresh fruit and vegetables Chronic esophagitis – Barrett's esophagus
B. Turkoman of the Caspian littoral (Iran)	Drinking hot beverages (tea, for its content of tannin and phenol) Opium (smoking or eating) Low consumption of fresh fruit Chronic vitamin deficiency (riboflavin, retinol, ascorbic acid)
C. Linxian population of north China	Nitrosamines contained in "dry wells" water; maize and other food contaminated with fungi/bacteria Consumption of pickled and fermented vegetables
D. Xhose tribes of Transkei (South Africa)	Nitrosamines contained in various foodstuffs (especially beer and maize) contaminated with fungi (*Fusarium*, *Aspergillus*) Zinc and molybdenum dificiency of the soil Cigarette and pipe smoking Poor nutritional status and vitamin deficiency

Clinical and Morphologic Features

Dysphagia, usually more pronounced for solid than for liquid foods, is the most common symptom of the disease, and is almost invariably associated with weight loss. In a minority of patients the onset of the disease may be characterized by dyspepsia, regurgitation, and gastroesophageal reflux. By the time symptoms develop, esophageal cancer is more often incurable, since dysphagia does not occur until 60% or more of the esophageal circumference is infiltrated with the neoplasm. If we divide the esophagus into three parts, the most frequent sites of cancer occurrence are the lower (40%–50% of the total) and the mid-third (30%–40%). Tumor spread occurs very early in the course of the disease by direct extension to the esophagus (both craniocaudal directions and circumferentially), invasion of the submucosa, and penetration of the muscular wall with direct mediastinal involvement. Mid- and lower third neoplasms spread to mediastinal and abdominal lymph nodes, while lesions of the upper third drain to deep cervical nodes. Liver, bones, lung, and brain are the most common sites of distant metastasis. Staging of esophageal cancer is difficult and no satisfactory classification has been developed; the diagnosis is based on upper endoscopy and a barium meal, while chest X-ray and especially computed tomography and endoscopic ultrasounds are valuable techniques for preoperative staging. Esophagoscopy is also important for dilating neoplastic strictures and inserting prosthetic tubes (Celestin or others) for palliation of dysphagia.

Squamous cell carcinoma and adenocarcinoma are by far the two commonest histologic types of esophageal cancer. Nearly half of the squamous cell lesions occur in the mid-esophagus, whereas the majority of adenocarcinomas develop in the lower third, and a large proportion of these are found with concomitant Barrett's esophagus [31]. It has been proposed that at least in Western countries, where the disease is relatively rare, the two main histologic types of esophageal cancer might have different etiologies; in particular, alcohol consumption and cigarette smoking seem to be more closely related to the development of squamous cell neoplasms, while gastroesophageal reflux and chronic esophagitis might predispose to both Barrett's esophagus and adenocarcinoma [32, 33].

Treatment and Prognosis

The overall prognosis of esophageal cancer is extremely poor, and the results of treatment remain discouraging with virtually no difference between the two main histologic subtypes. Earlam [34] recently reviewed the results of treatment in 90000 patients with esophageal carcinoma; the author concluded that overall 5-year survival was in the order of 6% for patients who received radiotherapy and of 4% for those who were treated with surgery. Although more favorable results have been reported, these regard only highly selected series of patients [35]. In individuals with cancer of the upper esophagus, radiotherapy is probably the treatment of choice, although surgery is also frequently carried out; for cancer of the mid and lower esophagus surgery is usually preferable, and the mobilized stomach is often used for reconstruction [36, 37]. Although various combined chemotherapy regimens have been proposed (mainly based on the use of 5-fluorouracil, mitomycin, vincristine, and/or cisplatin, and usually associated with radiation therapy), their benefit in terms of overall survival seems to be very limited [38, 39].

Preneoplastic Lesions and Biomarkers of Increased Susceptibility to Esophageal Cancer

Does esophageal cancer develop *ex novo* or does its natural history begin with preneoplastic lesions which gradually predispose the epithelium to the malignant phenotype? For the squamous cell carcinomas seen in Western countries there is no satisfactory answer to this question; however, since a history of esophagitis is infrequent in these patients, it is more likely that cancer develops from an apparently normal mucosa. In contrast, there is evidence indicating that adenocarcinomas, especially when localized in the lower third of the esophagus, might be related to longstanding inflammatory changes of the mucosa [32, 33]. Moreover, there are studies which support the hypothesis of a "multicentric carcinogenesis" in esophageal cancer development [40, 41].

The existence of precursor lesions and their pathogenetic role in esophageal cancer promotion have been well documented for some of the high-risk populations, especially in northern China and in the Caspian littoral. In 1982, Munoz et al. [42] reported the results of a large endoscopic survey involving more than 500 normal individuals living in Linxian county, most of whom were in the age group 35–54 years. Mild-moderate to severe esophagitis, usually not associated with symptoms; was found in 88% of males and in 70% of females; the mucosa appeared friable, edematous, and hyperemic, but without ulcerations; most changes were seen in the mid and lower third of the esophagus, while the precardial region appeared normal. These features are different from those of peptic esophagitis seen in Western countries, where erosions and ulcerations are commonly observed and the precardial region is also involved [32]. The endoscopic and histologic findings were surprisingly similar to those previously reported in the high-risk Turkoman of northern Iran [43]. This observation led the authors to hypothesize that in these regions the natural history of esophageal carcinoma begins with chronic esophagitis, which in a few presumably predisposed subjects progresses to dysplastic changes and eventually induces the development of the fully malignant phenotype [42]. The precise role of each of the putative etiologic factors listed in Table 1, in this sequence of events, remains unknown.

Subsequent studies by the same authors showed an elevated prevalence of esophagitis, in the high-risk areas of northern China, also among younger individuals; in fact, approximately 35%–40% of subjects in the age group 15–26 years had endoscopic and histologic evidence of esophagitis, the latter characterized by infiltration of the mucosa with inflammatory cells and superficial elongation of the vascular papillae [44, 45]. Multiple logistic regression analysis showed that the strongest risk factors for chronic esophagitis were drinking of beverages (especially tea) at burning hot temperature, low intake of fresh fruit and green vegetables, and presence of esophagitis among siblings; rather surprisingly, smoking and alcohol consumption were virtually unrelated to the disease.

In addition to inflammatory lesions, premorphologic changes have also been described in apparently normal esophageal mucosa of individuals living in areas at elevated risk for cancer of the esophagus. Modifications of epithelial cell proliferation and differentiation seem to be an early event in esophageal as well as in gastric and colorectal tumorigenesis [46]. Basically, available evidence suggests the existence of a disorder of cell cycle control mechanisms which leads to a continued DNA synthesis in maturing cells and to a delayed onset of terminal differentiation. Thus, the proliferative zone, normally situated only in the basal layer, expands from the deep portions of the epithelium to the most superficial compartments. It follows that immature S-phase cells may appear at the surface of esophageal mucosa, thus becoming more easily exposed to the possible mutagenic effect of various agents (i.e., nitrosamines, hot beverages, alcohol, and others) [46] (Fig. 2). Finally, changes in many other antigens (including keratins, beta-chorionic gonadotropin, placental lactogen, and alpha-fetoprotein) have also been described during the early phases of esophageal tumorigenesis [47].

In conclusion, esophagitis of various degrees of severity, atrophy or dysplasia of esophageal mucosa, and Barrett's esophagus – together with changes in cell replication and differentiation – represent the most common precursor lesions for cancer of the esophagus. If properly evaluated, these biological markers of increased susceptibility to the disease might be of great value for the identification, management, and follow-up of individuals at risk. Figure 3 illustrates the hypothetical sequence of events leading from a normal esophageal mucosa to carcinoma.

Familial Factors

In areas where the incidence of the disease is relatively low (i.e., many Western and industrialized countries), environmental agents are considered to be of major importance in the etiology of esophageal cancer, and little attention has been given to familial factors. In contrast, besides the undoubted importance of dietary habits and lifestyle (Table 1), the possible role of genetic factors in determining the susceptibility to esophageal carcinoma has been explored in more detail in the high-risk populations of northern China and Iran.

In 1951, Wu and Laucks [48] reported that among Chinese patients affected by esophageal cancer a positive family history of the same disease was much more frequent than in a control group (22% versus 5%, respectively). In another case-control study, Li et al. [49] compared familial aggregation of cancer in two regions of China with a markedly different incidence of the disease. Almost 60% of affected patients living in the high-risk region reported a positive family history for esophageal carcinoma as opposed to 43% of controls; these proportions were much lower in both cases and controls of the low-risk region. More recent epidemiologic surveys confirmed the marked familial aggregation of esophageal carcinoma in high-risk regions of north China [50, 51]. Moreover, in a large study carried out in Linxian county and involving 1244 patients with cancer of the esophagus and 1314 controls of similar age and sex, Li and colleagues [52] found an excess of esophageal or cardiac tumors among case relatives, and concluded that a positive family history for the disease was a significant risk factor (RR and confidence intervals: 1.7 and 1.4–2.0 for parents, 1.4 and 1.1–1.7 for siblings).

A similar familial aggregation of esophageal carcinoma has been reported by Ghadirian in the high-risk Iranian population of the Caspian littoral [53]. Detailed family histories were obtained from 602 patients with cancer of the

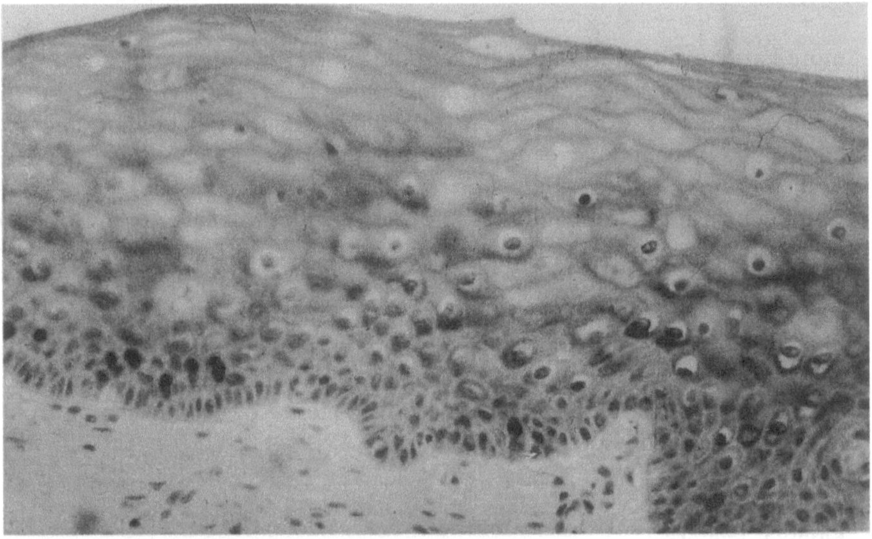
A

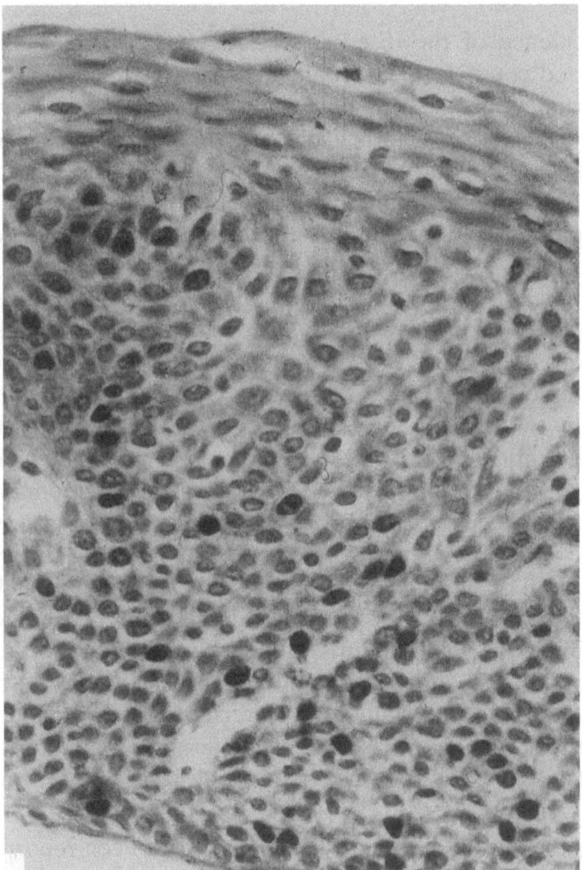
B

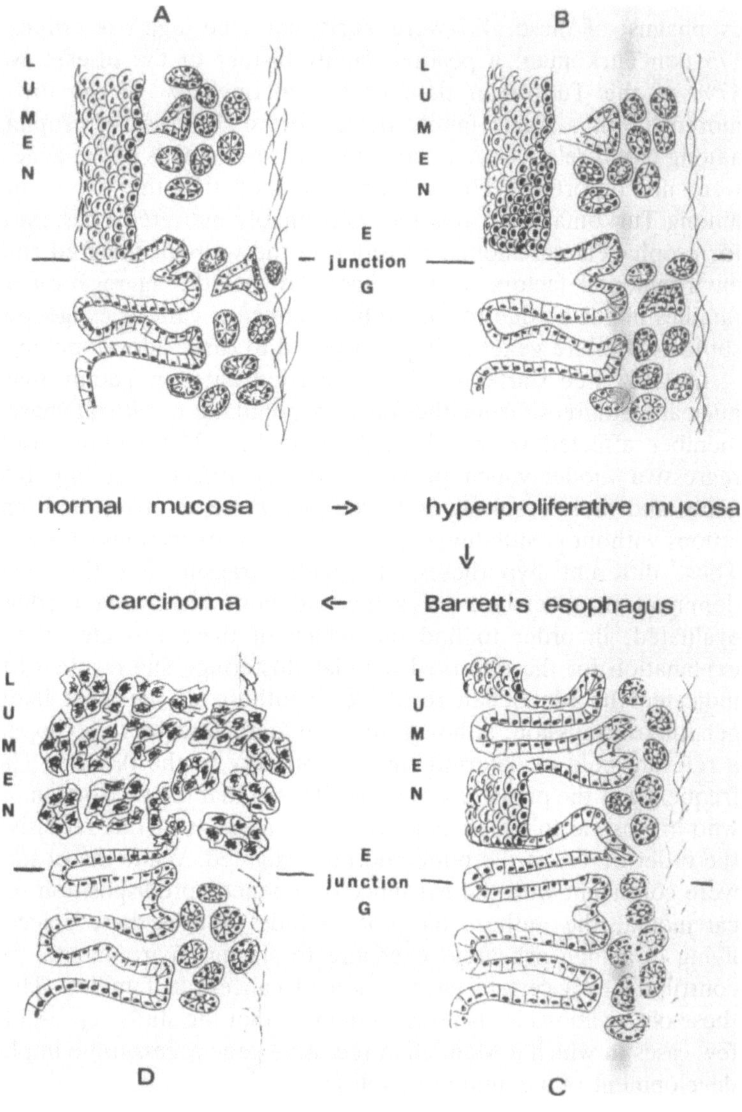

Fig. 3. Pathogenetic sequence from normal esophageal mucosa to carcinoma

◄

Fig. 2. A Normal esophageal mucosa. Cell proliferation evaluated with standard immunohistochemistry after incubation of tissue fragments with bromodeoxyuridine (×250, weak counterstaining with hematoxylin and eosin). Labeling (*dark nuclei*) is limited to the lower portions of the mucosa. **B** Example of expansion of the proliferative area to the most superficial portions of the esophageal mucosa (esophageal acanthosis). (Courtesy of Dr. Mauro Risio, Department of Pathology, Ospedale S. Giovanni Vecchio, Torino, Italy)

esophagus; of these, 427 were Turkoman (the high-risk ethnic group) and 175 non-Turkoman: a positive family history of the disease was found in 47% of the Turkoman patients but in only 2% of the low-risk group; moreover, in a single family there were eight cases of esophageal cancer among blood relatives (unfortunately, further details of the genealogical tree were not reported). The author concluded that this excess of neoplasms among Turkoman case relatives presumably indicates a certain familial risk for esophageal carcinoma; considering the well-documented role of several environmental factors, it was suggested that the aggregation of tumors in families might be due to the additive effect of various exogenous agents on subjects who are genetically predisposed to cancer development.

In 1992, Lee Carter et al. [54] carried out segregation analysis on 221 nuclear pedigrees, from the Linxian population, with at least one family member affected by esophageal carcinoma. The authors used a logistic regressive model which provided for the effects resulting from relevant genes and those resulting from complex patterns of residual familial correlations without postulating explicit genetic or exogenous causal mechanisms. Thus, different hypotheses of genetic transmission (i.e., monogenic – dominant or recessive; polygenic and nontransmission models) could be evaluated, in order to find out which of these provided the most likely explanation for the observed familial clustering. The results of this analysis indicated the Mendelian recessive hypothesis as the most likely model of genetic transmission, although residual familial factors also appeared to play a relevant role in determining susceptibility to the disease. The estimated frequency of the putative gene was 19%, so that the proportion of individuals who are prone to esophageal cancer as a result of this recessive gene is in the order of 4% of the population investigated. While the observed findings were consistent with the existence of a genetic predisposition to esophageal carcinoma, the authors did not exclude that in these selected families, living in a high-risk area, exposure to strong environmental factors might contribute to a certain aggregation of cancers in families. The interest of these observations is also due to the fact that the study represents one of the few cases in which a Mendelian recessive gene seems to be implicated in the development of a common neoplasm.

Pathogenesis of Esophageal Cancer as an Example of Interaction Between Environmental and Genetic Factors

In the previous sections, the relevant role of several environmental agents (Table 1), preneoplastic lesions (Fig. 3), and genetic factors in esophageal tumorigenesis has been reviewed. By combining all these clues, we are led to the conclusion that esophageal carcinoma represents another example of common neoplasm whose pathogenesis seems to be related to a close interaction between environment and genes. The evidence of this contention can be summarized as follows. First, chronic inflammation of the middle and lower third of the esophagus is extremely common in both male and female individuals of Linxian county, and its development has been related to various environmental factors [19–21, 47]. The presence of this precursor lesion was significantly associated, in this population, with a family history of esophageal carcinoma among first- and second-degree relatives [44]. Second, and not surprisingly, a significant "familiality" for the disease was also reported among close relatives of 1244 patients with esophageal carcinoma diagnosed between 1984 and 1985 in the same population of northern China. Moreover, a positive family history of esophageal cancer was observed in almost 50% of the affected patients in a different high-risk population (i.e., the Turkoman of northern Iran) [53]. Thus, it is likely that the various etiologic factors which have been related to esophageal cancer exert their carcinogenic effect mostly on individuals who are genetically predisposed to the development of the disease (at least in two high-risk areas). Finally, mutations of the *p53* tumor suppressor gene have been described in both esophageal carcinoma and preneoplastic lesions [55, 56]; as will be discussed in more detail in the next section, this gene is frequently mutated in germline cells of patients highly predisposed to develop specific tumors, and at the same time is the target of the effect of various carcinogens.

Biomolecular Changes in Esophageal Carcinoma and in Precursor Lesions

Advances in molecular biology over the last 2 decades indicated that cancer-associated loss of normal cell growth control is strictly related to specific genetic events at various chromosomal loci. Accordingly, several biomolecular changes have recently been reported in esophageal carcinoma and in some of its precursor lesions; as for many other tumors, the majority of these alterations consist of the activation of oncogenes, inactivation (by point mutation, rearrangements or allele deletion) of tumor suppressor genes, and altered expression of growth factors. Since the carcinogenic activity of *N*-nitroso compounds is due to their ability to generate highly reactive species that alkylate cellular DNA [57], and since nitrosamines seem to be closely related to esophageal cancer development, the study of genetic damage in these tumors is particularly attractive; indeed, recent observations revealed that in subjects living in high-risk areas (and, thus, exposed to increased amounts of *N*-nitroso compounds) levels of the DNA alkylation product *O*-6-methyldeoxyguanosine in esophageal mucosa were significantly higher than in low-risk populations [58].

Elevated levels of epidermal growth factor (EGF) receptor have been detected in many human tumors and in cultured cells of squamous-cell carcinoma [59, 60]. In 1987, Ozawa et al. [61] found a significantly higher EGF-binding activity in 22 out of 31 (71%) squamous-cell esophageal cancers than in adjacent normal mucosa; moreover, amplification of the EGF receptor and c-*myc* genes was frequently observed in DNA samples from Linxian patients operated on for esophageal carcinoma [62]. Rather surprisingly, similar changes were found in several samples of apparently normal esophageal mucosa from the same patients, thus indicating that amplification of these genes may occur at a very early stage of esophageal tumorigenesis, presumably in association with premorphologic abnormalities of cell replication and differentiation [46]. Moreover, recent studies showed coamplification of *hst-1* and *int-2* genes in 39%–52% of Japanese patients with cancer of the esophagus [63, 64], suggesting a possible role of these two closely related genes in tumor development. Finally, positive immunostaining for several oncogenes (including c-*erbB-2*, c-*src*, c-*jun*, c-*ras*, and c-*fos*) has recently been reported in 7%–73% of English patients with either esophageal cancer or Barrett's esophagus [60, 65].

In a recent report, restriction fragment length polymorphism analysis showed deletions at various loci on 13 out of 18 chromosomes in esophageal squamous-cell cancers [64]. However, only the frequency of allele loss on chromosome 17p (where the *p53* locus has been mapped) was significantly higher (i.e., 45%), whereas the low frequencies of loss of heterozygosity on other chromosomes (less than 22%) was more consistent with random rearrangements during tumor development. At variance with these results, Boyton et al. [66] reported loss of heterozygosity at the retinoblastoma (*Rb*) locus (*13q*) in 14 out of 26 (54%) squamous cell carcinomas and in 5 of 14 (36%) adenocarcinomas of the esophagus. These data suggest that allele deletions at *13q* are nonrandom events, and that loss of the *Rb* gene – or of a tumor suppressor gene near the *Rb* locus – might be involved in the pathogenesis of these tumors.

Point mutations of the *p53* gene have been detected in esophageal carcinoma cell lines, in human esophageal squamous cell carcinomas, and in precursor lesions [55, 56, 67, 68]. All these changes were located in the highly conserved region of the gene (exons 5 to 8), and in the majority of cases were missense mutations at G-C base pairs. These findings are highly suggestive of a possible role of the gene in the early stages of human esophageal tumorigenesis. Moreover, the possible involvement of *p53* in this process is particularly interesting if we consider that exposure to various mutagenic or carcinogenic compounds has frequently been associated with specific mutations or with altered expression of the gene [70, 71]. Finally, recent investigations [71] showed a "unique profile" of mutations of *p53* and *Rb* genes in esophageal carcinomas, thus suggesting that biomolecular changes in both genes might play a relevant role in the development and progression of these tumors.

References

1. Waterhouse J, Muir CS, Shanmugaratman K et al. (1976) Cancer incidence in five continents, vol III. Lyon, France (IARC scientific publication, no 42)
2. Levi F, Maisonneuve P, Filiberti R et al. (1989) Cancer incidence and mortality in Europe. Med Soc Prev 34[Suppl 2]:1–84
3. Day NE (1975) Some aspects of the epidemiology of esophageal cancer. Cancer Res 35:3304–3307
4. Sons HU (1987) Etiologic and epidemiologic factors of carcinoma of the esophagus. Surg Gynecol Obstet 165:183–190
5. Rose E (1973) Esophageal cancer in the Transkei: 1955–1969. JNCI 51:7–16
6. Joint Iran-IARC Study Group (1977) Oesophageal cancer studies in the Caspian littoral of Iran: results of population studies – a prodrome. JNCI 59:1127–1138
7. Yang CS (1980) Oesophageal cancer in China. Cancer Res 40:2633–2644
8. Warwick GP (1973) Some aspects of the epidemiology and aetiology of oesophageal cancer with particular emphasis on the Transkei, South Africa. Adv Cancer Res 17:81–229
9. Ghadirian P (1987) Thermal irritation and esophageal cancer in Northern Iran. Cancer 60:1909–1914
10. Sagar PM (1989) Aetiology of cancer of the esophagus: geographical studies in the footsteps of Marco Polo and beyond. Gut 30:561–564
11. Chang F, Syrjanen S, Wang L et al. (1992) Infectious agents in the etiology of esophageal cancer. Gastroenterology 103:1336–1348
12. Yu MC, Garabrant DH, Peters JM et al. (1988) Tobacco, alcohol, diet, occupation, and carcinoma of the esophagus. Cancer Res 48:3843–3848
13. Franceschi S, Talamini R, Barra S et al. (1990) Smoking and drinking in relation to cancers of the oral cavity, pharynx, larynx, and esophagus in Northern Italy. Cancer Res 50:6502–6507
14. Gray MR, Donnelly RJ, Kingsnorth AN (1993) The role of smoking and alcohol in metaplasia and cancer risk in Barrett's columnar lined esophagus. Gut 34: 727–731
15. Webb JN, Busuttil A (1978) Adenocarcinoma of the esophagus and of the esophagogastric junction. Br J Surg 65:475–479
16. Spechler SJ, Robbins AH, Rubins HB et al. (1984) Adenocarcinoma and Barrett's esophagus: an overrated risk? Gastroenterology 87:927–933
17. Ghadirian P, Stein GF, Gorodetzky C et al. (1985) Oesophageal cancer studies in the Caspian littoral of Iran: some residual results, including opium use as a risk factor. Int J Cancer 35:593–597
18. Kmet J, McLaren DS, Siassi F (1980) Epidemiology of oesophageal cancer with specific reference to nutritional studies among the Turkoman of Iran. Adv Mod Hum Nutr 1:343–365
19. Lu JB, Yand WX, Liu JM et al. (1985) Trends in morbidity and mortality for oesophageal cancer in Linxian county. Int J Cancer 36:643–645
20. Yang CS (1980) Research on esophageal cancer in China. Cancer Res 40:2633–2644
21. Singer GM, Chuan J, Roman J et al. (1986) Nitrosamines and nitrosamine precursors in foods from Linxian, China, a high incidence area for esophageal cancer. Carcinogenesis 7:733–736
22. Li M, Li P, Li B (1980) Recent progress in research on oesophageal cancer in China. Adv Cancer Res 33:173–246
23. Goff JS (1988) Infectious causes of esophagitis. Annu Rev Med 39:163–169
24. Wu Y, Chen J, Ohshima H et al. (1993) Geographic association between urinary excretion of *N*-nitroso compounds and esophageal cancer mortality in China. Int J Cancer 54:713–719

25. Marasas WFO, Jaskiewick K, Venter FS et al. (1988) Fusarium moniliforme contamination of maize in esophageal cancer areas in Transkei. S Afr Med J 74:110–114
26. Silber W (1985) Carcinoma of the esophagus: aspects of epidemiology and etiology. Proc Nutr Soc 44:101–110
27. Rose EF (1981) A review of the factors associated with cancer of the esophagus in Transkei. Prog Clin Biol Res 53:67–75
28. Williamson AI, Jaskiesick K, Gunning A (1991) The detection of human papillomavirus in oesophageal lesions. Anticancer Res 11:263–266
29. McKay JS, Day DW (1982) Herpes simplex oesophagitis. Histopathology 7:409–420
30. Furihata M, Ohtsuki Y, Ogoshi S et al. (1993) Prognostic significance of human papillomavirus genome and aberrant expression of p53 protein in human esophageal cancer. Int J Cancer 54:226–230
31. Spechler SJ, Goyal RK (1986) Barrett's esophagus. N Engl J Med 315:362–371
32. Wand HH, Antonioli DA, Goldman H (1986) Comparative features of esophageal and gastric adenocarcinomas. Hum Pathol 17:482–487
33. Yang PC, Davis S (1988) Incidence of cancer of the esophagus in the US by histologic type. Cancer 61:612–617
34. Earlam R, Cunha-Melo JR (1980) Oesophageal squamous cell carcinoma: I. A critical review of surgery. II. A critical review of radiotherapy Br J Surg 67:381–389, 457–463
35. Launois B, Paul JL, Lygidakis NJ et al. (1983) Results of the surgical treatment of carcinoma of the esophagus. Surg Gynecol Obstet 156:753–760
36. Smithers D (1956) Adenocarcinoma of the esophagus. Thorax 11:257–267
37. Cederquist C, Nielson J, Berthelsen A (1980) Adenocarcinoma of the esophagus. Acta Chir Scand 146:411–415
38. Resbeut M, Le Prise-Fleury E, Ben-Hassel M et al. (1985) Squamous cell carcinoma of the esophagus. Cancer 56:1246–1250
39. Coia LR, Paul AR, Engstrom PF (1988) Combined radiation and chemotherapy as primary management of adenocarcinoma of the esophagus and gastroesophageal junction. Cancer 61:643–649
40. Kuwano H, Matsuda H, Matsouka H et al. (1987) Intra-epithelial carcinoma concomitant with esophageal squamous cell carcinoma. Cancer 59:783–787
41. Tsutsui S, Kuwano H, Mori M et al. (1991) Comparison of cell nuclear DNA contents between intraepithelial and invasive components of oesophageal squamous cell carcinoma. Eur J Cancer 27:620–624
42. Munoz N, Crespi M, Grassi A et al. (1982) Precursor lesions of oesophageal cancer in high-risk populations in Iran and China. Lancet I:876–879
43. Crespi M, Munoz N, Grassi A et al. (1979) Oesophageal lesions in Northern Iran: a premalignant condition? Lancet II:217–221
44. Wahrendorf J, Chang-Cluude J, Liang QS et al. (1989) Precursor lesions of oesophageal cancer in young people in a high-risk population of China. Lancet II:1239–1241
45. Chang-Claude JC, Wahrendorf J, Liang QS et al. (1990) An epidemiological study of precursor lesions of esophageal cancer among young persons in a high-risk population in Huixian, China. Cancer Res 50:2268–2274
46. Lipkin M (1988) Biomarkers of increased susceptibility to gastrointestinal cancer. Cancer Res 48:235–245
47. Burg-Kurland CL, Purnell DM, Combs JW et al. (1986) Immunocytochemical evaluation of human esophageal neoplasms and preneoplastic lesions for beta-chorionic gonadotropin, placental lactogen, alpha-fetoprotein, carcinoembryonic antigen, non-specific cross-reacting agent. Cancer Res 46:2936–2943

48. Wu YK, Laucks HH (1951) Carcinoma of the oesophagus or cardia of the stomach. Ann Surg 134:946–956
49. Li KH, Kao JC, Wu YK (1962) A survey of prevalence of carcinoma of the esophagus in North China. Chin Med J 81:489–494
50. Wu M, Hu N, Wang X (1989) Genetic factors in the etiology of esophageal cancer and the strategy for its prevention in high-risk incidence areas in Northern China. In: Lynch HT, Hirayama T (eds) Genetic epidemiology of cancer. CRC Press, Boca Raton, pp 187–200
51. Wu M, Hu N, Wang X (1985) Familial aggregation of esophageal cancer in high incidence areas of North China: a strategy of control through genetic analysis. In: Muller HJ, Weber W (eds) Familial cancer. Karger, Basel, pp 48–57
52. Ji JY, Ershow AG, Chen ZJ et al. (1989) A case-control study of cancer of the esophagus and gastric cardia in Linxian. Int J Cancer 43:755–761
53. Ghadirian P (1985) Familial history of esophageal cancer. Cancer 56:2112–2116
54. Lee Carter C, Hu N, Lin PZ et al. (1992) Segregation analysis of esophageal cancer in 221 high-risk Chinese families. JNCI 84:771–776
55. Hollstein MC, Metcalf RA, Welsh JA et al. (1990) Frequent mutation of the p53 gene in human esophageal cancer. Proc Natl Acad Sci USA 87:9958–9961
56. Bennett WP, Hollstein MC, Metcalf RA et al. (1992) p53 mutation and protein accumulation during multistage human esophageal carcinogenesis. Cancer Res 52:6092–6097
57. Doerfler W (1983) DNA methylation and gene activity. Annu Rev Biochem 52:93–124
58. Umberhauer D, Wild CP, Montesano R et al. (1985) 0-6-Methyldeoxyguanosine in oesophageal DNA among persons at high risk of oesophageal cancer. Int J Cancer 36:661–665
59. Yamamoto T, Kamata N, Kawano H et al. (1986) High incidence of amplification of the epidermal growth factor receptor gene in human squamous carcinoma cell lines. Cancer Res 46:414–416
60. Al-Kasspooles M, Moore JH, Orringer MB et al. (1993) Amplification and overexpression of the EGFR and erbB-2 genes in human esophageal adenocarcinomas. Int J Cancer 54:213–219
61. Ozawa S, Ueda M, Ando N et al. (1987) High incidence of EGF receptor hyperproduction in esophageal squamous-cell carcinomas. Int J Cancer 39:333–337
62. Lu SH, Hsieh LL, Luo PC et al. (1988) Amplification of the EGF receptor and c-myc genes in human esophageal cancers. Int J Cancer 42:502–505
63. Tsuda T, Tahara E, Kajiyama G et al. (1989) High incidence of hst-1 and int-2 genes in human esophageal carcinomas. Cancer Res 49:5505–5508
64. Wagata T, Ishikazi K, Imamura M et al. (1991) Deletion of 17p and amplification of the int-2 gene in esophageal carcinoma. Cancer Res 51:2113–2117
65. Jankowski JJ, Coghill D, Hopwood D et al. (1992) Oncogenes and onco-suppressor gene in edenocarcinoma of the esophagus. Gut 33:1033–1038
66. Boyton FR, Huang Y, Blount PL et al. (1991) Frequent loss of heterozygosity at the Rb locus in human esophageal cancer. Cancer Res 51:5766–5769
67. Wagata T, Shibagachi I, Imamura M et al. (1993) Loss of 17p, mutations of p53, and overexpression of p53 protein in esophageal squamous cell carcinoma. Cancer Res 53:846–850
68. Wang LD, Hong JY, Qiu SL et al. (1993) Accumulation of p53 protein in human esophageal precancerous lesions. Cancer Res 53:1783–1787
69. Ohgaki H, Hard GC, Hirota N et al. (1992) Selective mutation of codons 204 and 213 of the p53 gene in rat tumors induced by alkylating N-nitroso compounds. Cancer Res 52:2995–2998

70. Makino H, Ishikaza Y, Tsujimoto A et al. (1992) Rat p53 gene mutations in primary zymbal gland tumors induced by a food mutagen. Proc Natl Acad Sci USA 89:4850–4854
71. Huang Y, Meltzer SJ, Yin J et al. (1993) Altered messanger RNA and unique mutational profile of p53 and Rb in human esophageal carcinoma. Cancer Res 53:1889–1894

Genetic Predisposition and Environmental Factors in Gastric Carcinoma

Gastric carcinoma is estimated to be the world's second most common cancer. Although the dramatic decline in the incidence of gastric carcinoma in the United States and Western Europe over the past 50 years has led some to proclaim an "unplanned triumph", in much of Latin America and Asia the incidence remains very high.

(J. PARSONNET et al. 1991)

Introduction

The biology of gastric carcinoma remains poorly understood and rather mysterious, often eludeing not only any rational explanation but also common sense. Thus, a decline in the incidence of gastric cancer has been reported in most countries over the last 5–6 decades; however, no satisfactory explanation for this trend has been provided; moreover, the fall in incidence concerns mainly antral carcinomas but not cancer of the cardia (whose frequency is increasing), and is more marked for the "intestinal" histologic type. Second, incidence and mortality rates show a large geographic variation, which ranges from values as low as 3 to more than 100 new cases/100 000 per year; this might not be surprising, since it has been observed for many other malignancies – the characteristic of gastric cancer is that a wide variation in mortality can be detected even within small countries such as Belgium, where rather curiously the disease is much more frequent among the Flemish than the Walloon population. Third, it has been suggested that fresh fruit and vegetables exert a protective effect against the development of these tumors; however, there is evidence indicating that the disease is more frequent in rural areas, where we should reasonably expect a larger consumption of green vegetables and several fruits. Finally, recent investigations favor a pathogenetic link between *Helicobacter pylori* infection and gastric carcinogenesis; however, despite the interest of these observations, one should not forget that owing to the diffusion of this infection most individuals positive for *Helicobacter pylori* will never develop gastric cancer.

Various studies have suggested that genetic factors might also be of importance in the pathogenesis of gastric tumors. Thus, gastric cancer occurs more frequently among close relatives of affected individuals than in the general population; moreover, some of the most common precancerous lesions (i.e., gastric metaplasia and pernicious anemia) seem to be genetically determined. Gastric tumors are also relatively frequent in Lynch syndrome II and, in addition, "gastric cancer families" as well as the occurrence of these tumors in identical twins have been reported. Finally, biomolecular studies have shown the frequent occurrence of genetic alterations in a large proportion of gastric carcinomas; these include loss of alleles at various chromosomal loci (*17p*, *18q*), inactivating mutations of tumor suppressor genes (*p53*, *APC*), and activation and/or overexpression of dominant oncogenes (*ras*, *myc*, c-*erbB-2*). It is likely therefore that despite several inexplicable aspects of its biology and epidemiology, gastric carcinoma represents an interesting and rewarding model for the study of the interaction between environment and genes in tumor induction and progression.

General Aspects

Descriptive Epidemiology

In spite of the declining incidence and mortality rates, gastric carcinoma is still the second most common fatal cancer in the world, with about 650000 new cases/year [1]. It was estimated that in 1989 approximately 20000 gastric cancers were diagnosed in the United States, and that 14000 Americans died of the disease; similarly, 10000–15000 persons die annually of gastric carcinoma in countries such as Italy and the United Kingdom [1, 2]. In the United States and western Europe, the disease was a leading cause of neoplastic mortality in 1930 [3], with rates of 30–40 deaths/100000 per year; since then, incidence and mortality have decreased steadily, and at present in North America no more than 5–10 cases/100000 are seen in whites [4], and similar changes were observed in almost all countries [5]. Although the reasons for this "unexpected success" remain unclear, hypothetical factors possibly contributing to the declining incidence of gastric carcinoma include: (a) better preservation of food, with widespread use of refrigerators in all socioeconomic classes [5]; (b) consequent gradual elimination of salt as a method of food preservation [6]; (c) general improvement of nutritional status and increased availability (again, in all social classes) of fruits, vegetables, and other "protective" nutrients [7]; (d) refinement in recognition and cure of precancerous lesions; and (e) decrease, over time, of *Helicobacter pylori* infection (and, thus, reduction in the prevalence of chronic gastritis) [8]. At variance with the decreasing occurrence of gastric cancer, several observations have shown a rise in the incidence of carcinoma of the cardia [9, 10]; once again, the underlying reasons for this trend remain unclear.

Besides temporal trends, gastric cancer shows marked geographic variations, with incidence rates ranging, in males, from 3–4 new cases/100000 per year in some African countries to more than 100 in Japan [11]. Other areas with high incidence rates include China, Colombia, Chile, and other Latin American countries, while those with the lowest rates are India and North America [12]. The scenario becomes more complex if we consider various ethnic groups within countries; thus, for example, in the United States incidence and mortality rates in blacks, Japanese, Chinese, and American Indians are higher than those reported for whites [13]; moreover, temporal trends differed among ethnic groups during the period 1958–1982, with a rather unexpected increase in mortality rates in American Indians [14]. Similarly, wide variations in the frequency of gastric carcinoma were reported in France, Spain, Switzerland, Belgium, Holland, and Italy [15]. Although the reasons for these regional and racial variations remain unknown, two more aspects deserve some comment: First, in many countries an inverse socioeconomic gradient in the risk of gastric neoplasms has been observed, with lower classes having about 2.5 times the risk of more wealthy classes; second, urbanization tends to be associated with a lower risk of the disease [12]. At variance with these observations, a rather paradoxical geographic pattern of gastric cancer occurrence was observed in Italy, where the lowest rates occur in the southern areas, which are the poorest, less industrialized, and more rural parts of the country; in contrast, high incidence and mortality rates are usually recorded in the more wealthy and developed northern regions [16, 17]. Moreover, in a few provinces of northern and central Italy the frequency of this tumor is appreciably higher than the national average [18].

Etiology and Pathogenesis

Although temporal trends and geographic variation in gastric tumor occurrence led to the formulation of various hypotheses on the etiopathogenesis of this common malignancy [12], cancer of the stomach remains an enigmatic disease, not associated with any strong causative environmental or genetic factor, as in the case of other neoplasms, such as lung or colonic carcinoma, respectively (see the chapters on "Genetic Factors in Lung Cancer," "Hereditary and Familial Colorectal Cancer," and "Hereditary Gastrointestinal Polyposis Syndrome").

An interesting model of gastric carcinogenesis was proposed by Correa and collaborators [19, 20]. This appealing hypothesis can be summarized as follows (Fig. 1): In the first phase, chronic gastritis develops owing to genetic factors or exogenous agents (i.e., *Helicobacter pylori*); gastritis may result in atrophy of the mucosa, hypochlorhydria, further bacterial colonization, and consequent reduction (by bacteria) of dietary nitrate to nitrite; in

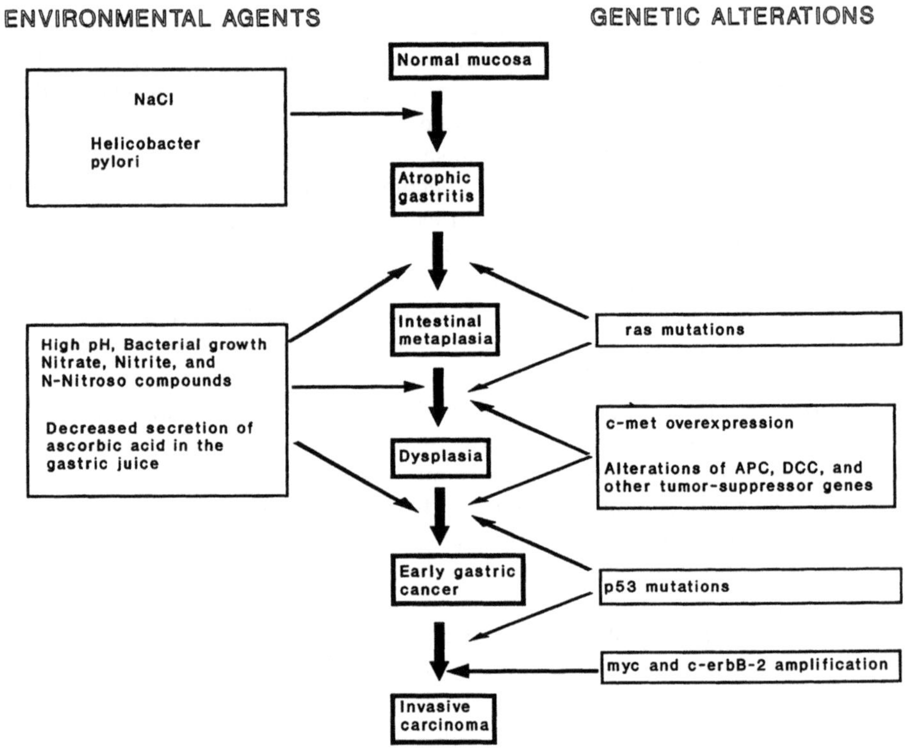

Fig. 1. General hypothesis of gastric carcinogenesis which takes into consideration the main environmental and genetic factors

addition, chronic inflammation may induce the appearance of intestinal metaplasia and of dysplastic lesions, together with a generalized hyperproliferative state of the gastric mucosa. In the second phase, nitrite reacts with certain protein substrates (amines, amides, and urea) to generate *N*-nitroso compounds; the presence of these carcinogens together with precancerous dysplastic alterations in the mucosal cells may result in the development of malignancy. In line with this model, serial endoscopic examinations in patients with atrophic gastritis have shown replacement of the usual gastric mucosa by intestinal-type cells and various other dysplastic changes. However, other observations were not consistent with this hypothesis; thus, various investigators found that some populations at risk of gastric cancer may have lower exposure to nitrate than populations at low risk [21, 22]. In other studies, patients with gastric cancer were less exposed to nitrate than controls [23]; moreover, in some countries (including France and the United Kingdom) nitrate content of the drinking water does not seem to be correlated with the occurrence of gastric cancer [24, 25]. These and other observations do not imply that the hypothesis is wrong, but simply indicate that more careful studies are needed to prove or disprove the proposed model. As recently suggested by Hill [26],

> "In the life history of a hypothesis there is a stage when the available evidence strongly supports it, followed by a period of confusion, followed by either rejection of the hypothesis or its acceptance in a modified and usually more complex form. Studies on the role of gastric microenvironment and the role of bacterial metabolites in gastric carcinogenesis are in the middle stage of this sequence".

Finally, it is worth noting that this hypothesis of gastric cancer development is much more closely related to intestinal type carcinomas, whereas it is still unclear whether the model can be extended to the "diffuse" (or "infiltrative") histologic type [26, 27].

Several etiologic factors have been associated with the risk of gastric cancer, but not without controversy. These include a high intake of salty foods and starch [28, 29], low consumption of fruits and fresh vegetables [30, 31], alcohol ingestion and cigarette smoking [32], irregularity of eating [33], and chronic ingestion of gastric "irritants" (i.e., nonsteroid antiinflammatory drugs) [27], long-term use of H_2-receptor antagonists (gastric hypoacidity induced by these drugs might favor bacterial growth in the stomach and, thus, formation of *N*-nitroso compounds; in addition, diagnosis might be delayed due to better control of symptoms) [34], previous surgery for peptic ulcer [35], blood group A, and hypertrophic gastritis.

Various lines of evidence indicate that certain substances act as "protectors," presumably by creating obstacles to the process of gastric tumorigenesis. Fresh fruits, vegetables, vitamins C and E, beta-carotene, and selenium [7, 20, 27, 36] all appear to play a protective role against tumor development, and the frequency of their ingestions (or serum levels, for micronutrients) seems to be inversely related to gastric cancer risk [37, 38]. These findings support the potential relevance of fruits and vegetables in reducing the risk of gastric malignancies, and this contention has been further documented by more recent studies carried out in populations with different incidences of gastric tumors [39, 40].

Finally, the recent identification of *Helicobacter pylori* and the definition of its role in chronic gastritis (and peptic ulcer) [20, 41] stimulated a growing interest in the potential role of this microorganism in gastric carcinogenesis. *Helicobacter pylori* can colonize the gastric mucosa for years, and its presence is associated with chronic, superficial, diffuse gastritis of the fundus and antrum; this process may progress over decades to chronic atrophic gastritis [42], which is a precursor lesion of gastric carcinoma [12]. In two recent studies [43, 44], 84%–94% of patients with gastric carcinoma had a positive test for *Helicobacter pylori* antibodies, as opposed to 60%–76% of the controls; moreover, the risk of gastric cancer was closely related to the antibody levels. The authors suggested that infection with *Helicobacter pylori* seems to be strongly associated with the risk of subsequent gastric carcinoma, and that the bacteria might be a cofactor in gastric tumorigenesis; however, the presence of a positive test in a large proportion of controls [45] clearly indicates that *Helicobacter pylori* alone is not sufficient for the induction of the neoplastic phenotype. Several other observations lend further support to the possible etiologic role of these bacteria in gastric cancer development, especially in the case of intestinal-type tumors localized in the body and the antrum [46–50]. Besides chronic inflammation, there is evidence that *Helicobacter pylori* infection reduces the concentration of ascorbic acid in the gastric juice, thus impairing one of the main defensive mechanisms against oxidative DNA damage [51, 52].

Morphology

More than 90% of gastric malignancies are adenocarcinomas arising in the distal stomach or in the lesser curvature; other histologic types include carcinoids, lymphomas, and leiomyosarcomas. Microscopically, one of the most useful subdivisions is made between diffuse (or infiltrative) and intestinal (or expansive) types [53–55]. The diffuse type of gastric carcinoma is composed of isolated or small groups of cells with only occasional glandular formation; cell cohesion is poor, so that individual cells tend to infiltrate the stomach wall. The intestinal type shows cohesive neoplastic cells forming tubular structures similar to intestinal neoplasms, with moderately differentiated glands lined by goblet and absorptive cells. The main problem of this classification is that the two subtypes of gastric carcinoma are separated on the basis of different parameters, largely morphologic for intestinal tumors, mostly "functional" for the diffuse type [56]. Despite these drawbacks, the Laurèn-Ming classification has been found to be a valuable tool in clinical and epidemiologic investigations; thus, while the incidence of diffuse tumors is similar in most populations, the intestinal subtype tends to be more prevalent in populations at high risk for gastric cancer [27]. Moreover, there is evidence that genetic factors are more closely related to diffuse carcinomas than to the intestinal type [27].

Gastric tumors are usually classified by staging into four main categories according to the TNM system [56]. In stage I, tumors are limited to the mucosa or submucosa ("early gastric cancer"); when the disease is recognized at this pathologic stage, prognosis is excellent, with 5-year survival in the order of 86%–98% [57, 58]. Unfortunately, only 10%–20% of all gastric malignancies are diagnosed at this favorable stage, although there is evidence that mass screening and surveillance may increase consistently the proportion of these early lesions [59]. In stage II, tumors extend to muscular wall or through the serosa, but without lymph node involvement; stage III and IV tumors are characterized by metastases in the lymph nodes or other organs, respectively. Blood-borne metastases are particularly frequent in the liver and lung, but relatively uncommon in the bones and central nervous system; local spread through the stomach wall may involve the omentum, liver, and pancreas, whereas peritoneal invasion can cause malignant ascites and Krukenberg's tumors of the ovary.

Precancerous lesions can be defined as morphologic alterations associated with an increased risk of malignant transformation; the possible role of atrophic gastritis in gastric tumorigenesis has already been discussed [1, 12, 26, 27]. Other precancerous conditions include pernicious anemia (which is associated with chronic gastritis, polyps, and dysplasia), gastric polyps, Ménétrier's disease, and gastric ulcer; despite the undoubted preneoplastic role of all these lesions, their precise contribution to the total burden of gastric cancer remains uncertain [60]. Interestingly, recent studies showed that in a province of China with one of the highest incidence rates of gastric cancer, chronic gastritis, intestinal metaplasia, and other precancerous lesions were seen in almost all the 3433 residents aged 35–64 years who received endoscopic examinations [61].

Clinical Features

Early gastric cancer usually produces few symptoms and is therefore difficult to diagnose. As the tumor progresses symptoms may appear, but they are usually mild, insidious and indefinite. Patients may complain of upper abdominal discomfort or postprandial fullness, which are commonly referred to as "gastritis" or "dyspepsia." Persistent anorexia, nausea, and steady abdominal pain are also frequent on presentation, but it is not rare to see patients who are diagnosed when there is a large, palpable epigastric mass, or when there is malignant ascites, both signs of advanced disease with little or no prospect of cure. Difficulties in swallowing are typical of tumors involving the cardiac region, while vomiting and weight loss are prominent with tumors of the antropyloric region; since bleeding is not rare, iron deficiency anemia is another relatively common presentation of the disease.

Although double-contrast radiographic examination was the standard diagnostic procedure for many years, there is no doubt that gastroscopy – together with multiple biopsies and brush cytology of suspected lesions – has led to a definite improvement in accuracy of diagnosis. Chest X-ray, hepatic ultrasounds, and computed tomography are of great help for preoperative staging and detection of metastasis; moreover, laparoscopy appears to be an extremely valuable technique for diagnosing liver metastases and peritoneal dissemination of the disease [62]. There is no evidence that tumor markers are of help in early diagnosis or management of gastric carcinoma, though some studies suggest a possible use of these markers for identifying individuals with chronic gastritis (and, thus, at risk of the disease) [63, 64].

Prognosis and Treatment

Prognosis of gastric carcinoma is closely related to the pathologic staging. Penetration of the tumor through the gastric wall, involvement of regional lymph nodes, and vascular invasion are found in the majority of patients, at least in Western countries. Thus, in European and American series only 50%–60% of patients undergoing operation have a resectable disease; of these, 20%–30% will be alive at 5 years, giving an overall 5-year survival of 10%–15% [65]. In sharp contrast to these discouraging results, Japanese studies showed resectability rates of 70%–80%, with 5-year survival of 46% in patients with advanced carcinoma and of 89% for early gastric cancer [66, 67]. The reasons for these discrepancies remain unclear, and do not seem to be entirely dependent on the presence of a large proportion of early tumors in the Japanese series.

Various indicators of the clinical outcome have been investigated in gastric carcinoma, including DNA ploidy, flow cytometric determination of the S-phase fraction, in vitro labeling of proliferating cells with [^{3}H]thymidine or bromodeoxyuridine, immunostaining for the Ki-67 antigen and the proliferative-associated nuclear antigen p105 (which are expressed in the G-1, S, G-2, and M phases of the replicative cycle, but not in the G-O phase), and AgNor count [68–75]. Although univariate and multivariate analysis showed a prognostic significance for some of these biomarkers [71, 74], in our opinion the overall results are still insufficient to recommend a more general use of these indicators in daily clinical practice.

Surgical resection represents the only chance of cure for patients with gastric carcinoma. The most radical approach (total gastrectomy) involves the removal of the entire stomach, the greater omentum, part of the duodenum, the spleen, and for proximal tumors the lower portion of the esophagus. Since the morbidity of total gastrectomy is considerable, subtotal resection is often preferred in patients with distal neoplasms [76]. Gastric cancer is basically a radioresistant tumor, and the major role of radiation therapy is usually limited to palliation of pain and other symptoms [77]. The clinical effect of cytotoxic drugs in patients with advanced cancer is still unsatisfactory; although objective response (i.e., reduction of the tumor mass) can be seen in 30%–50% of the patients, this effect is usually transient, complete disappearance remains extremely rare, and there is no evidence that survival can be prolonged by the use of drugs [78, 79]. Similarly, the role of adjuvant chemotherapy [the most widely used regimens are combinations of 5-fluorouracil, adriamycin, and mitomycin C (FAM) or etoposide, adriamycin, and cisplatin (EAP)] continues to be an unsettled issue, and conflicting results have been reported [80, 81]. The general impression is that chemotherapy is effective in a small proportion only of the patients, and is not associated with a substantial improvement in the length or quality of life [82, 83].

Preneoplastic Lesions and Biomarkers of Increased Susceptibility to Gastric Cancer

The normal gastric mucosa is covered by mucinous epithelial cells which extend into gastric pits. In the deep portions of the mucosa these cells proliferate more rapidly and then migrate to the superficial areas, where they differentiate into mature cells (Fig. 2); in physiological conditions, replacement of the gastric epithelial surface takes about 1 week [84]. Replication and maturation of surface lining cells are modulated by several factors, including gastrin, bombesin, somatostatin, epidermal growth factor, and some intestinal peptides [85].

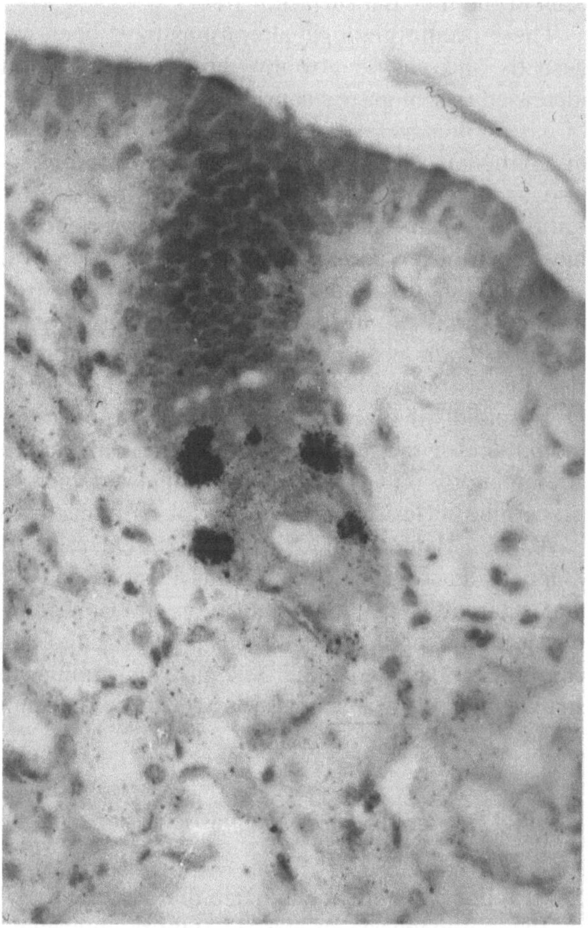

Fig. 2. Representative example of cell proliferation in normal gastric mucosa evaluated by histoautoradiography. S-phase cells (covered by silver grains) are limited to the deep portions of gastric pits

In premalignant conditions, the development of cancer is preceded by changes in the normal pattern of cell replication and differentiation. First, the absolute number of proliferative cells tends to increase. Second, replicating cells fail to differentiate normally as they migrate to the surface, so that immature cells line the gastric mucosa and directly contact the gastric content and the various carcinogens (*N*-nitroso compounds) which may be present; this is of particular importance if we consider that DNA-synthesizing cells are particularly susceptible to DNA damage and mutations [86]. Third, the proliferative compartments tend to expand from the deep to the most superficial portions of the gastric mucosa. The net result of these changes is an overall increase in cell replication, with a shift of the replicative zone to the upper portions of the gastric pits, and presence of immature epithelial cells in the mucosal surface.

These premorphologic alterations have been well documented in chronic gastritis and gastric atrophy, both clinical conditions associated with an increased risk of gastric cancer [87, 88]. Moreover, a hyperproliferative state of gastric mucosa, expansion of the proliferative compartments, and failure of epithelial cells to undergo normal differentiation and maturation have also been reported in individuals with longstanding gastritis living in some Latin American countries where high incidence rates of gastric carcinoma have been observed [85]. Similarly, expansion of the proliferative zone and accumulation of abnormally replicating cells are frequent findings in the remaining gastric mucosa after partial resection of the stomach for peptic diseases, again a condition which is epidemiologically related to an increased risk of gastric neoplasia [35, 89]. Finally, flow cytometric assessment of DNA ploidy in precancerous lesions or conditions represents a valuable biomarker of cancer susceptibility; in Barrett's esophagus and in colonic adenomatous polyps – two of the most common and largely investigated preneoplastic lesions of the digestive organs – aneuploid cell populations have been demonstrated in 5%–30% of cases [90, 91] (see chapters on "Genetic Factors in Prccancerous Lesions and Cancer of the Esophagus" and "Hereditary and Familial Colorectal Cancer"). In accordance with these observations, preliminary studies [92] indicated that peaks of aneuploid cells can also be detected in chronic gastritis, though the clinical and prognostic significance of these changes has yet to be determined.

Familial Occurrence of Preneoplastic Lesions and Gastric Carcinoma

Several lines of evidence indicate that genetic factors might be of importance in the pathogenesis of gastric tumors; however, the available literature suggests that genetic susceptibility to gastric malignancies is not as strong as for colonic or breast tumors. The main findings favoring the existence of hereditary factors in gastric tumorigenesis can be summarized as follows.

First, some of the most common precancerous conditions of gastric neoplasms seem to be genetically determined. Second, gastric cancer tends to occur more frequently among relatives of affected patients than in the general population. Third, gastric tumors are relatively frequent in Lynch syndrome II (hereditary nonpolyposis colorectal cancer, see next chapter), and "gastric cancer families" have also been described. Finally, there is anecdotal evidence for the almost simultaneous occurrence of these tumors in monozygotic twins.

In pernicious anemia, the basic lesion is chronic atrophic gastritis, mainly located in the body of the stomach, which impairs intrinsic factor secretion with consequent malabsorption of vitamin B_{12}. Several studies showed that gastric cancer is three to four times more frequent among patients with pernicious anemia [88, 93]; in addition, these patients seem to be at higher risk of other neoplasms, including esophageal and pancreatic carcinoma, colorectal tumors, myeloid leukemia, and myeloma [88]. Although most cases of pernicious anemia are usually attributed to exogenous (i.e., autoimmune) factors, pedigree analysis showed a marked aggregation of this trait in a subset of families showing atrophic gastritis in two or more successive generations [94, 95]. Thus, there is evidence that in families with pernicious anemia a distinct subpopulation can be identified in which severe atrophic gastritis shows a striking vertical transmission consistent with an autosomal dominant type of inheritance [96].

Gastric polyps are frequent in adenomatosis coli (or familial polyposis), a genetically determined disease characterized by the occurrence of adenomatous lesions in the large bowel, the periampullary region, and the jejunum (see chapter on "Hereditary Gastrointestinal Polyposis Syndromes"). Besides familial polyposis, Santos and Magalhaes [97] described a large Portuguese kindred in which several individuals had multiple polyps dispersed in the corpus and antrum of the stomach, but without colorectal lesions. Rather interestingly, although most polypoid lesions were classified as "hyperplastic" (i.e., a type of lesion usually not considered premalignant), several family members developed gastric carcinoma. Assuming that polyps and cancer were the expression of the same genetic alteration, the authors suggested an autosomal dominant pattern of transmission of this trait. An updated report of the same family [98] confirmed all these findings and reinforced the contention of a Mendelian inheritance; in addition, eight members of this family were affected by psoriasis.

Various studies showed the frequent occurrence of gastric tumors among family members of patients with clinical diagnosis of cancer of the stomach, especially when histology showed a diffuse carcinoma. Thus, Macklin [99] evaluated the frequency of gastric cancer among 1429 relatives of 167 index patients; 62 gastric tumors were reported, and this was significantly higher than the 41.4 expected cases. Since no simple pattern of inheritance could be observed, it was concluded that the familial basis of gastric cancer is likely to reflect a multifactorial type of transmission. A similar excess of gastric carcinoma among relatives of probands was reported by Woolf, and by Videbaek and Moshbech [100, 101].

Lehtola [102] analyzed a large series of 341 cases of gastric carcinoma (diagnosed in the Finnish province of Uusimaa) and a total of 2243 case relatives; the occurrence of cancer among these was compared with that of a suitable control group matched for age and sex to the index cases. An overall relative risk of 1.5 was found, which was of borderline significance; however, in the subgroup of probands with diffuse carcinoma, the relative risk of gastric cancer among relatives was actually 7.0 ($P < 0.005$), whereas no increased risk could be found in patients with intestinal type or with undifferentiated carcinoma. The author concluded that the role of familial factors in gastric tumor development was much more evident when the patients were subdivided into two major groups according to the current morphologic classification [53, 54]; familial factors seem to be of possible etiologic significance only for diffuse carcinomas. A significant excess in the occurrence of gastric cancer among family members of affected patients was also documented in other populations characterized by high incidence rates of cancer of the stomach, such as the Hungarians and the San Marinese [103, 104].

At variance with the above-mentioned studies, Zanghieri et al. [105] evaluated the familial occurrence of gastric cancer through a population-based approach. The authors examined family trees of 154 patients with gastric carcinoma registered in 1986–1987 in a Health Care District of northern Italy. Thirty cases of gastric cancer were recorded among first-degree relatives of the registered patients versus 15 cases found in a matched control group (odds ratio: 3.14, $P < 0.01$); no other type of tumor developed more frequently among case families; moreover, the familial occurrence of gastric cancer tended to be more frequent in patients with diffuse carcinoma than in individuals with intestinal-type tumors. Since a family history for tumors of the stomach was observed in about 10%–15% of the registered cases, it was concluded that "familiality" for gastric carcinoma suggests the possible existence of a genetic susceptibility to these tumors, at least in a fraction of these patients, and especially for diffuse-type carcinomas. La Vecchia et al. [106] assessed the familial aggregation of gastric neoplasms in a series of 628 histologically confirmed carcinomas of the stomach and in a suitable control group; the risk of gastric cancer was significantly associated with a positive family history for the same disease (RR, 2.6; CI, 1.9–3.7), while the occurrence of several other common neoplasms among family members did not differ appreciably between cases and controls. The authors estimated that in terms of population attributable risk approximately 8% of gastric carcinomas would be related to this familial component, thus confirming that genetic factors seem to be of etiologic importance in a small proportion of these neoplasms.

Gastric tumors are commonly observed in hereditary nonpolyposis colorectal cancer (or Lynch syndrome, see next chapter); indeed, in the first

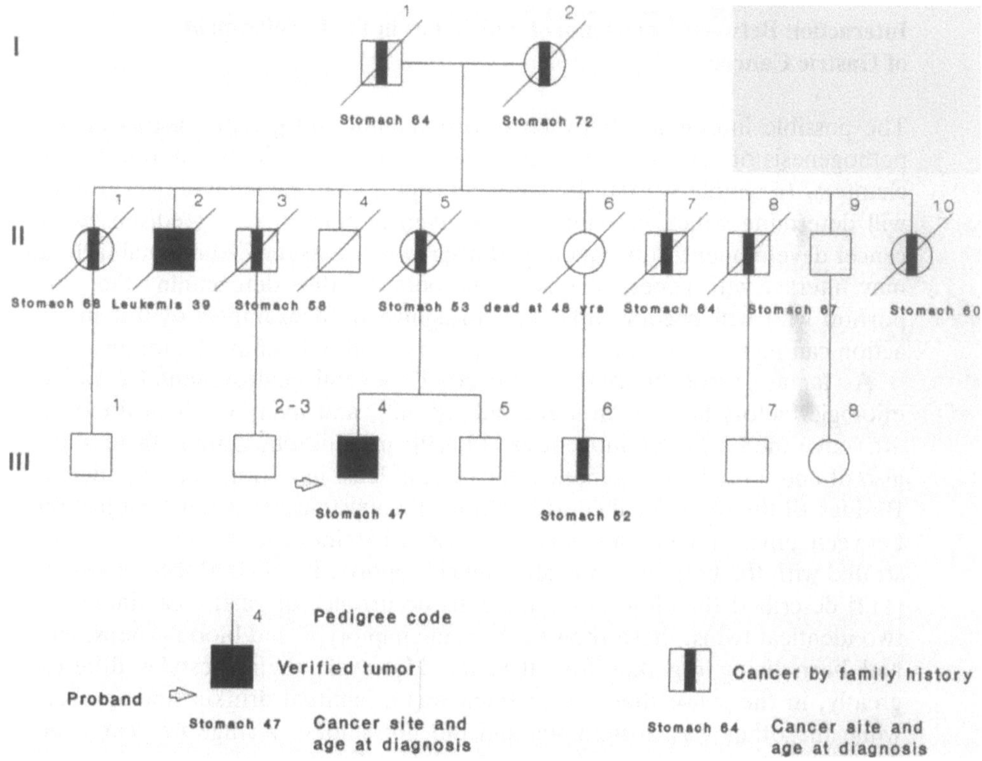

Fig. 3. Representative example of a extended genealogical tree showing a striking aggregation of gastric cancer in three different generations, and often with early onset. Unfortunately, in most cases the information was obtained only by family history

report of this syndrome [107] cancer of the stomach was actually diagnosed more often than colorectal neoplasms. More recent series [108, 109] showed that gastric carcinomas are the second or third most common malignancy in the tumor spectrum of Lynch syndrome, and one of the most frequent neoplasms observed in the follow-up of high-risk individuals in these families [110]. Reports of true "gastric cancer families" are rare; a remarkable familial aggregation of five gastric and one colorectal neoplasm spanning two generations was reported by Farinati et al. [111]. Interestingly, chronic atrophic gastritis and intestinal metaplasia were frequently detected in both affected and unaffected members of this family. However, at variance with the most common hereditary cancer syndromes, none of the affected individuals showed early onset or multiple tumors. A representative example of a family with a marked aggregation of tumors spanning two generations and virtually limited to gastric cancer is shown in Fig. 3.

Interaction Between Environment and Genes in the Development of Gastric Cancer

The possible interaction between environmental and genetic factors in the pathogenesis of several malignancies has already been discussed in previous chapters. In simple words, the basic concept is that the genetic background will determine which individuals in a given population are predisposed to cancer development; subsequently, during many years, environmental factors may interact with genes, in susceptible persons, thus determining the proportion who will become affected. Straightforward examples of this interaction can be seen in esophageal, mammary, and pulmonary tumorigenesis.

As far as gastric tumors are concerned, several environmental putative etiologic factors have been identified [28–42], and many of them fitted an attractive model of carcinogenesis [19, 20]; in addition, genetic factors are also of undoubted pathogenetic relevance, at least in a subgroup of patients. Besides all the theoretical considerations, the existence of a clear interaction between environment and genes in gastric carcinogenesis can be demonstrated with the help of two recent clinical reports. In 1988, Matsukura et al. [112] described the almost simultaneous occurrence of gastric carcinoma in two identical twins; these showed the same haplotype and blood groups, and had been living together for 40 years. However, their lifestyles differed greatly, in the sense that one of them was a habitual drinker and smoker, while the other was abstemious and did not smoke. At age 47 years, the former brother presented with epigastric complaints, nausea, and vomiting; clinical examination showed an advanced gastric carcinoma invading the serosa, and the patient died within 2 months of palliative subtotal gastrectomy. The noncancerous gastric mucosa showed diffuse and severe intestinal metaplasia. The other twin was advised to undergo clinical studies after the operation of his brother; although he was completely asymptomatic, an early gastric cancer of the lesser curvature was found. At laparotomy, no serosal involvement or lymphonodal metastases were seen, and a curative subtotal gastrectomy was carried out; only spotty metaplastic areas were seen in the noncancerous gastric mucosa. It is likely therefore that environmental agents (i.e., smoking and drinking) determined the different clinical course of the disease in two individuals with an identical genetic complexion which rendered them particularly susceptible to the development of gastric cancer. The second example is the large family described by Farinati et al. [111] with a striking aggregation of gastric tumors and chronic atrophic gastritis (with intestinal metaplasia). Although a genetic predisposition to cancer intuitively seemed likely from a simple inspection of the family tree, detailed epidemiologic investigations showed some peculiar dietary habits in many members of the family. These included a very low intake of fruits and fresh vegetables (with consequent low intake of vitamin C), high intake of homemade, salttreated pork meat, and an elevated consumption of wine and other alcoholic beverages, which in one case represented more than

50% of total caloric intake. Once again, it is tempting to speculate that a close interaction between genetic and environmental factors determined this striking aggregation of precancerous lesions and of gastric carcinoma.

Oncogenes, Tumor Suppressor Genes, and Gastric Cancer

As for all other common malignancies, the basic biology of gastric carcinoma has been extensively investigated in the last few years, though a lot remains to be explored in the molecular pathogenesis of this enigmatic disease. Before describing in more detail specific alterations of oncogenes and tumor suppressor genes, a few general points deserve some comment. First, it is becoming clear that a close similarity exists between the molecular events underlying colorectal and gastric tumorigenesis; thus, for example, *ras* oncogene mutations, allele losses at chromosomes 5q, 17p, and 18q, and mutations of various tumor suppressor genes (including *p53* and *APC*) are frequently observed in both types of tumors. These similarities are undoubtedly surprising if we consider the biological and epidemiologic pecularities of colorectal and gastric neoplasms; on the other hand, it is also plausible that all cancers of the digestive organs maintain some pathogenetic steps in common, and that the different behavior of these tumors is determined by other molecular alterations which are still unknown or poorly defined. Second, various biomolecular investigations revealed differences between intestinal and diffuse type carcinomas; this clearly indicates that in spite of its limits the Laurèn-Ming classification [53, 54] is able to distinguish, on a simple morphologic basis, tumors with different biologic characteristics. Third, some of the biomolecular changes observed in gastric carcinoma have also been found in precancerous lesions (for example, *ras* overexpression in metaplastic lesions of the stomach); these findings further emphasize the true premalignant nature of dysplasia and intestinal metaplasia; in addition, they suggest the involvement of specific cancer-related genes in the early phases of gastric tumorigenesis. Finally, although there are studies indicating the possible prognostic significance of some genetic alterations (i.e., c-*erbB-2* overexpression), the general impression is that it is still premature to recommend a direct application of molecular techniques in routine clinical practice.

Oncogenes and Growth Factors

Increased expression or mutational activation of the *ras* genes have frequently been reported in early as well as in advanced gastric carcinomas [113–115]; in contrast, other investigators were unable to find a significant rate of *ras* alterations [116, 117]. In addition, positive immunostaining for the *ras* gene product (p21 protein) has also been reported in dysplastic and metaplastic lesions and in normal gastric mucosa around the tumor [114, 118], while in some studies p21 expression seemed to be related to metastatic diffusion and poor clinical outcome [119].

Amplification and/or increased expression of the c-*myc* gene have been found in 5%–23% of gastric carcinomas [117, 120]; in one of these studies, patients with c-*myc*-protein-positive tumors had a significantly poorer prognosis, thus suggesting the possible use of c-*myc* expression as a marker of tumor aggressiveness. Several other studies showed amplification of the c-*erbB-2* oncogene in 5%–20% of gastric tumors [117, 121–123], the incidence of c-*erbB-2* amplification in metastatic lesions was significantly higher than that of primary tumors, suggesting that this alteration represents a late event in the temporal development of gastric neoplasia. In one of these studies [123], patients with positive immunoreactivity for the c-*erbB-2* protein showed a 5-year survival of 11%, as opposed to much more favorable outcome (50% at 5 years) of patients with a negative test; moreover, by multivariate analysis, c-*erbB-2* status revealed itself as an independent prognostic parameter (together with the presence of distant metastasis, nodal status, and serosal invasion).

The human c-*met* oncogene encodes a transmembrane tyrosine kinase showing structural and functional features of a growth factor receptor [124]; this oncogene was found to be amplified and overexpressed in human gastric carcinoma cell lines [125]; more recently, a monoclonal antibody has been used to investigate the distribution of the c-*met* protein in normal and neoplastic tissues. Preliminary observations showed positive immunostaining in the majority (11 out of 12) of gastric carcinomas [126]; however, positive immunoreactivity was also observed for several other tumors and in many normal tissues (including gastric and colonic mucosa). Thus, although there is some evidence indicating a direct involvement of the c-*met* gene in gastric cancer development, the precise role of this gene in the multistep process of gastric tumorigenesis remains undefined.

Abnormalities of several other concogenes, growth factors, and their receptors have often been detected in gastric tumors. These include amplification or rearrangement of *hst* and c-*mos* genes [117], amplification of *int-2* or K-*sam* [122, 127], overexpression of the epidermal growth factor receptor (EGFR), and of transforming growth factor alpha [127]. EGFR is overexpressed more frequently in intestinal-type carcinomas than in diffuse or undifferentiated tumors. The contribution of all these changes in the pathogenesis of cancer of the stomach remains to be elucidated.

Cytogenetics and Tumor Suppressor Genes

Chromosomal studies in gastric carcinoma were not as frequent as for other common solid tumors, and indeed a recent review on cytogenetics of epithelial malignant lesions did not mention gross chromosomal abnormalities in this disease [128]. However, other investigators found frequent breakpoints at chromosome 3p21 [129], or translocations and deletions at 11p13 in gastric malignancies [130]; interestingly, similar alterations were also observed in adenocarcinomas of the lower esophagus, lending further support to the view of a similar pathogenesis for these two types of tumor [127].

Restriction fragment length polymorphism analysis allowed a more precise definition of the chromosomal losses involved in tumorigenesis. As far as gastric cancer is concerned, allelic deletions were frequently found at chromosomes 5q, 13q, 17p, and 18q. Thus, Sano et al. recently reported a high incidence of loss of heterozygosity on chromosomes 17p and 5q in neoplasms of the stomach [131]; moreover, similar results were also obtained by other authors [132]. Since the 5q site corresponds to two genes closely involved in colorectal tumorigenesis (*APC*, which is the gene of adenomatosis coli, and *MCC*, a gene frequently mutated in sporadic colorectal carcinoma), it is tempting to speculate that loss or rearrangements of these genes might represent a key event in the pathogenesis of tumors of the gastrointestinal tract. This contention was further reinforced by the recent finding of APC mutations (exon 15) in a small fraction of gastric carcinomas (3 out of 44, all of the diffuse histologic type) in which one-half of the coding region of the gene was examined by RNase protection analysis [133].

Various authors found allele loss on chromosome 17p, at the site of the *p53* tumor suppressor gene [127, 131, 132]. Sequence analysis, however, showed a low frequency of *p53* mutation (0%–13%) in primary gastric tumors, whereas the gene was often mutated in metastases and in cell lines established from gastric cancer metastases [134, 135], thus suggesting that *p53* alterations preferentially occur in the advanced stages of gastric tumorigenesis. At variance with these observations, Brito et al. [136] found positive immunoreactivity for the p53 protein (indicative of the presence of a mutated allele) in early gastric cancer and in precancerous lesions. Uchino et al. [137] examined loss of heterozygosity on various chromosomes in a large series of intestinal type gastric cancers; while allelic deletions at 18q were found in 62% of the cases and without any apparent relation to tumor invasion, the incidence of allele loss on 17p (42% of all cases) was appreciably higher in locally infiltrative tumors. These findings led the authors to speculate that inactivation of tumor suppressor genes located on chromosomes 17p and 18q – *p53* and *DCC* (for "deleted in colorectal carcinoma, see next chapter), respectively – might be of critical importance in the development of many gastric cancers, and that alterations of these two genes are probably involved in different phases of gastric tumorigenesis. Finally, loss of alleles at loci on chromosomes 13q [138] and 8p [138] has also been reported in some 40%–50% of gastric carcinomas; the clinical relevance of these or other gene deletions on chromosomes 1q, 6q, 7q, and 22q [127, 131, 137] remains to be elucidated.

References

1. Parkin DM, Laara E, Muir CS (1988) Estimates of the worldwide frequency of 16 major cancers in 1980. Int J Cancer 41:184–197
2. Cipriani F, Buiatti E, Palli D (1991) Gastric cancer in Italy. Ital J Gastroenterol 23:429–435
3. American Cancer Society (1991) Cancer facts and figures, vol 3. American Cancer Society, Atlanta
4. Devesa SS, Silverman DT, Young LY et al. (1987) Cancer incidence and mortality trends among whites in the USA. JNCI 79:701–770
5. Joossens JV, Geboers J (1984) Diet and environment in the etiology of gastric cancer. In: Levin B, Riddell RH (eds) Frontiers in gastrointestinal cancer. Elsevier, Amsterdam, pp 167–183
6. Joossens JV, Geboers J (1981) Nutrition and gastric cancer. Nutr Cancer 2:250–261
7. Buiatti E, Palli D, Decarli A et al. (1990) A case-control study of gastric cancer and diet in Italy. Int J cancer 45:896–901
8. Rios-Castellanos E, Sitas F, Shepherd NA et al. (1992) Changing pattern of gastric cancer in Oxfordshire. Gut 33:1312–1317
9. Weyers WC, Damiano RJ, Postlethwait RW et al. (1987) Adenocarcinoma of the stomach: changing pattern over the last four decades. Ann Surg 205:1–8
10. Golematis B, Tzardis P, Hatzikostas P et al. (1990) Changing pattern of distribution of cancer of the stomach. Br J Surg 77:63–64
11. Waterhouse J, Muir C, Shanmugaratnam K et al. (1982) Cancer incidence in five continents, vol 4. International Agency for Research on Cancer, Lyon, pp 706–707 (IARC scientific publication, no 42)
12. Correa P (1986) Epidemiology of gastric cancer. In: Filipe MI, Jass JR (eds) Gastric carcinoma. Churchill Livingstone, New York, pp 1–10
13. Holm J, Asire A, Young JL et al. (1984) SEER program: cancer incidence and mortality in the United States 1973–81. National Cancer Institute, Bethesda (NIH publication, no 85.1837)
14. Wigging CL, Becker TM, Rey CR et al. (1989) Stomach cancer among New Mexico's American Indians, Hispanic whites, and non-Hispanic whites. Cancer Res 49:1595–1599
15. Tuyns AJ, Kaaks R, Haelterman M et al. (1992) Diet and gastric cancer. A case-control study. Int J Cancer 51:1–6
16. Decarli A, La Vecchia C (1985) Cancer mortality in Italy, 1979. Tumori 71:519–528
17. Facchini U, Camnasio M, Cantaboni A et al. (1985) Geographic variation of cancer mortality in Italy. Int J Epidemiol 14:538–548
18. Decarli A, La Vecchia C, Cislaghi C et al. (1986) Descriptive epidemiology of gastric cancer in Italy. Cancer 58:2560–2569
19. Correa P, Haenszel W, Cuello C et al. (1975) A model for gastric cancer epidemiology. Lancet II:58–60
20. Correa P (1992) Human gastric carcinogenesis. Cancer Res 52:6735–6740
21. Forman D, Al-Dabbagh SA, Doll R (1985) Nitrates, nitrites and gastric cancer in Great Britain. Nature 313:620–625
22. Fontham E, Zavala D, Correa P et al. (1986) Diet and chronic atrophic gastritis. JNCI 76:621–627
23. Risch HA, Jain M, Choi NW et al. (1985) Dietary factors and the incidence of cancer of the stomach. Am J Epidemiol 122:947–959
24. Beresford SA (1985) Is nitrate in the drinking water associated with the risk of stomach cancer in the urban UK? Int J Epidemiol 14:57–63

25. Vincent P, Dubois G, Leclerc H et al. (1986) Nitrates dans l'eau de boisson et mortalitè par cancer. Br J Int Med 43:507–515
26. Hill MJ (1986) Aetiologic and micro-environment of gastric cancer. In: Filipe MI, Jass JR (eds) Gastric carcinoma. Churchill Livingstone, New York, pp 11–19
27. Correa P (1988) A human model of carcinogenesis. Cancer Res 48:3554–3560
28. Ramòn JM, Serra L, Cerdò C et al. (1993) Dietary factors in gastric cancer risk. Cancer 71:1731–1735
29. Trichopoulos D, Ouranos G, Day NE et al. (1985) Diet and cancer of the stomach. Int J Cancer 36:291–297
30. Correa P, Fontham E, Pickle LW et al. (1985) Dietary determinants of gastric cancer in South Louisiana inhabitants. JNCI 75:645–654
31. La Vecchia C, Negri E, Decarli A et al. (1987) A case-control study of gastric cancer in Northern Italy. Int J Cancer 40:484–489
32. Hoey J, Montvernay C, Lambert R (1981) Wine and tobacco: risk factors for gastric cancer in France. Am J Epidemiol 113:668–674
33. Graham S, Lilienfeld AM, Tidings JE (1967) Dietary and purgation factors in the etiology of gastric cancer. Cancer 20:2224–2234
34. Moller H, Lindvig K, Klefter R et al. (1989) Cancer occurrence in a cohort of patients treated with cimetidine. Gut 30:1558–1562
35. Moller H, Toftgaard C (1991) Cancer occurrence in a cohort of patients surgically treated for peptic ulcer. Gut 32:740–744
36. Chyuo PH, Nomura AMY, Hankin JH et al. (1990) A case-cohort study of diet and stomach cancer. Cancer Res 50:7501–7504
37. Tajima K, Tominaga S (1985) Dietary habits and gastrointestinal cancer. Jpn J Cancer Res (Gann) 76:705–716
38. You W, Blot W, Chang Y et al. (1988) Diet and high risk of stomach cancer in Shandong, China. Cancer Res 48:3518–3523
39. Forman D (1991) The etiology of gastric cancer. In: O'Neill IK, Chen J, Bartsch H (eds) Relevance to human cancer of N-nitroso compounds, tobacco smoke and mycotoxins. IARC, Lyon, pp 22–32
40. Buiatti E, Palli D, Bianchi S et al. (1991) A case-control study of gastric cancer and diet in Italy. Int J Cancer 48:369–374
41. Marshall BJ, Warren JR (1984) Unidentified curved bacilli in the stomach of patients with gastritis and peptic ulceration. Lancet I:1311–1315
42. Siurala M, Sipponen P, Kekki M (1985) Chronic gastritis: dynamic and clinical aspects. Scand J Gastroenterol [Suppl] 109:69–76
43. Parsonnet J, Friedman GD, Vandersteen DP et al. (1991) Helicobacter pylori infection and the risk of gastric carcinoma. N Engl J Med 325:1127–1131
44. Nomura A, Stemmermann GN, Chyou PH et al. (1991) Helicobacter pylori infection and gastric carcinoma among Japanese Americans in Hawaii. N Engl J Med 325:1132–1136
45. Kuipers EJ, Gracia-Casanova M, Pena As et al. (1993) Helicobacter pylori serology in patients with gastric carcinoma. Scand J Gastroenterol 28:433–437
46. Talley NJ, Zinsmeister AR, Weaver A et al. (1991) Gastric adenocarcinoma and Helicobacter pylori infection. JNCI 83:1734–1739
47. Parsonnet J, Vandersteen D, Goates J et al. (1991) Helicobacter pylori infection in intestinal and diffuse type gastric adenocarcinoma. JNCI 83:640–643
48. Kneller RW, Guo WD, Hsing AW et al. (1992) Risk factors for stomach cancer in 65 Chinese counties. Cancer Epidemiol Biomarkers Prev 1:113–118
49. Guarner J, Mohar A, Parsonnet J et al. (1993) The association of Helicobacter pylori with gastric cancer and preneoplastic gastric lesions in Chipas Mexico. Cancer 71:297–301

50. The Eurogast Study Group (1993) An international association between Helicobacter pylori infection and gastric cancer. Lancet 341:1359–1362
51. Sobala GM, Schorah CJ, Shires S et al. (1990) Gastric ascorbic acid concentration and acute Helicobacter pylori infection. Rev Esp Enferm Dig 78[Suppl 1]:63
52. Forman D (1991) Helicobacter pylori infection: a novel risk factor in the etiology of gastric cancer. JNCI 83:1702–1703
53. Laurèn P (1965) The two histologic main types of gastric carcinomas: diffuse and so-called intestinal-type carcinoma: an attempt at a histoclinical classification. Acta Microbiol Immunol Scand 63:31–49
54. Ming SC (1977) Gastric carcinoma: a pathobiologic classification. Cancer 39: 2475–2485
55. Laurèn PA, Nevalainen TJ (1993) Epidemiology of intestinal and diffuse types of gastric carcinoma. Cancer 71:2929–2923
56. Ming CS (1986) Classification of gastric carcinoma. In: Filipe MI, Jass JR (eds) Gastric carcinoma. Churchill Livingstone, New York, pp 197–216
57. Biasco G, Paganelli GM, Azzaroni D et al. (1987) Early gastric cancer in Italy. Dig Dis Sci 32:113–120
58. Sue-Ling HM, Martin I, Griffith J et al. (1992) Early gastric cancer: 46 cases treated in one surgical department. Gut 33:1318–1322
59. Kawai K (1978) Screening for gastric cancer in Japan. Clin Gastroenterol 7:605–622
60. Sipponen P, Kekki M, Siurala M (1986) Precancerous conditions. In: Filipe MI, Jass JR (eds) Gastric carcinoma. Churchill Livingstone, New York, pp 152–171
61. You WC, Blot WJ, Li JY et al. (1993) Precancerous gastric lesions in a population at high risk for stomach cancer. Cancer Res 53:1317–1321
62. Possik RA, Eduardo LF, Pires DR et al. (1986) Sensitivity, specificity and predictive value of laparoscopy for the staging of gastric cancer and for the detection of liver metastases. Cancer 58:1–6
63. Farinati F, Nitti D, Cardin F et al. (1988) CA 19.9 determination in gastric juice: role in identifying gastric cancer and high risk patients. Eur J Cancer Clin Oncol 24:923–927
64. Palli A, Decarli A, Cipriani F et al. (1991) Plasma pepsinogen, nutrients, and diet in areas of Italy at varying gastric cancer risk. Cancer Epidemiol Biomarkers Prevention 1:45–50
65. Weed TE, Nuessle W, Ochsner A (1981) Carcinoma of the stomach: why are we failing to improve survival? Ann Surg 193:407–413
66. Nakamura K, Ueyama T, Yao T et al. (1992) Pathology and prognosis of gastric carcinoma. Cancer 70:1030–1037
67. Bollschweiler E, Bottcher K, Hoelscher AH et al. (1993) Is the prognosis for Japanese and German patients with gastric cancer really different? Cancer 71:2918–2925
68. Amadori D, Bonaguri C, Volpi A et al. (1993) Cell kinetics and prognosis in gastric cancer. Cancer 71:1–4
69. Sowa M, Yoshino H, Kato Y et al. (1988) An analysis of the DNA ploidy pattern in gastric cancer. Cancer 62:1325–1330
70. Wyatt JI, Quirke P, Ward DC et al. (1989) Comparison of histopathological and flow cytometric parameters in prediction of prognosis in gastric cancer. J Pathol 158:195–201
71. Ohyama S, Yonemura Y, Miyazaki I (1990) Prognostic value of S-phase fraction and DNA ploidy studied with in vivo administration of bromodeoxyurudine on human gastric cancers. Cancer 65:116–121

72. Yonemura Y, Ohoyama S, Kimura H et al. (1991) The expression of proliferative-associated nuclear antigen p105 in gastric carcinoma. Cancer 67:2523–2528
73. Kakeji Y, Korenaga D, Tsujitani S et al. (1991) Predictive value of Ki-67 and AgNor for lymph node metastasis in gastric cancer. Cancer Res 51:3503–3506
74. Ohyama S, Yonemura Y, Miyazaki I (1992) Proliferative activity and malignancy in human gastric cancers. Cancer 69:314–321
75. Johnson H, Belluco C, Masood S et al. (1993) The value of flow cytometry analysis in patients with gastric cancer. Arch Surg 128:314–317
76. Douglas HO, Nava HR (1985) Gastric adenocarcinoma: management of the primary disease. Semin Oncol 12:32–41
77. Gunderson LL, Martin JK, O'Connell MJ et al. (1985) Residual, recurrent and unresectable gastrointestinal cancer. Cancer 55:2250–2258
78. The Gastrointestinal Tumor Study Group (1984) A randomized study of combination chemotherapy in unresectable gastric cancer. Cancer 53:13–17
79. Wils J, Bleiberg H, Dalesio O et al. (1986) An EORTC gastrointestinal group evaluation of the combination of sequential methotrexate and 5-FU combined with adriamycin in advanced measurable gastric cancer. J Clin Oncol 4:1799–1803
80. Wilke H, Preusser P, Fink U et al. (1990) New developments in the treatment of gastric carcinoma. Semin Oncol 17[Suppl 2]:61–70
81. Saini A, Waxman J (1992) Chemotherapy for gastric cancer. Gut 33:1153–1154
82. Kornek G, Schulz F, Depisch D et al. (1993) A phase I-II study of Epirubicin, 5-FU, and Leucovorin in advanced adenocarcinoma of the stonach. Cancer 71:2177–2180
83. Hermans J, Bonekamp JJ, Boon MC et al. (1993) Adjuvant therapy after curative resection for gastric cancer: meta-analysis of randomized trials. J Clin Oncol 11:1441–1447
84. Lipkin M, Bell B, Sherlock P (1963) Cell proliferation kinetics in the gastrointestinal tract of men. J Clin Invest 42:767–776
85. Lipkin M (1988) Biomarkers of increased susceptibility to gastrointestinal cancer. Cancer Res 48:235–245
86. Offerhaus GJA, van de Stadt J, Samson G et al. (1985) Cell proliferation kinetics in the gastric remnant. Eur J Cancer Clin Oncol 21:73–79
87. Bell B, Almy TP, Lipkin M (1967) Cell proliferation kinetics in the gastrointestinal tract of man. JNCI 38:615–628
88. Hsing AW, Hansson LE, McLaughlin JK et al. (1993) Pernicious anemia and subsequent cancer. Cancer 71:745–750
89. Hansen OH, Larsen JK, Svendsen LB (1978) Changes in gastric mucosa cell proliferation after antrectomy or vagotomy in man. Scand J Gastroenterol 13:947–952
90. Borkje B, Hostmark J, Skagen DW et al. (1988) Flow cytometry of biopsy specimens from ulcerative colitis, colorectal adenomas and carcinomas. Scand J Gastroenterol 22:1231–1237
91. Fennerty MB, Sampliner RE, Way D et al. (1989) Discordance between flow cytometry abnormalities and dysplasia in Barrett's esophagus. Gastroenterology 97:815–820
92. Capurso L, Teodori L, DeVita R et al. (1982) DNA content as a marker of precancerous lesions of the digestive tract. Gastroenterology 82:1029
93. Brinton LA, Gridley G, Hrubec Z et al. (1989) Cancer risk following pernicious anemia. Br J Cancer 59:810–813

94. Varis K, Kekki M, Ihamaki T et al. (1985) Familial behavior of chronic gastritis. In: Muller HJ, Weber W (eds) Familial cancer. Karger, Basel, pp 60–62
95. Varis K, Ihamaki T, Harkonan M et al. (1979) Gastric morphology, function and immunology in first-degree relatives of probands with pernicious anemia and in controls. Scand J Gastroenterol 14:123–129
96. Varis K (1981) Family behaviour of chronic gastritis. Ann Clin Res 13:123–129
97. Santos JG, Magalhaes J (1980) Familial gastric polyposis: a new entity. J Genet Hum 28(3):293–297
98. Seruca R, Carneiro F, Castedo S et al. (1991) Familial gastric polyposis revisited. Cancer Genet Cytogenet 53:97–100
99. Macklin MT (1960) Inheritance of cancer of the stomach and large intestine in man. JNCI 24:551–571
100. Woolf CM (1950) Investigation of genetic aspects of carcinoma of the stomach. Am J Hum Genet 8:102–108
101. Videbaek A, Mosbech J (1954) The aetiology of gastric carcinoma elucidated by a study of 302 pedigrees. Acta Med Scand 149:137–159
102. Lehtola J (1978) Family study of gastric carcinoma; with special reference to histological types. Scand J Gastroenterol 13[Suppl 50]:11–54
103. Juhàsz L (1985) Familial occurrence of stomach cancer and precancerous lesions in North-East Hungary. In: Muller HJ, Weber W (eds) Familial cancer. Karger, Basel, pp 63–65
104. Jackson CE, Schouman BM, Salerno Mele P et al. (1985) Familial factors in the high incidence of gastric cancer in San Marino: gastroscopic findings. In: Muller HJ, Weber W (eds) Familial cancer. Karger, Basel, pp 66–69
105. Zanghieri G, Di Gregorio C, Sacchetti C et al. (1990) Familial occurrence of gastric cancer in the 2-year experience of a population-based registry. Cancer 66:2047–2051
106. La Vecchia C, Negri E, Franceschi S et al. (1992) Family history and the risk of stomach and colorectal cancer. Cancer 70:50–55
107. Warthin AS (1913) Heredity with reference to carcinoma. Arch Intern Med 12:546–555
108. Vasen HFA, Offerhaus GJA, den Hartog Jager FCA et al. (1990) The tumor spectrum in HNPCC: a study of 24 kindreds in the Netherlands. Int J Cancer 46:31–34
109. Watson P, Lynch HT (1993) Extracolonic cancer in HNPCC. Cancer 71: 677–685
110. Benatti P, Sassatelli R, Roncucci L et al. (1993) Tumour spectrum in HNPCC and in families with suspected HNPCC. A population-based study in Northern Italy. Int J Cancer (in press)
111. Farinati F, Cardin F, Di Mario F et al. (1989) Genetic, dietary and environmental factors in the pathogenesis of gastric cancer. Ital J Gastroenterol 19: 321–324
112. Matsukara N, Onda M, Tokunaga A et al. (1988) Simultaneous gastric cancer in monozygotic twins. Cancer 62:2430–2435
113. Fujita K, Ohuchi N, Tsuneyoshi Y et al. (1987) Frequent overexpression, but not activation by point mutation, of ras genes in primary human gastric cancer. Gastroenterology 93:1339–1345
114. Czerniak B, Herz F, Gorczyca W et al. (1989) Expression of ras oncogene p21 protein in early gastric carcinoma and adjacent gastric epithelia. Cancer 64: 1467–1473
115. Deng G, Liu X, Wang J et al. (1991) Correlation of mutation of oncogene c-Ha-ras at codon 12 with metastases and survival of gastric cancer patients. Oncogene Res 6:33–38

116. Victor T, du Toit R, Jordaan AM et al. (1990) No evidence for point mutations in codon 12, 13 and 61 of the ras gene in a high incidence area for esophageal and gastric cancer. Cancer Res 50:4911–4914
117. Ranzani GN, Pellegata NS, Previderè C et al. (1990) Heterogeneous proto-oncogene amplification correlates with tumor progression and presence of metastases in gastric cancer patients. Cancer Res 50:7811–7814
118. Yoshida K, Yasuii W, Taniyama K et al. (1988) Preparation of anti-ras Mr 21 000 protein monoclonal antibody and immunohistochemical on expression of ras genes in human stomach and thyroid cancer. Cancer Res 48:5503–5509
119. Tahara E, Yasui W, Taniyama K et al. (1986) Ha-ras oncogene product in human gastric carcinoma. Jpn J Cancer Res 77:517–522
120. Ninomiya I, Yonemura Y, Matsumoto H et al. (1991) Expression of c-myc gene product in gastric carcinoma. Oncology 48:149–153
121. Park JB, Rhim JS, Park SC et al. (1989) Amplification, overexpression and rearrangement of the erbB-2 protooncogene in primary human stomach carcinoma. Cancer Res 49:6605–6609
122. Tsujino T, Yoshida K, Nakayama H et al. (1990) Alterations of oncogenes in metastatic tumours of human gastric carcinomas. Br J Cancer 62:226–230
123. Yonemura Y, Ninomiya I, Ohoyama S et al. (1991) Expression of c-erbB-2 oncoprotein in gastric carcinoma. Cancer 67:2914–2918
124. Park M, Dean M, Kaul K et al. (1987) Sequence of met protooncogene cDNA has features characteristic of the tyrosine kinase of growth factors receptors. Proc Natl Acad Sci USA 84:6379–6383
125. Giordano S, Ponzetto C, di Renzo MF et al. (1989) Tyrosine kinase receptor indistinguishable from the c-met protein. Nature 399:155–156
126. Prat M, Narsimhan RP, Crepaldi T et al. (1991) The receptor encoded by the human cMet oncogene is expressed in hepatocytes, epithelial cells and solid tumors. Int J Cancer 49:323–328
127. Wright PA, Williams GT (1993) Molecular biology of gastric carcinoma. Gut 34:145–147
128. Pathak S (1992) Cytogenetics of epithelial malignant lesions. Cancer 70:1660–1670
129. Ochi H, Douglas HO, Sandberg AA (1986) Cytogenetic studies in primary gastric cancer. Cancer Genet Cytogenet 22:295–307
130. Rodriguez E, Rao PH, Ladanyi M et al. (1990) 11p13–15 is a specific region of chromosome rearrangement in gastric and esophageal carcinoma. Cancer Res 50:6410–6416
131. Sano T, Tsujino T, Yoshida K et al. (1991) Frequent loss of heterozygosity on chromosomes 1q, 5q and 17p in human gastric carcinoma. Cancer Res 51:3231–3233
132. Neuman WL, Wasylyshyn ML, Jacoby R et al. (1991) Evidence for a common molecular pathogenesis in colorectal, gastric and pancreatic cancer. Genes Chromos Cancer 3:468–473
133. Horii A, Nakatsuru S, Miyoshi Y et al. (1992) The APC gene, responsible for FAP, is mutated in human gastric cancer. Cancer Res 52:3231–3233
134. Yamada Y, Yoshida T, Hayashi K et al. (1991) p53 gene mutations in gastric cancer metastases and in gastric cancer cell lines derived from metastases. Cancer Res 51:5800–5805
135. Seruca R, David L, Holm R et al. (1992) p53 mutations in gastric carcinoma. Br J Cancer 65:708–710
136. Brito MJ, Filipe MI, Lane D et al. (1992) p53 overexpression in early gastric carcinoma and precancerous lesions. J Pathol 167:95A
137. Uchino S, Tsuda H, Noguchi M et al. (1992) Frequent loss of heterozygosity at the DCC locus in gastric cancer. Cancer Res 52:3099–3102

138. Motomura K, Nishisho I, Takai SI et al. (1988) Loss of alleles at loci on chromosome 13 in human primary gastric cancer. Genomics 2:180–184
139. Wasylyshyn ML, Neuman WL, Angriman I et al. (1991) Evidence for a new tumor suppressor gene involved in gastrointestinal malignancies. Surgery 110: 265–269

Hereditary and Familial Colorectal Cancer

Large bowel cancer has complex, multifactorial etiologic factors, each of which play a major or minor role, through specific mechanisms, in the overall prolonged process leading to clinically overt cancer. Some factors may be directly causative, others may enhance or promote, and still others may be protective or inhibiting.

(J.H. WEISBURGER and E.L. WYNDER 1987)

Introduction

Colorectal cancer is a major cause of death in Western countries and one of the neoplasms in which the contribution of heritable factors has been investigated in more detail, in terms of both genetic epidemiology and molecular biology.

The factors leading or predisposing to colorectal cancer are still unclear. There are, however, at least three major aspects which together differentiate this tumor from other neoplastic disorders. First, at variance with tumors of many other organs, a definite fraction of colorectal cancers may be considered hereditary; the main features of this subgroup of tumors include: (a) frequent location in the proximal colon; (b) early age of onset (<50 years); (c) excess of multiple primaries (both in the large bowel and in other organs); and (d) vertical transmission and aggregation in accordance with an autosomal dominant type of inheritance. In addition, familial clusters of colorectal tumors but without clinical features of monogenic transmission are frequently observed. Second, environmental agents are similarly important in the development of colorectal carcinoma; the impact of exogenous factors is exemplified by the study of Japanese immigrants to the United States: after one generation the incidence rate of this neoplasm approaches the rate observed in the host country. Third, various lines of evidence suggest that a large proportion (if not all) of colorectal cancers develops from benign precursor lesions of the large intestine (i.e., adenomatous polyps). The best clinical evidence of the "adenoma-carcinoma sequence" is provided by adenomatosis coli (and related syndromes, see next chapter), an inherited condition in which the entire large bowel is carpeted with polyps; if untreated, a malignant tumor develops, usually in the distal colon, virtually in all cases.

Finally, the molecular biology of large bowel tumors has received particular attention in the last few years. Recent observations showed that the various steps of colorectal tumor formation seem to depend on the accumulation of genetic alterations involving both oncogenes and tumor suppressor genes. Hypomethylation of DNA, mutations of the K-*ras* oncogene, and allelic losses in chromosome 5q appear as early events, associated with the induction of a hyperproliferative state of colonic mucosa and with the appearance of small adenomas. Subsequently, loss of genetic material at 17p, 18q, and various other chromosomal loci probably represents late events, mainly implicated in the progression of large adenomas or localized tumors to infiltrating carcinomas.

General Aspects

Epidemiology and Etiology: One Tumor or Four?

Colorectal cancer is one of the most threatening neoplastic diseases, and a major cause of cancer incidence and mortality especially in developed and industrialized countries. Each year between 130000 and 150000 North Americans are affected and approximately half of them will die of this disease [1]. Similar figures can be found in Europe, where in countries such as France, Italy, and the United Kingdom data from cancer registries suggest that we should expect 20000–40000 new cases/year [2, 3]. About one-third of these neoplasms are located in the rectum [1]. Incidence rates of colorectal cancer show large variations between countries, from 0.5–5.0 new cases/100000 per year in poor and less-industrialized countries, such as Senegal and India, to more than 50/100000 in North America and Europe (especially Scotland and many central-northern regions) and New Zealand [1, 4, 5]. Temporal trends have shown little change in the overall incidence and mortality rates over the last 30–40 years in most Western countries [4, 6, 7]. The situation is more complex if we consider various sites in the large bowel; thus, cancer of the rectum tended to decrease in both sexes, at least in the United States [1], while the steady increase in incidence rate observed in countries such as Japan has to be almost entirely attributed to a sharp rise in cancer of the left colon [8]; moreover, a trend towards a decline in incidence of left-side cancer and an increase in proximal colonic tumors has been reported, especially in North America [9, 10].

The International Classification of Diseases for Oncology (ICD-O) considers colonic and rectal tumors as different nosologic entities [11]. Although there are also reasons for considering colonic and rectal neoplasms as a single disease (the structure and the main function of the two tracts are rather similar), more recently the distinction between proximal and distal colonic cancers has received particular attention. After a careful review of the literature, Weisburger and Wynder came to the conclusion that we are actually dealing with three different types of large bowel neoplasms: cancer of the right colon, cancer of the left colon, and cancer of the rectum [1]. This contention is mainly based on the following considerations: (a) tumors at these three sites tend to occur with different incidence and mortality rates in diverse areas of the world, thus suggesting that different etiologic agents might be implicated; (b) neoplasms of the various colonic subsites show a specific age and sex relationship (for example, tumors of the right colon tend to be more frequent in young females, while those of the left colon tend to be more frequent in elderly males) [12, 13]; (c) as already discussed, temporal trends showed a shift of incidence between right and left colonic tumors [8–10], again suggesting the possible existence of different etiologic and risk factors. The principal features of these three types of large bowel cancer can be summarized as follows:

1. Cancer of the proximal colon (cecum, ascending, transverse, and flexures) is relatively common in some geographic areas with a low incidence of colorectal neoplasms, and is the most common cancer in some hereditary neoplastic disorders of the large bowel (see later).
2. Cancer of the distal colon (descending, sigmoid, and rectosigmoid region) is particularly frequent in Western countries, and is epidemiologically related to most of the environmental risk factors known for this tumor.
3. Cancer of the rectum (i.e., located within 8 cm from the anal verge) does not seem to be related to well-known risk factors, and its epidemiology differs from that of the two other types of tumors.

Since the pathogenesis and risk factors for anal cancer are different from those of the other large bowel tumors (i.e., the disease is frequent in homosexuals, and is often associated with genital warts, a relationship which implicates a possible role of human papillomavirus; moreover, these tumors are strongly related to cigarette smoking) [14, 15], these neoplasms might represent a fourth type of large bowel malignancy [13].

As for other tumors of the digestive organs, a plethora of investigations (mostly case control studies) explored the possible relevance of dietary factors in the etiopathogenesis of colorectal neoplasms. The results of these studies were frequently discordant, the observed relative risks usually low, and no strong causative dietary factor could be detected; however, the available experimental evidence can be summarized in these general terms. First, dietary consumption of fat (especially from an animal source), meat, alcohol, and total energy intake seem to be positively correlated with the incidence of colorectal cancer [1, 4, 16–21]; moreover, animal experiments showed that diets containing 40% of the calories as saturated or unsaturated fat are associated with a higher incidence of colorectal neoplasms as compared to diets with a low fat content irrespective of the type of carcinogen used in the study [1, 22]. Second, a high intake of dietary fiber, fresh fruits, vegetable, and calcium was found to be associated with a reduced risk of colorectal malignancies [4, 16, 23–27]; this protective effect might be due, at least in part, to many potentially anticarcinogenic substances contained in vegetables, such as vitamins A, C, and E, flavonoids, protease inhibitors, and others [1, 16, 28]. In addition, fiber may be protective against colorectal cancer through other mechanisms, including a decrease in intestinal transit time (thus reducing the contact time of putative carcinogens with mucosal cells), a "bulky" effect with consequent "dilution" of the large bowel content, and the possible interaction with carcinogens present in the gut lumen [29]. Finally, calcium feeding seems to be protective by reducing the abnormal pattern of cell replication frequently observed in colonic crypts of individuals at risk of colorectal cancer [30, 31]. Third, a further confirmation of the role of diet (presumably together with other undefined factors related to lifestyle) in colorectal tumorigenesis derives from the already mentioned "migrant studies"; thus, migrants from countries with a low incidence of colorectal cancer – such as Japan or South America – to areas with a higher risk – such as North America – show a rapid increase in the incidence rates of this neoplasm usually after only one generation [1, 32]. Conversely, migrants from a high-risk area for cancer of the large bowel to a country at lower risk may show a reduction of incidence [33]. In addition, "special populations" [1], such as the Mormons or Seventh Day Adventists, with peculiar dietary habits are at lower risk for colorectal neoplasms than the general population [34].

Although not limited to the prevention of one type of tumor, the recently published recommendations of the American Cancer Society are in close agreement with the putative effect of dietary factors in colorectal cancer development. These suggestions can be summarized as follows [35]: (a) avoid obesity, reaching and maintaining the ideal body weight; (b) reduce total fat intake; (c) include a variety of fruits and vegetables in the daily diet; (d) eat more high-fiber food; (e) limit the consumption of alcoholic beverages; and (f) limit the consumption of smoked or salt-cured foods (Table 1).

Besides diet, a few other exogenous factors have been etiologically related to colorectal cancer development. Thus, evidence has been provided

Table 1. Summary of the dietary recommendations of the American Cancer Society for the primary prevention of cancer [35]

1. Avoid obesity (approximately 25% of adults are overweight, and 10% severely overweight)
2. Include a variety of fresh vegetables and fruits in the daily diet (especially those rich in vitamins A and C)
3. Reduce total fat intake (especially of an animal source)
4. Increase consumption of high-fiber foods, such as whole grain cereals, vegetables, and fruits
5. Limit consumption of alcoholic beverages (distilled spirits, wine, and beer)
6. Reduce consumption of smoked, salt-cured, and nitrite-cured foods

that a low level of physical exercise is associated with an excess risk of colonic cancer in both sexes, while the risk seems to decrease stepwise for jobs requiring a higher level of physical activity [36–38]; however, more recent findings failed to confirm these findings [39]. Occupation has rarely been documented to play a role in the pathogenesis of tumors of the large bowel [1]; moreover, the close similarity of incidence rates observed in men and women virtually exclude the presence of major risk factors related to sex. Finally, an increased risk for large bowel cancer has been documented for patients with inflammatory bowel diseases [40, 41], with diverticular disease [42], after colecystectomy [43] (but not without controversy), and for patients using antihypertensive drugs or sedatives [44].

Clinical and Morphologic Features

The clinical onset of colorectal carcinoma is often insidious, with vague and nonspecific symptoms which may be referred to chronic conditions, such as hemorrhoids, "colitis," or irritable bowel disease. Rectal bleeding, changes in bowel habits, abdominal pain, anemia, and weight loss are the most common of these symptoms, for either proximal or distal tumors; in addition, cancer of the rectosigmoid may present with acute bowel obstruction or perforation with peritonitis. Although early diagnosis based on symptom appearance is theoretically appealing, various studies indicated that when symptoms develop the disease is often in an advanced stage; it follows that one of the main objectives in colorectal cancer research is to reach a diagnosis before the appearance of symptoms, when the chances of finding a large adenomatous polyp or a stage I carcinoma should be higher [45–47]. Rectal examination, sigmoidoscopy, and double contrast enema have been for many years the standard diagnostic procedures; at present, pancolonoscopy represents the technique of choice, mainly because this procedure allows the direct exploration of the entire large bowel, giving the opportunity to biopsy any suspected lesion. Intrarectal ultrasonography, computed tomography, and magnetic nuclear imaging are particularly valuable for tumors localized in the rectosigmoid, in order to assess the spread of tumor beyond the muscular wall into the perirectal fat.

Adenocarcinoma is the most common histologic type of large bowel cancer; mucinous carcinomas represent 10%–20% of all tumors [48] and tend to be more frequent in hereditary nonpolyposis colorectal cancer (see below). The degree of differentiation (the most common classification distinguishes "well," "moderately," and "poorly" differentiated tumors) shows large variations even within a single neoplasm, and does not seem to be closely related to invasiveness and prognosis. The staging system proposed by Cuthbert Dukes in 1932 [49] is still widely employed and easy to apply; unfortunately the issue became more complex owing to the modifications introduced by several authors [50]. A universal staging system has recently been proposed by Hutter and Sobin [51], in which a close correspondence between TNM and Dukes' staging can be observed; this staging system follows simple physiopathologic considerations and eliminates ambiguities and confusion consequent to the numerous revisions of the Dukes' staging. Thus, stage I tumors (corresponding to Dukes A) are confined within the muscular wall, so that malignant polyps are usually included in this subgroup: in stage II (i.e., Dukes B), the neoplasm spreads beyond the smooth muscle and may infiltrate perirectal (or pericolic) tissues and organs. In stage III tumors (or Dukes C), lymphonodal metastases are present, whereas in stage IV (corresponding to the D class of other classifications), the tumor diffuses through the blood, giving metastases to the liver, lung, and other organs [52].

Management and Prognosis

Overall 5-year survival for patients operated on for colorectal cancer is about 40%. Survival, however, is strongly related to pathologic stage at diagnosis, ranging from 70% to 80% in stage I–II to less than 10% for stage IV patients [47, 53]. In patients undergoing resection for cure (approximately 60%–70% of total incident cases) 5-year survival is in the order of 50%–60% [54, 55]. Local recurrences (more frequent after excision of rectal carcinoma) are responsible for failure of treatment in 5%–30% of all cases, usually within 2–3 years from the operation [56–58]; liver and lung metastases are also frequent in the follow-up of patients undergoing curative resections, especially in Dukes C cancers.

Besides staging, several other clinical and morphologic variables have been proposed as potential biological indicators of prognosis; however, the results often appear controversial, and despite the undoubted interest of some biomarkers, the available evidence does not favor their routine clinical application. Thus, for example, Kemeny and Braun reported that lactic dehydrogenase levels, performance status, and lung involvement were the best predictors of survival in patients with advanced colorectal carcinoma [59], while Hannisdal and Thorsen showed that a high erythrocyte sedimentation rate and leukocyte count were important prognostic indicators in addition to stage [60]. Similarly, the prognostic relevance of other clinical variables has also been suggested [61, 62]. The effect of age on survival of patients with colorectal cancer is also controversial, with some authors suggesting a more favorable outcome for younger patients, others a more severe prognosis, and others no age-related difference [63–66]. The clinical importance of various histologic and grade-related parameters is even less clear. Thus, Jass et al. [67] found that three morphologic variables (lymphocytic infiltration, tubular configuration, and pattern of growth) maintained an independent prognostic value in patients with rectal cancer, while Stahle et al. were unable to confirm these findings [68]. Moreover, other reports suggest the possible prognostic significance of variables such as degree of differentiation [69], eosinophil infiltration [70], tumor morphology [71], and venous invasion [72].

The DNA content of tumor cell populations has been found to be of some prognostic relevance in several tumors; consequently, in patients with colorectal cancer, DNA index by flow cytometry (see the chapter on "Biomarkers of Increased Susceptibility to Cancer") became the objective of many investigations. Although, once again, the results were not entirely concordant, there is a general consensus on a more severe prognosis for aneuploid tumors [73–76]. Other investigators assessed the role of cell proliferation as a possible indicator of the clinical outcome in these patients; despite the availability of techniques of great biological interest (tritiated thymidine or bromodeoxyuridine incorporation, immunostaining with Ki-67 or PCNA, determination of S-phase parameters by flow cytometry), the prognostic significance of all these biomarkers is still questionable [77–80].

The current approach to treatment of colorectal cancer remains primarily surgical. Ample resections (right or left hemicolectomy) are usually considered the technique of choice, whereas abdominoperineal resections (Miles procedure) are required for tumors of the lower rectum which cannot be removed through the abdominal route. Some surgeons recommend a more radical approach for the management of colorectal cancer; more specifically, subtotal colectomy with ileorectal anastomosis has been suggested, with the main objective of reducing the development of metachronous tumors [81, 82]. Adjuvant systemic treatment with 5-fluorouracil plus either levamisole or folinic acid provided a significant advantage in overall and disease-free survival for stage III (or Dukes C) colon cancer, whereas the impact of these regimens in rectal cancer and in colonic neoplasms of other stages remains unproven [83–85]. As far as tumors of the rectum are concerned, some surgeons prefer preoperative or postoperative radiation therapy to prevent metastatic spread; in a recent review, Mohiuddin and Marks [86] concluded that adjunctive radiation therapy represents an attractive new option in the treatment of rectal cancer, and that its judicious use may be followed by a reduction of local recurrences and an improved overall survival.

Precancerous Lesions and Conditions

Colorectal Polyps and the "Adenoma Carcinoma" Sequence

At variance with tumors which develop "ex novo" or in the absence of well-grounded precancerous changes, there is considerable clinical, biological, and pathologic evidence implicating precursor lesions in the pathogenesis of colorectal cancer; adenomatous polyps of the large bowel are the most common of these lesions. Colorectal adenomas can be defined as well-demarcated, circumscribed lumps of epithelial dysplasia, and can be classified into three major histologic types: tubular, villous, and tubulovillous. These three types, however, are not sharply separable from one another, being only different manifestations of a spectrum of abnormal tissue architecture [87]. A marked geographic variation in the frequency of colorectal adenomas can be observed; thus, these lesions are uncommon in Africa and in some Asian countries (such as the Philippines), but extremely common in Europe and North America [88, 89]. Colorectal adenomas are rare under the age of 30 years, but their prevalence increases with increasing age, being present in 30%–40% of people over the age of 50 years in many Western countries. There is no obvious reason to expect a different frequency of polyps in the two sexes, yet a certain male prevalence has been observed in most series [88]. Although adenomatous polyps can be observed in all tracts of the large bowel, their distribution tends to parallel that of colorectal cancers, so that approximately 70% of either lesions are localized in the left colon [90]. The large majority of colorectal adenomas (80%–90%) are under 1 cm in diameter [91]; larger adenomas often show a villous pattern and are more frequently associated with malignant changes [87, 88]. Besides adenomatous lesions, polyps of the large bowel may also be of other types, such as "hamartomatous," "inflammatory," or "hyperplastic"; although the biological significance of these lesions remains unclear, there is no firm evidence of their malignant potential [88, 92].

Several observations indicate that adenomatous polyps may become cancerous; this fact, however, does not mean that all polyps undergo malignant changes, neither does it exclude the possibility of "de novo" (i.e., without precursor lesions) colorectal tumorigenesis [93]. The evidence that adenomatous polyps may transform into carcinomas stems from several clinical, biological, and epidemiologic observations, which can be summarized as follows. *First*, adenomatous areas are frequently observed in specimens of colorectal carcinoma; in a series of malignancies examined at St. Mark's hospital, 14.2% of all tumors showed varying proportions of adenomatous tissue [94]. Conversely, malignant changes – either confined above the muscularis mucosae or invading into the submucosa – can be seen in approximately 5% of all polyps [95]. *Second*, in adenomatosis coli – an autosomal dominant disease in which a myriad of adenomatous polyps of different dimensions are scattered in the various large bowel tracts (see next chapter) – malignant colorectal tumors develop virtually in 100% of untreated cases, usually around the age of 35–40 years [88]. *Third*, after a 25-year study of periodic sigmoidoscopy and polyp removal in a group of more than 18 000 patients, Gilbertsen [96] was able to demonstrate a significant reduction in the expected number of invasive carcinomas; these findings not only give further support to the adenoma-carcinoma sequence, but also represent the first experimental evidence that periodic endoscopic screening might lower the mortality rate for colorectal carcinoma. More recent studies, which included a control group, confirmed these preliminary and uncontrolled observations [97, 98]. *Fourth*, in a series of 226 patients in whom colorectal polyps larger than 10 mm could not be excised, clinical follow-up showed the occurrence of 21 invasive carcinomas, with a cumulative risk of cancer at the polyp site, after 20 years, of 24% [99]; in line with this report, a recent study [100] showed that mortality from colorectal cancer was significantly higher in a large group of individuals with polyps than in the general population. *Fifth*, adenomatous polyps are seen in approximately 35% of all resected specimens for intestinal tumors; moreover, there is evidence that in patients with synchronous colorectal tumors the proportion of cases with associated adenomas is more than double (75%) [101], thus suggesting that the simultaneous presence of carcinomas and adenomas is not a chance event. *Sixth*, age-specific incidence rate of colorectal polyps shows an earlier rise than cancer, with a peak of incidence which anticipates by 5 years that of malignant tumors [90]; since the carcinomatous change of a benign adenoma usually takes years [99], this pattern of incidence seems to suggest a sequence between polyps and cancer. *Seventh*, polyps and cancers tend to have a similar distribution in the various large bowel tracts [13, 88, 90], with a maximum frequency in the rectosigmoid region. *Eighth*, both patients with colorectal cancer and polyps share a similar, highly significant frequency of tumors of the large bowel among first-degree relatives [90]. *Finally*, a recent study [102] suggested that the risk of developing colorectal polyps seems to be associated with the same dietary factors which have been related to the risk of colorectal malignancies and, particularly, with a high intake of animal fat and low consumption of fruits and vegetables [1, 4]; rather intuitively, it can be stated that if polyps and cancers share the same etiologic factors, it is likely that they represent two different clinical phases of the same disorder. The main elements favoring the adenoma-carcinoma sequence in the large bowel have been summarized in Table 2.

Table 2. Main data favoring the existence of the "adenoma-carcinoma" sequence in large bowel tumorigenesis [85–101]

A. Adenomatous areas are frequently observed in colorectal carcinomas
B. Apparently benign adenomas may contain malignant changes
C. Adenomatosis coli is almost invariably associated – when untreated – with the development of colorectal cancer
D. Routine polypectomy seems to reduce colorectal cancer occurrence and mortality
E. If large polyps are not removed, part of them becomes malignant
F. Colorectal cancer mortality rates are higher in individuals with colonic adenomas
G. Adenomas can be observed in 30%–40% of intestinal specimens resected for cancer, and in over 70% of patients with synchronous colorectal malignancies
H. The peak of age-specific incidence for colonic polyps occurs approximately 5 years prior to the peak incidence of colorectal cancer
I. Adenomas and carcinomas tend to have a similar distribution in the various large bowel tracts
J. Patients with either colorectal cancer or adenoma show an elevated frequency of colorectal malignancy among first-degree relatives
K. The same dietary factors seem to be epidemiologically related to either adenomas or carcinomas of the large bowel
L. Geographically, the prevalence of adenomas closely reflects that of carcinomas

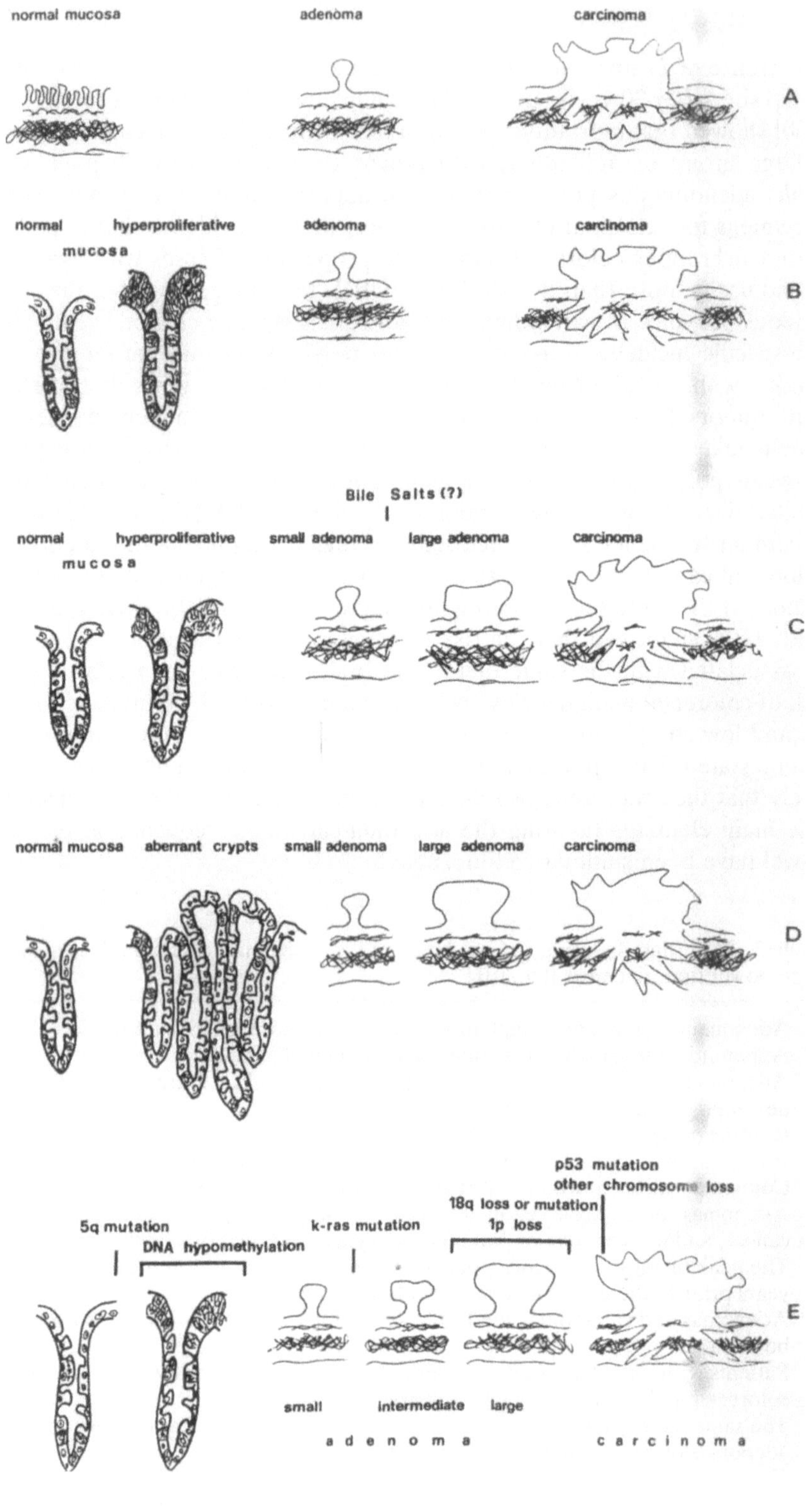
normal mucosa
adenoma
carcinoma
A
normal
hyperproliferative
mucosa
adenoma
carcinoma
B
Bile Salts (?)
normal
hyperproliferative
small adenoma
large adenoma
carcinoma
mucosa
C
normal mucosa
aberrant crypts
small adenoma
large adenoma
carcinoma
D
p53 mutation
other chromosome loss
18q loss or mutation
1p loss
5q mutation
k-ras mutation
DNA hypomethylation
E
small
intermediate
large
a d e n o m a
c a r c i n o m a

The adenoma-carcinoma sequence was initially proposed by Morson and coworkers mainly on the basis of morphologic observations [87, 88]; as already discussed, subsequent studies basically confirmed and reinforced the original intuition of Morson; however, at the same time (and almost inevitably) the sequence leading from a normal colorectal mucosa to invasive carcinoma became more complex, involving putative pathogenetic determinants (bile acids, oncogenes, tumor suppressor genes) and various intermediate stages (hyperproliferative mucosa, aberrant crypts, polyps of various dimensions, and degree of differentiation) [103, 104]. Many of these aspects will be discussed in the following sections; moreover, Fig. 1 illustrates the "evolution" of the concept of "adenoma-carcinoma" sequence, from a merely morphologic phenomenon to a complex chain of biomolecular events still under active investigation.

Cell Replication and Differentiation in Colorectal Mucosa

Several lines of evidence suggest that before the appearance of adenomatous polyps other premorphologic or preneoplastic alterations can be detected in the apparently normal mucosa of the large bowel, thus suggesting that the process of colorectal tumorigenesis begins with a generalized disorder of cell proliferation and differentiation that antedates and then accompanies the development of morphologic lesions [105]. Through a proper assessment of these premorphologic changes, individuals at increased risk for colorectal neoplasms might be identified; moreover, measurement of cell replication in the large bowel mucosa as well as evaluation of other preneoplastic alterations (i.e., aberrant crypt foci) can serve as "intermediate biomarkers" for studying the effect of dietary intervention or chemoprevention in colorectal tumorigenesis [106].

The normal human colorectal mucosa is covered by mucinous and columnar cells; the proliferative zone is normally confined to the lower three-fourths of the colonic crypts; cells migrate towards the upper portions of the glands and then are extruded from the mucosal surface; the whole process takes 4–6 days [107]. In the early stages of colorectal carcinogenesis, colonic epithelial cells become unable to repress DNA synthesis during migration from the base to the surface of the crypt, and develop an enhanced capacity to proliferate [108]; consequently, the proliferative zone expands,

Fig. 1A–E. The adenoma-carcinoma sequence over the last 20 years. **A** The sequence in its simplest formulation; **B** the concept of "hyperproliferative mucosa" as an intermediate step to adenoma formation; **C** small and large adenomas, and the possible cocarcinogen effect of secondary bile acids; **D** the possible "alternative way" which includes aberrant crypt foci; **E** genetic events associated with the development of polyps and cancer of the large bowel

and S-phase cells are observed throughout the whole length of the gland. Two stages of alteration have been defined in flat mucosa; in the first, proliferative cells are seen in the whole crypt, but the area of higher proliferation is still confined to the lower portions; in the second, the zone of maximal kinetic activity is shifted to the upper portions of the crypts (stage I and II abnormalities, respectively) [106, 108]. An abnormal pattern of cell replication has been characterized in several clinical conditions associated with an increased risk of colorectal malignancy; these include patients with adenomatosis coli [108], members of families with inherited tumors [109], patients with sporadic adenomas [106, 110, 111], and ulcerative colitis [112], normal individuals older than 65 years [113], and patients with previous surgery for cancer of the large bowel [114].

Besides alterations of the replicative activity, intestinal cells progressing through different stages of premalignancies may show lack of terminal differentiation and modified gene structure or expression [106]; examples of these changes include an increased expression of Lewis antigens and of other blood-group-related antigens [115], an abnormal expression of K-*ras* and c-*myc* oncogenes [116, 117], and a modified response of cells to growth factors or tumor promoters [118].

A new preneoplastic lesion has recently been described by Bird et al. [119]. During experimental carcinogenesis, 2 or more weeks after treatment with azoxymethane or other carcinogens, darkly stained, enlarged, and slightly elevated crypts can be observed over the background of normal colorectal crypts after staining the mucosa with methylene blue. These "aberrant crypt foci" are relatively rare in human colorectal mucosa from normal individuals, while their number increases significantly in flat mucosa of patients with adenomatosis coli or, to a lesser extent, with sporadic colorectal cancer [120]. Since most aberrant crypts show evidence of dysplasia, the term "microadenoma" is frequently used to designate these lesions [121]. Recent animal studies [122] showed that the administration of retinoic acid reduces the number and the multiplicity of aberrant crypts in colonic mucosa, thus suggesting the possible use of these lesions as intermediate biomarkers in chemoprevention studies. Moreover, the kinetic properties of aberrant crypt foci in patients with colorectal neoplasms have recently been characterized with the in vivo administration of bromodeoxyuridine (a thymidine analogue) [123]. Thus, the available evidence suggests that aberrant crypt foci might represent a precursor lesion in the development of adenomatous polyps, and probably a valuable biomarker of increased susceptibility to colorectal cancer.

Interaction Between Environmental and Genetic Factors

One of the reasons which make the pathogenesis of colorectal cancer of particular interest when compared to many other neoplasms is the complex interaction between environmental and genetic factors. The importance of environment stems from various epidemiologic investigations [32, 33], animal experiments [1, 4], and case control studies [16–29], which focused on specific dietary components and different styles of life. On the other hand, the relevance of genetic factors was suggested by several observations indicating that colorectal cancer occurs more often in close relatives of affected patients than in the general population. Pedigree analysis has shown that there are syndromes in which colorectal tumors aggregate in families, and that transmission from one generation to another is consistent with an autosomal dominant pattern of inheritance. This has been described in hereditary nonpolyposis colorectal cancer and in adenomatosis coli, two genetically determined diseases where environmental agents presumably play a minor role in tumor development (see later sections, and next chapter). Apart from these well-defined syndromes – which account for a relatively modest fraction of all colorectal malignancies – tumor aggregation in families suggests that even some apparently sporadic forms of colorectal cancer may involve a genetic component; however, since no Mendelian pattern of inheritance could be discerned, the most likely type of transmission seems to be multifactorial [90, 124], which implicates a close interaction between exogenous agents and several genes for the full expression of a given trait (in this case, colorectal tumor).

Several studies showed a positive family history for colorectal neoplasms in 10%–20% of probands with either cancer or polyps of the large bowel [125, 126]. Thus, Woolf [127] compared the mortality rates in first-degree relatives of colorectal cancer patients with the rates of a matched control group; 26 deaths from large bowel cancer were observed among case relatives versus 8 deaths in control relatives (a 3.2 times higher mortality). Though using a slightly different experimental design, similar conclusions were also drawn by Macklin [128] and, subsequently, Lovett [129]. In a population-based study, Ponz de Leon et al. [90] found 37 cases of colorectal cancer among 1069 first-degree relatives of probands versus 5 cases in 1051 control relatives (relative risk, RR: 7.0; $P < 0.001$); moreover, the same excess of colorectal cancers among close relatives was also observed in patients with adenomatous polyps (35 versus 11 in controls; RR, 3.0, $P < 0.001$). Similarly, an increased risk of developing carcinomas of the large bowel in individuals with a positive family history of colorectal cancer has been reported by several other authors [130–133]. All these studies seem to suggest that if we exclude the small proportion of genetically determined colorectal tumors (3%–5% of the total) and the much larger fraction of "truly sporadic" carcinomas, then approximately 10%–20% of the commonly observed cancers of the large bowel might be attributed to polygenic inheritance [134]. This view has been challenged by Burt et al. [135, 136], who recently showed evidence suggesting a possible dominant inheritance also for patients with colonic neoplasms without features of Lynch syndrome. The authors carried out a systematic screening for colorectal neoplasms using flexible sigmoidoscopy; their findings, initially limited to a single large kindred, were subsequently extended to 34 families, with virtually identical results. The importance of these observations is primarily due to the fact that for the first time a Mendelian basis was suggested to explain the susceptibility to the commonly observed colorectal tumors. Similar conclusions were recently reached by Ponz de Leon et al. [137], who suggested that predisposition to cancer of the large bowel may be the result of a dominant gene with greatly reduced penetrance. The authors applied classical segregation analysis to the data of a population-based colorectal cancer registry; rather surprisingly, the study showed that colorectal carcinoma could be attributed to at least two genetically heterogeneous entities; in a small proportion of cases (4.6%, corresponding to hereditary nonpolyposis cancer families) inheritance was compatible with an autosomal dominant type of transmission with high penetrance; the remaining fraction (95.4%, representing sporadic plus "familial" cases) showed features of dominant transmission with greatly reduced penetrance. The possible genetic basis of virtually all cases of colorectal cancer does not exclude the role of environmental factors in the pathogenesis of the disease. It has already been discussed that several dietary factors together with lifestyle and various other conditions are closely related to these tumors; thus, we might assume that the genetic background determines which individuals in the general population are prone to develop cancer of the large bowel; subsequently, over the course of many years, environmental factors may interact with genes in susceptible persons determining the fraction of them who will become affected.

Hereditary Nonpolyposis Colorectal Cancer (Lynch Syndrome)

In hereditary nonpolyposis colorectal cancer (HNPCC) genetic factors are of major importance, while the role of environmental factors, if any, remains to be elucidated. Being relatively frequent in almost all populations, this syndrome poses several important problems concerning (a) its recognition and biological characterization, (b) the identification of susceptible individuals, (c) optimal treatment and follow-up of affected patients, and (d) choice of the most appropriate screening and surveillance program for subjects at risk of tumors.

Definition, History, and Clinical Features

Hereditary nonpolyposis colorectal cancer, or Lynch syndrome, is an autosomal dominant disease characterized by early appearance of tumors usually of the right colon, common occurrence of synchronous or metachronous neoplasms of the large bowel, and the frequent association with malignancies of other organs (in particular, endometrium, stomach, and skin). HNPCC was reported for the first time by Warthin, in 1913 [138]; the author described some families with multiple occurrence of gastric and colorectal carcinomas spanning three generations; cancers of the mouth, lip, uterus, and breast were also commonly observed; moreover, the tendency for these neoplasms to develop at an earlier age than that of sporadic tumors was also noticed. Some of these families were "revisited" 20 years later by Hauser and Waller [139], and subsequently by Lynch and Krush [140, 141], who described in great detail the clinical and genetic features of the syndrome. Because of the continued efforts of Henry T. Lynch, during the last 25 years, in expanding and updating the genealogical trees, and in promoting basic and clinical research on HNPCC virtually in all possible directions, the disease is also commonly referred to as Lynch syndrome.

In more detail, the main clinical features of Lynch syndrome can be summarized as follows. First, the disease shows aggregation of cancers and vertical transmission consistent with an autosomal dominant mode of inheritance; "skipped" generations are rare. Second, onset of cancer before the age of 45–50 years is particularly frequent in this syndrome, although this does not exclude the possible occurrence of tumors at an older age. Third, colorectal tumors are by far the most common malignancy in HNPCC, and approximately 70% of the cases are located in the proximal colon. Fourth, multiple tumors are extremely frequent (synchronous and/or metachronous lesions of the large bowel); in addition, colorectal tumors are often associated with malignancies of other organs. HNPCC may be further divided into: (a) "hereditary site-specific colorectal cancer" (Lynch syndrome type I), when colorectal tumor is the only cancer type observed and (b) "Lynch syndrome type II," when tumors of other organs (especially endometrium, stomach, skin, and a few others) are also present in a given family [142]. Other authors, however, did not find clinical evidence for this subdivision [143]. Representative pedigrees of families with Lynch syndrome I and II are shown in Figs. 2 and 3.

Although in many "typical" cases the diagnosis of Lynch syndrome can be reached without difficulty, in many other families the identification of HNPCC is extremely complex; this may be due to the fact that none of the above-mentioned criteria are definitive or discriminatory, and that no biochemical, morphologic, or genetic biomarkers are available. In addition, the usual small size of most modern families and the presence of phenocopies further complicate the identification of the disease. To obviate – at least in part – all these difficulties, a panel of experts recently suggested the following minimum criteria which should be met for a proper definition of HNPCC [144]: (a) At least three relatives should have histologically verified colorectal cancer, and one of them should be a first-degree relative to the other two; adenomatosis coli should be excluded. (b) At least two successive generations should be affected. (c) In one of the relatives colorectal cancer should be diagnosed under the age of 50 years. Despite some obvious

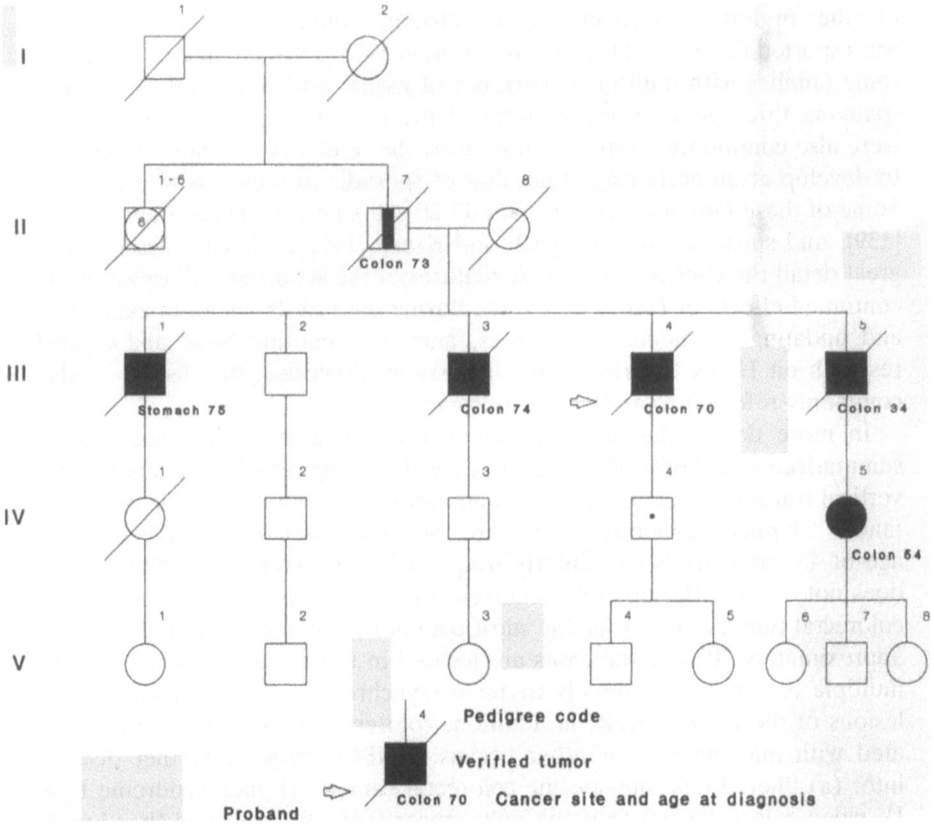

Fig. 2. Genealogical tree of a family with clinical features of Lynch syndrome I. Gastric cancer in *III-1* presumably represents a phenocopy, though two colonic cancers also developed after the age of 70 years

limitations (one might argue, for example, that these criteria are much more suitable for diagnosing Lynch syndrome I than Lynch syndrome II), the "Amsterdam criteria" (the panel of experts met in Amsterdam, The Netherlands, August 1990) appear of great help especially for studies of early detection and follow-up of HNPCC patients, whereas more extended pedigrees are usually needed for linkage studies.

Frequency of HNPCC

Although HNPCC has been described in many races and populations (white Americans, Europeans, and Australians, but also Japanese, Filipinos, and Indian Americans) [145–148], the real prevalence of the syndrome remains undefined. Mecklin et al. [149, 150] assessed the frequency of HNPCC

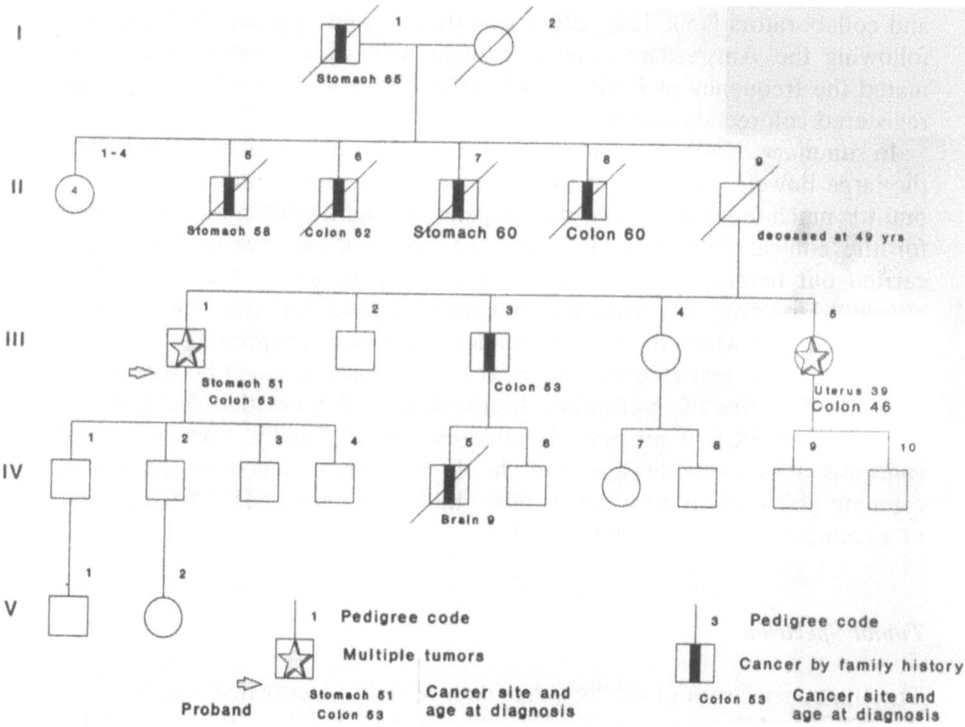

Fig. 3. Representative pedigree of a family with Lynch syndrome II. Two members of the same generation had multiple, verified malignancies at an early age of onset. Besides colonic cancer, gastric and endometrial carcinomas have aggregated in this family

through the data of the Finnish Cancer Registry (relative to a county of 250000 inhabitants, in middle Finland) during the period 1970–1979; according to their estimates, HNPCC was strongly suspected in 3.8%–5.5% of all patients with cancer of the large bowel. Westlake et al. [151] estimated a 3.4% frequency of Lynch syndrome among 390 colorectal cancer patients under the age of 50 years in southern Alberta (Canada). In this study, the diagnosis of HNPCC was established if colorectal cancer was present in at least three first-degree relatives from the same side of the family, and with the proband of less than 50 years; by using less strict criteria, 25 additional families could be included, increasing the overall frequency to 9.5% of all colorectal neoplasms. Rather surprisingly, Kee and Collins [152] found only 13 families with 3 or more members affected by colorectal cancers (including a proband of less than 55 years at diagnosis) out of 1241 cases of cancer of the large bowel diagnosed in Northern Ireland during the study period; these findings, therefore, correspond to a frequency of HNPCC ranging between 1% and 2% of all colorectal malignancies. Finally, Ponz de Leon and collaborators [153, 154] with a slightly different approach but basically following the Amsterdam criteria (though with some modifications) estimated the frequency of HNPCC in Northern Italy to be 3.4%–4.5% of all registered colorectal cancers.

In summary, HNPCC seems to account for 1%–5% of all malignancies of the large bowel; variations in the estimate might reflect ethnic differences, but it is much more likely that they depend on slightly different criteria used for the clinical definition of Lynch syndrome (these investigations were carried out before or immediately after the definition of the Amsterdam criteria). However, it is without doubt that "single cases" (i.e., those due to new mutations, which in the case of adenomatosis coli represent 20%–40% of all cases, see next chapter) escape our attention and might be recognized only with the use of appropriate biomarkers; it follows that the real frequency of HNPCC is presumably underestimated. Finally, since colorectal cancer is a frequent disease, one should not forget that even the lowest estimate (1%) would mean some 1000–1500 new cases of HNPCC per year in a country such as the United States.

Tumor Spectrum

The tumor spectrum of HNPCC has been widely investigated, especially in American and European series. Fitzgibbons et al. [155] examined the distribution of 334 cancers diagnosed in 10 extended families with Lynch syndrome; they found that colorectal tumors represented 55% of all cancers (183 out of 334) and endometrial carcinoma 14% (45 cases); both these tumor types were markedly more frequent than the rates expected in the general population. Gastric and skin tumors were also slightly more prevalent in HNPCC, whereas breast and especially lung tumors occurred less frequently. The study confirmed several other features of HNPCC: the mean age of onset of colorectal cancer was 45.6 years, and 69% of these were located in the right colon (proximally to the splenic flexure); in addition, synchronous and metachronous lesions of the large bowel occurred in 18% and 24% of patients, respectively. Vasen et al. [156] described the tumor spectrum of 24 Dutch families with HNPCC; as expected, colorectal cancers were by far the most frequent malignancies (mean age of onset, 46 years), and the only type of cancer observed in four families. Among extracolonic tumors, endometrial, gastric, and urinary tract carcinomas were found more frequently than expected, leading the authors to conclude that these cancer types were integral to the hereditary tumor spectrum of Lynch syndrome. A similar spectrum was reported by Mecklin et al. [157] in 22 Finnish HNPCC kindreds; in this survey, the mean age of onset of colorectal cancer was 41 years, with 54% of these neoplasms being localized in the proximal colon; moreover, multiple tumors were detected in 24% of the patients. Slightly different results were reported by Benatti et al. [154] in an

Italian series of 28 HNPCC families; colorectal cancer was by far the most common neoplasm (146 out of 245, or 59%), followed by gastric and endometrial carcinomas, respectively, whose frequency was not markedly different from that expected in the general population; in 3 families (10.7%) colorectal cancer was the only type of tumor. The mean age of onset of cancer of the large bowel was 56 years, with only 42% of these lesions being localized in the proximal colon; finally, multiple tumors were seen in 12% of the patients. In another large Italian kindred, Cristofaro et al. [158] reported a marked excess of gastric carcinoma (almost as frequent as colorectal cancer and with an early onset in all cases) and of chronic atrophic gastritis confined to the antrum. More recent studies showed the occurrence, in some HNPCC families, of early onset laryngeal carcinomas [159], bile duct tumors (cholangiocarcinoma), cancers of the urinary tract, and early onset pancreatic tumors [160, 161]. Finally, the frequency of specific types of cancer has been analyzed in members of 23 HNPCC families from the Omaha series [162]. The authors compared the observed numbers of cancers to the expected rates from tumor registries. The results showed that tumors of the stomach, small intestine, hepatobiliary system, kidney, uterus, and ovary all occurred significantly more often (odds ratio ranging from 3.2 for neoplasms of the kidney to 25 for small bower cancer) in high-risk HNPCC family members than in the general population.

In summary, tumor spectrum in HNPCC is not limited to a few neoplasms (i.e., colon-rectum, endometrium, skin, stomach) as shown in initial reports; indeed, the close observation of these families over many years revealed the frequent occurrence of many other unsuspected neoplasms, raising the possibility of a marked genetic heterogeneity of this syndrome. From a practical point of view, this progressively extending neoplastic spectrum complicates the clinical management and the surveillance program of HNPCC family members.

Biological Characterization

Among the features of Lynch syndrome there is the impression that the clinical course of the disease might be different from that of sporadic carcinomas, for the tendency to a more favorable prognosis. The suggestion of a better clinical outcome is mainly based on unchecked historical data [147, 163], and not on careful survival studies. Moreover, a recent study showed that a positive family history for colorectal cancer did not influence the prognosis of patients with large bowel tumors [164]. Two recent flow cytometric studies, however, showed a definite prevalence of diploid neoplasms in HNPCC patients, thus suggesting that this might be one of the features of colorectal carcinoma in Lynch syndrome [165, 166]. Since diploid tumors are usually associated with a better prognosis than aneuploid neoplasms [73, 74], predominance of the diploid pattern might partially explain the proposed more favorable outcome of colorectal malignancies in HNPCC. The issue, however, is much more complex and rather paradoxical, since various other morphologic features usually associated with a more aggressive clinical course seem to be more frequent in HNPCC; these include mucinous histologic type (present in approximately 40% of HNPCC patients in some series, versus 15%–20% of common colorectal carcinoma) and a poor degree of differentiation [147, 167, 168].

The fact that Lynch syndrome is designated as "nonpolyposis" colorectal cancer underlines the concept that the disease is different from adenomatosis coli, but does not imply the absolute absence of adenomas in the large bowel. Indeed, recent studies showed that the prevalence of adenomatous polyps in HNPCC is greater than in an unselected reference group (30% versus 11% in controls), and that polyps tend to be located more proximally, thus corresponding to the site of cancer distribution observed in HNPCC [169]. Moreover, Jass and Stewart [148] showed that adenomas can be found in 30%–40% of these patients, and that the lesions are often large and with a villous configuration. Taken together, these findings support the contention that adenomatous polyps represent premalignant lesions in HNPCC as well as in sporadic colorectal cancer.

Genetics of HNPCC

Since the gene responsible for HNPCC has not yet been identified, the clinical diagnosis of Lynch syndrome is still based on a careful evaluation of the family tree. In typical cases, vertical transmission and aggregation of early onset cancer can be observed in these families, in accordance with an autosomal dominant type of inheritance often with a high penetrance. To elucidate the role of a single gene in colorectal cancer susceptibility, segregation analysis was carried out in 11 extended families with HNPCC [170]; the results showed that there is no significant deviation from the Mendelian autosomal hypothesis, while both recessive model and absence of intergenerational transmission were rejected. The estimated gene frequency of the putative susceptibility allele was 0.015. Similar results were reported by Ponz de Leon et al. [137] in 28 families with a strong clinical suspicion of Lynch syndrome; maximum likelihood analysis showed that the observed segregation ratio was consistent with the hypothesis of autosomal dominant transmission, while other hypotheses were rejected. Burt et al. [135, 136] carried out a segregation analysis in 34 Utah kindreds (with a total of 670 individuals) characterized by clusters of close relatives with common colorectal cancer and/or adenomatous polyps; again, the results showed that an autosomal dominant type of inheritance could explain the susceptibility to both polyps and cancer. Besides the selection of families, the characteristic of this approach is that the authors gave the same relevance to the observed cancers and to adenomatous polyps; although this might appear logical (on the basis of the adenoma-carcinoma sequence) it is also true that only a small proportion of polyps undergo malignant transformation, while the majority remain benign or disappear.

The autosomal dominant transmission of HNPCC is further confirmed by anecdotal reports. In one of these [171], an asymptomatic "obligate carrier" was identified in a large family with all the clinical features of Lynch syndrome; the father of this patient had multiple tumors (colon and bladder), while the son developed colonic cancer at age 28 years; when this obligate carrier underwent colonoscopy, a partially obstructing neoplasm of the transverse colon was found.

Treatment and Follow-up

Following the suggestion of Lynch and collaborators [155], most investigators recommend subtotal colectomy with ileorectal anastomosis for newly diagnosed colonic cancer in HNPCC, although right (or left) hemicolectomy with careful endoscopic surveillance may appear as a reasonable alternative. In addition, the high risk of endometrial cancer suggests prophylactic hysterectomy at the time of surgery for large bowel cancer or, alternatively, biannual pelvic (or intravaginal) ultrasounds and annual endometrial aspiration biopsy. After the operation, patients should be monitored with frequent (biannual) endoscopic controls of the remaining large bowel; moreover, an individualized surveillance program should be developed on the basis of the tumor spectrum observed in each specific family.

Subjects at risk of cancer in HNPCC families should be screened and followed up at regular intervals; however, no standard protocol has been developed, and the strategies adopted by various centers may be different, in relation to: (a) availability of resources, (b) medical and cultural traditions, (c) observed tumor spectrum [155, 172–175], (d) pattern of cancer occurrence in the follow-up [176, 177], and (e) biological features of the neoplasms. As an example, these are the major guidelines proposed by the Colorectal Cancer Study Group of the University of Modena, Italy, for the follow-up of high-risk subjects in HNPCC families [154]:

1. Pancolonoscopy remains the most important investigation, and should be recommended to all individuals at risk, usually beginning at the age of 25 years and then repeating the examination every 2–3 years.
2. Gastroscopy is suggested only to those families in which cases of gastric cancer have been reported, especially if at an early onset or developed during the last 20 years.
3. Gynecologic investigation and lower abdominal ultrasounds are suggested for all women at risk, but especially in families with cases of endometrial or other gynecologic cancers.
4. More specific procedures (such as urography, cholangiography, or computed tomography) are proposed more rarely, and in a few families only.

5. Finally, since the genetic nature of the disease does not exclude the possible role of environmental factors, the authors recommend modification of dietary habits (by increasing the amount of fiber, vegetables, and fruit, and reducing the intake of animal fat and meat), to avoid obesity, and to spend more time in physical activity.

Genetic Alterations in Colorectal Cancer Progression

The clinical, biological, and epidemiologic observations which support the existence of an adenoma-carcinoma sequence in colorectal tumorigenesis have already been discussed in detail (Fig. 1). It is worth noting that unlike the situation for other common malignancies, colorectal cancer development appears as an ordered multistep process in which tumors of various stages of progression – from very small polyps to invasive carcinoma – can be obtained for investigation; this particular biological behavior provided an excellent system for analyzing the genetic abnormalities involved in tumor formation.

Studies over the past 10 years allowed the formulation of a genetic model for colorectal tumorigenesis [104, 178], interpreted as a multistep process in which the various phases of tumor development seem to be the consequence of genetic alterations, involving mutational activation of oncogenes coupled with mutation or loss of tumor suppressor genes (Fig. 1). According to this model, a small number of genetic changes might be sufficient for inducing the appearance of benign adenomas, whereas five to six mutations (or even more) would be required for the full manifestation of the malignant phenotype. Moreover, although these alterations seem to follow a preferred sequence, it is the overall accumulation of genetic changes, more than their ordered sequence, which is responsible for cancer development and for determining the biological characteristics of the neoplasm.

The majority of the biomolecular investigations have been carried out in apparently sporadic colorectal cancer; more recent studies, however, seem to suggest that some genetic changes and their biological sequence might be different in sporadic and in hereditary tumors; consequently, common neoplasms of the large bowel and tumors occurring in Lynch syndrome will be discussed separately.

Sporadic Colorectal Tumors

Various cytogenetic studies showed that chromosome 5q, 17p, and 18q were frequently altered in colorectal carcinoma in both numerical and structural aspects, while abnormalities of other chromosomes were observed less frequently [179–181]. These findings are of considerable interest, since they represent a further demonstration that the simple morphologic observation of chromosome structure may provide valuable information on the presumable localization of oncogenes and tumor suppressor genes involved in tumorigenesis. Partial or complete monosomy 18, deletion of the short arm of chromosome 17, reciprocal translocation between chromosomes 5 and 17, pericentric inversion, and other rearrangements of chromosome 5 were the most frequent of these karyotypic changes [179–182].

Oncogenes frequently altered in colorectal tumorigenesis include K-*ras*, c-*myc*, c-*erbB-2*, c-*myb*, and c-*src* [183]. Point mutations in codon 12, 13, or 61 of K-*ras* have been found in 40%–70% of colorectal malignancies and in about 40% of adenomas [178, 184–186]; although K-*ras* mutations might be the initiating event in a fraction of colorectal tumors, small adenomas may progress to large adenomas and to invasive cancer also without *ras* mutations [10]. Amplification, overexpression, or rearrangements of other oncogenes have also been frequently reported in colorectal tumors [183, 187, 188]; however, the available evidence does not suggest a major role for changes of these genes in colorectal cancer formation [104].

Tumor suppressor genes more directly involved in colorectal cancer development include *APC* and *MCC* (located on chromosome 5q), *p53* (chromosome 17p), and *DCC* (chromosome 18q). *APC* is abnormal in the germline cells of patients with adenomatosis coli [189, 190], so that the syndrome is likely to be determined by point mutations (or other changes) of this gene (see next chapter). Moreover, recent sequence analysis [191] showed point mutations of the *APC* gene in 63% of sporadic colorectal adenomas; since these mutations were found in tumors as small as 5 mm and, more important, tended to remain stable during tumor progression from adenoma to carcinoma, these findings strongly indicate that *APC* mutations might play a determinant role in the early phases of colorectal tumorigenesis.

MCC (for "mutated in colorectal carcinoma") is a large gene, localized on the long arm of chromosome 5 (5q21, close to *APC*), which has been implicated in the pathogenesis of sporadic colorectal cancer [192]. Various alterations of *MCC* – including point mutations and deletions – have been found in more than 50% of large bowel cancers [183, 193], although it is not yet clear if they represent early or late events in colorectal tumorigenesis. In addition, loss of heterozygosity of both *APC* and *MCC* has recently been reported in a large proportion of lung cancers and in the majority of human esophageal carcinomas [194, 195], thus suggesting that inactivation of these genes (or of a linked gene on chromosome 5q) might play a role also in the development of other types of tumors, and should not be viewed as genetic events exclusively associated with colonic cancer and familial polyposis.

DCC (for "deleted in colorectal carcinoma") is a putative tumor suppressor gene which has recently been identified on the long arm of chromosome 18 [196]. Deletions affecting the gene locus were detected in about 70% of colorectal carcinomas but only in a low proportion of adenomas of various size [178]; it follows that these genetic alterations represent late events in colorectal tumorigenesis, presumably associated with the development of locally invasive or metastatic carcinoma. In keeping with these observations, Yanoshita et al. [197] showed that mRNA transcripts of the *DCC* gene are present in normal colonic mucosa and in adenomas, while the gene is frequently unexpressed in invasive colorectal cancer. Rather interestingly, the *DCC* gene product specifies a protein with sequence similarities to neural cell adhesion molecules, which indicates a possible role of this gene product in regulating cell-environment interaction.

p53 is the tumor suppressor gene more frequently mutated in human tumors [198], and colorectal carcinoma is not an exception. Thus, several authors showed loss of heterozygosity at *17p* and mutations of *p53* in a large proportion of colorectal cancers [178, 198–200]. The usual pattern is point mutations of one allele (more often in the evolutionary conserved region of the gene) coupled with loss of the remaining wild-type allele [201, 202]. It has been hypothesized that *p53* inhibits tumor growth, and that mutation of one allele followed by deletion of the remaining wild-type allele leads to the inactivation of the gene, which cannot suppress further tumor progression. Alternatively, but with a similar ultimate result, the expression product of the mutated gene can bind the normal p53 protein and sequester it in a biologically inactive product, thus preventing its normal interaction with other cellular constituents [104]. The frequency of *p53* mutations in infiltrating colorectal carcinoma [201, 202] contrasts with the rarity of mutations in adenomas (about 5% of the total) [203] and with the lack of reports on germline *p53* alterations in patients with large bowel tumors; it follows that these mutations presumably represent late events in tumorigenesis, which seem more closely related to tumor progression and to the acquisition of the invasive pattern of growth, than to the development of early neoplastic lesions (i.e., aberrant crypt foci and adenomas). In line with this contention, two recent studies [204, 205] showed that allelic deletion on the short arm of chromosome 17 was an independent indicator of poor clinical outcome in patients with Dukes' B or C colorectal carcinoma.

Finally, in addition to the genetic alterations which occur more frequently in colorectal neoplasms (i.e., *ras* mutations, losses, and/or mutations of *APC*, *MCC*, *DCC*, and *p53*), other genetic abnormalities might play a certain role in deregulating tumor cell growth or in promoting metastases. These include: (a) allelic deletions at several other chromosomal loci, including 1q, 8p, 11q, 13q, and 14q [206–211]; (b) overexpression of the c-*met* oncogene [212]; (c) deletions of the *nm23* gene, which seem to be strongly related to the development of the metastatic phenotype [213]; and (d) amplification and overexpression of the cyclin genes [214].

Hereditary Nonpolyposis Colorectal Cancer

Owing to the difficulty of identifying Lynch syndrome in the general population, there are only few studies on the biological characterization and the molecular biology of hereditary colorectal tumors. Aaltonen et al., however, recently reported that mutations in K-*ras*, *p53*, and *APC* genes occurred with the same frequency in sporadic and hereditary colorectal tumors [215]. Many of the genetically determined neoplasms, however, showed widespread alterations in short repeated DNA sequences, indicating that various replication errors had occurred during tumor development, and suggesting that a certain genetic instability is presumably a component of the hereditary cancer phenotype. Although these observations are still preliminary and should therefore be interpreted with caution, they might be of major practical interest for the characterization of hereditary tumors and, more generally, for the identification of subjects at genetic risk of colorectal neoplasms.

The search for the gene responsible for HNPCC has been in vain for many years. Thus, Peltomaki et al. [216], by linkage analysis, excluded that the *DCC* gene could be considered as the HNPCC susceptibility locus in five large Finnish families with the classical clinical features of Lynch syndrome. One year later, the same authors found no evidence that the *MCC-APC* gene region, on chromosome 5q21, could be the site for a putative *HNPCC* gene [217]. Similarly, Bhagirat et al. [218] were unable to find constitutional *p53* mutations in patients meeting the clinical criteria of HNPCC. At variance with these negative results, more recent studies [215, 219] in two large families with HNPCC found a close linkage of the disease to a microsatellite marker (*D2S123*), which had been mapped to chromosome 2p15–16 by in situ hybridization. However, no linkage was found in various other families with clinical features of HNPCC; in addition, no loss of heterozygosity for chromosome 2 markers could be detected. Thus, preliminary results seem to indicate that the gene responsible for HNPCC (*COCA1*) might be located on the short arm of chromosome 2, at least in some of these families.

References

1. Weisburger JH, Wynder EL (1987) Etiology of colorectal cancer with emphasis on mechanisms of action and prevention. In: Devita VT, Hellman S, Rosenberg SA (eds) Important advances in oncology. Lippincott, Philadelphia, pp 197–200
2. Zanetti R, Crosignani P (1992) Cancer in Italy: incidence data from cancer registries 1983–1987. Lega Italiana per la Lotta contro i Tumori, Torino
3. Waterhouse J, Muir C, Shanmugaratnam K et al. (1982) Cancer in five continents. International Agency for Research on Cancer, Lyon, pp 680–681, 710–713 (IARC scientific publication, no 42)
4. Weisburger JH (1991) Causes, relevant mechanisms, and prevention of large bowel cancer. Semin Oncol 18:316–336
5. Doll R, Peto R (1981) The causes of cancer: quantitative estimates of avoidable risk of cancer in the United States today. JNCI 66:1191–1308
6. Devesa SS, Chow WH (1993) Variation in colorectal cancer incidence in the USA by subsite and origin. Cancer 71:3819–3826
7. Johansen C, Mellemgaard A, Skov T et al. (1993) Colorectal cancer in Denmark 1943–1988. Int J Colorectal Dis 8:42–47

8. Tajima K, Hirose K, Nakagawa N et al. (1985) Urban-rural difference in the trend of colorectal cancer mortality with special reference to the subsites of colon cancer in Japan. Gann 76:717–728
9. Beart RW, Melton LJ, Maruta M et al. (1983) Trends in right and left-sided colon cancer. Am Soc Colon Rect Surg 26:393–398
10. Cady B, Stone MD, Wayne J (1993) Continuing trends in the prevalence of right-sided lesions among colorectal carcinomas. Arch Surg 128:505–509
11. World Health Organization (1986) Statistic annals, 1979–85. World Health Organization, Geneva
12. Moller Jensen O (1984) Different age and sex relationship for cancer of subsites of the large bowel. Br J Cancer 50:825–829
13. Ponz de Leon M, Sacchetti C, Sassatelli R et al. (1990) Evidence for the existence of different types of large bowel tumor: suggestions from the clinical data of a population-based registry. J Surg Oncol 44:35–43
14. Daling JR, Weiss NS, Hislop TG et al. (1987) Sexual practices, sexually transmitted diseases, and the incidence of anal cancer. N Engl J Med 317: 973–977
15. Daniell HW (1985) Causes of anal carcinoma. JAMA 254:358
16. Levin B (1992) Nutrition and colorectal cancer. Cancer 70:1723–1726
17. Steinmetz KA, Potter JD (1993) Food group consumption and colon cancer risk in the Adelaide case-control study. Int J Cancer 53:720–727
18. Kreger BE, Anderson KM, Schatzkin A et al. (1992) Serum cholesterol levels, body mass index, and the risk of colon cancer. Cancer 70:1038–1043
19. Min-Lee I, Paffenbarger RS (1992) Quetelet's index and risk of colon cancer in college alumni. JNCI 84:1326–1331
20. Choi SY, Kahyo H (1991) Effect of cigarette smoking and alcohol consumption in the etiology of cancers of the digestive tract. Int J Cancer 49:381–386
21. Winawer SJ, Shike M (1992) Dietary factors in colorectal cancer and their possible effects on earliest stages of hyperproliferation and adenoma formation. JNCI 84:74–75
22. Sakaguchi M, Minoura T, Hiramatsu Y et al. (1986) Effect of dietary saturated and unsaturated fatty acids on colon carcinogenesis induced by azoxymethane in rats. Cancer Res 46:61–65
23. Steinmetz KA, Potter JD (1993) Food-group consumption and colon cancer risk in the Adelaide study: vegetables and fruit. Int J Cancer 53:711–719
24. Little J, Logan RFA, Hawtin PG et al. (1993) Colorectal adenomas and diet: a case-control study of subjects participating in the Nottingham programme. Br J Cancer 67:177–184
25. Benito E, Stiggelbout A, Bosch FX et al. (1991) Nutritional factors in colorectal cancer risk: a case-control study in Majorca. Int J Cancer 49:161–167
26. Bidoli E, Franceschi S, Talamini R et al. (1992) Food consumption and cancer of the colon and rectum in North-Eastern Italy. Int J Cancer 50:223–229
27. Arbman G, Axelson O, Ericsson-Begodzki AB et al. (1992) Cereal fiber, calcium, and colorectal cancer. Cancer 69:2042–2048
28. Macquart-Moulin G, Riboli E, Cornee J et al. (1986) Case-control study on colorectal cancer and diet in Marseilles. Int J Cancer 38:183–191
29. Ponz de Leon M, Biasco G (1987) Polyps of the large bowel: can their recurrence be prevented? Ital J Gastroenterol 19:164–167
30. Lipkin M, Newmark H (1985) Effect of added dietary calcium on colonic epithelial cell proliferation in subjects at high risk for familial colonic cancer. N Engl J Med 313:1381–1384
31. Bresalier RS, Kim YS (1985) Diet and colon cancer. N Engl J Med 313:1413–1414

32. Haenszel W (1982) Migrant studies. In: Schottenfeld D, Fraumeni JF (eds) Cancer epidemiology and prevention. Saunders, Philadelphia, pp 194–207
33. McMichael AJ, McCall MG, Hartshorne JM et al. (1980) Patterns of gastro-intestinal cancer in European migrants to Australia: the role of dietary changes. Int J Cancer 25:431–437
34. Phillips R, Snowdon DA (1985) Dietary relationship with fatal colorectal cancer among Seventh-Day Adventists. JNCI 74:307–317
35. Bal DG, Foerster SB (1991) Changing the American diet. Cancer 67:2671–2680
36. Garabrant DH, Peters JM, Mack TM et al. (1984) Job activity and colon cancer risk. Am J Epidemiol 119:1005–1014
37. Gehardsson M, Norell SE, Kiviranta H et al. (1986) Sedentary job and colon cancer. Am J Epidemiol 123:775–780
38. Gerhardsson M, Steineck G, Hagman U et al. (1990) Physical activity and colon cancer: a case-referent study in Stockholm. Int J Cancer 46:985–989
39. Min-Lee I, Paffenbarger RS, Hsieh CC (1991) Physical activity and risk of developing colorectal cancer among college alumni. JNCI 83:1324–1329
40. Hamilton SR (1985) Colorectal carcinoma in patients with Crohn's disease. Gastroenterology 89:398–407
41. Langholz E, Munkholm P, Davidsen M et al. (1992) Colorectal cancer risk and mortality in patients with ulcerative colitis. Gastroenterology 103:1444–1451
42. Stefànsson T, Ekbom A, Sparèn P et al. (1993) Increased risk of left sided colon cancer in patients with diverticular disease. Gut 34:499–502
43. Lowenfels AB, Domellòf L, Lindstrom CG et al. (1982) Cholelithiasis, chole-cystectomy and cancer. Gastroenterology 83:672–676
44. Suadicani P, Hein HO, Gyntelberg F (1993) Is the use of antihypertensives and sedatives a major risk factor for colorectal cancer? Scand J Gastroenterol 28:475–481
45. Gerard A, Bleiberg H (1987) Delay in diagnosis of colorectal cancer. Eur J Cancer Clin Oncol 23:1089–1090
46. Robinson E, Mohilever J, Zidan J et al. (1986) Colorectal cancer: incidence, delay in diagnosis and stage of disease. Eur J Cancer Clin Oncol 22:157–161
47. Ponz de Leon M, Sant M, Micheli A et al. (1992) Clinical and pathologic prognostic indicators in colorectal cancer. Cancer 69:626–635
48. Minsky BD, Mies C, Rich TA et al. (1987) Colloid carcinoma of the colon and rectum. Cancer 60:3103–3112
49. Dukes CE (1932) The classification of cancer of the rectum. J Pathol Bacteriol 35:1489–1494
50. Cooper HS, Slemmer JR (1991) Surgical pathology of carcinoma of the colon and rectum. Semin Oncol 18:367–380
51. Hutter RVP, Sobin LH (1986) A universal staging system for cancer of the colon and rectum. Arch Pathol Lab Med 110:367–368
52. Niederhuber JE (1993) Colon and rectum cancer: pattern of spread and implications for workup. Cancer 71:4187–4192
53. Kune GA, Kune S, Field B et al. (1990) Survival in patients with large bowel cancer. Dis Colon Rectum 33:938–946
54. Griffin MR, Bergstralh EJ, Coffey RJ et al. (1987) Predictors of survival after curative resection of carcinoma of the colon and rectum. Cancer 60:2318–2324
55. Orkin BA, Dozois RR, Beart RW et al. (1989) Extended resection for locally advanced primary adenocarcinoma of the rectum. Dis Colon Rectum 32: 286–292
56. Michelassi F, Vannucci L, Ayala JJ et al. (1990) Local recurrence after curative resection of colorectal carcinoma. Surgery 108:787–793

57. Pheils MT, Chapuis PH, Newland RC et al. (1983) Local recurrence following curative resection for carcinoma of the rectum. Dis Colon Rectum 26:98–102
58. Amato A, Pescatori M, Butti A (1991) Local recurrence following abdominoperineal excision and anterior resection for rectal carcinoma. Dis Colon Rectum 34:317–322
59. Kemeny N, Braun DW Jr (1983) Prognostic factors in advanced colorectal carcinoma. Am J Med 74:786–796
60. Hannisdal E, Thorsen G (1988) Regression analyses of prognostic factors in colorectal cancer. J Surg Oncol 37:109–112
61. Wiggers T, Arends JW, Schutte B et al. (1988) A multivariate analysis of pathologic prognostic indicators in large bowel cancer. Cancer 61:386–395
62. Wiggers T, Arends JW, Volovics A et al. (1988) Regression analysis of prognostic factors in colorectal cancer after curative resection. Dis Colon Rectum 31:33–41
63. Rigby CS, Subramony C, Kukora JS (1983) Carcinoma of the colon and rectum in adolescents and young adults. Surg Gastroenterol 2:283–288
64. Chapuis PH, Dent OF, Fisher R et al. (1985) A multivariate analysis of clinical and pathologic variables in the prognosis after resection of large bowel cancer. Br J Surg 72:698–702
65. Svendsen LB, Sorensen C, Kjersgaard et al. (1989) The influence of age upon the survival after curative operation for colorectal cancer. Int J Colorectal Dis 4:123–127
66. Isbister WH, Fraser J (1990) Large bowel cancer in the young: a national survival study. Dis Colon Rectum 33:363–366
67. Jass JR, Atkin WS, Cuzic J et al. (1986) The grading of rectal cancer: historical perspectives and a multivariate analysis of 447 cases. Histopathology 10: 437–459
68. Stahle E, Enblad P, Pàhlman L et al. (1989) Can mortality from rectal and rectosigmoid carcinoma be predicted from histopathological variables in the diagnostic biopsy? APMIS 97:513–522
69. Halvorsen TB, Seim E (1988) Degree of differentiation in colorectal adenocarcinoma: a multivariate analysis of the influence on survival. J Clin Pathol 41:532–537
70. Fisher ER, Rockette H, Jones J et al. (1989) Prognostic significance of eosinophils and mast cells in rectal cancer. Hum Pathol 20:159–163
71. Shepherd NA, Saraga EP, Love SB et al. (1989) Prognostic factors in colonic cancer. Histopathology 14:613–620
72. Moore PA, Dilawari RA, Fidler WJ (1984) Adenocarcinoma of the colon and rectum in patients less than 40 years of age. Am Surg 50:10–14
73. Armitage NC, Robins RA, Evans DF et al. (1985) The influence of tumor cell DNA abnormalities on survival in colorectal carcinoma. Br J Surg 72:828–830
74. Emdin SO, Stenling R, Roos G (1987) Prognostic value of DNA content in colorectal carcinoma. Cancer 60:1282–1287
75. Goh HS, Jass JR, Atkin WS et al. (1987) Value of flow cytometry determination of ploidy as a guide to prognosis in operable rectal cancer. Int J Colorectal Dis 2:17–21
76. Giaretti W, Danova M, Geido E et al. (1991) Flow cytometry DNA index in the prognosis of colorectal carcinoma. Cancer 67:1921–1927
77. Meyer JS, Prioleau PG (1981) S-phase fraction of colorectal carcinomas related to pathologic and clinical features. Cancer 48:1221–1228
78. Schutte B, Reynders MMJ, Wiggers T et al. (1987) Retrospective analysis of the prospective significance of DNA content and proliferative activity in large bowel carcinoma. Cancer Res 47:5494–5496

79. Johnston PG, O'Brien MJ, Dervan PA et al. (1989) Immunohistochemical analysis of cell kinetic parameters in colonic adenocarcinomas, adenomas, and normal mucosa. Hum Pathol 20:696–799
80. Al-Sheneber IF, Shibata HR, Sampalis J et al. (1993) Prognostic significance of PCNA expression in colorectal cancer. Cancer 71:1954–1959
81. Polk HC (1972) Extended resection for selected adenocarcinomas of the large bowel. Ann Surg 175:892–899
82. Brief DK, Brener BJ, Goldenkranz B et al. (1983) An argument for increased use of subtotal colectomy in the management of carcinoma of the colon. Am Surg 49:66–72
83. Moertel CG, Fleming TR, MacDonald JS et al. (1990) Levamisole and fluorouracil for adjuvant therapy of resected colon carcinoma. N Eng J Med 322: 352–358
84. Kane MJ (1991) Adjuvant systemic treatment for carcinoma of the colon and rectum. Semin Oncol 18:421–442
85. Metzger U (1990) Adjuvant therapy for colon and rectal cancer. Eur J Cancer 26:753–755
86. Mohiuddin M, Marks G (1991) Adjuvant radiation therapy for colon and rectal cancer. Semin Oncol 18:411–420
87. Morson BC, Dowson IM (1979) Gastrointestinal pathology, 2nd edn. Blackwell Scientific, Oxford
88. Morson BC, Bussey HJR, Day WD et al. (1983) Adenomas of the large bowel. Cancer Surv 2:451–477
89. Cajucom CC, Barrios GG, Cruz L et al. (1992) Prevalence of colorectal polyps in Filipinos. Dis Colon Rectum 35:676–680
90. Ponz de Leon M, Antonioli A, Ascari A et al. (1987) Incidence and familial occurrence of colorectal cancer and polyps in a Health Care District of Northern Italy. Cancer 60:2848–2859
91. Williams AR, Balasooriya BAW, Day DW (1982) Polyps and cancer of the large bowel: a necroscopy study, in Liverpool. Gut 23:835–842
92. Jass JR, Young PJ, Robinson EM (1992) Predictors of presence, multiplicity, size and dysplasia of colorectal adenomas. A necroscopy study in New Zealand. Gut 33:1508–1514
93. Bedenne L, Faivre J, Boutron MC et al. (1992) Adenoma-carcinoma sequence or "de novo" carcinogenesis? Cancer 69:883–888
94. Muto T, Bussey HJR, Morson BC (1975) The evolution of cancer of the colon and rectum. Cancer 36:2251–2270
95. Kyzer S, Bègin LR, Gordon PH et al. (1992) The care of patients with colorectal polyps that contain invasive adenocarcinoma. Cancer 70:2044–2050
96. Gilbertsen VA (1974) Proctosigmoidoscopy, polypectomy and rectal cancer. Cancer 34:936–939
97. Selby JV, Friedman GD, Queensberry CJ et al. (1992) A case-control study of screening sigmoidoscopy and mortality from colorectal cancer. N Engl J Med 326:653–657
98. Atkin WS, Cuzick J, Northover JMA et al. (1993) Prevention of colorectal cancer by once-only sigmoidoscopy. Lancet 341:736–740
99. Stryker SJ, Wolff BG, Culp CE et al. (1987) Natural history of untreated colonic polyps. Gastroenterology 93:1009–1013
100. Simons BD, Morrison AS, Lev R et al. (1992) Relationship of polyps to cancer of the large intestine. JNCI 84:962–966
101. Heald RJ, Bussey HJR (1975) Clinical experience at St Mark's hospital with multiple synchronous cancers of the colon and rectum. Dis Colon Rectum 18:6–10

102. Giovannucci E, Stampfer MJ, Colditz G et al. (1992) Relationship of diet to risk of colorectal adenoma in men. JNCI 84:91–98
103. Hill MJ, Morson BC, Bussey HJR (1978) Aetiology of adenoma-carcinoma sequence in large bowel. Lancet 1:245–247
104. Fearon ER, Vogelstein B (1990) A genetic model for colorectal tumorigenesis. Cell 61:759–767
105. Deschner EE (1980) Cell proliferation as a biomarker in human colorectal neoplasia. In: Winawer S, Schottenfeld D, Sherlock P (eds) Colorectal cancer: prevention, epidemiology and screening. Raven, New York, pp 133–142
106. Lipkin M (1988) Biomarkers of increased susceptibility to gastrointestinal cancer: new application to studies of cancer prevention in human subjects. Cancer Res 48:235–245
107. Lipkin M, Bell B, Sherlock P (1963) Cell proliferation kinetics in the gastrointestinal tract of men. I. Cell renewal in colon and rectum. J Clin Invest 42:767–776
108. Deschner EE, Lipkin M (1975) Proliferative pattern in colonic mucosa in familial polyposis. Cancer 35:413–418
109. Lipkin M, Blattner WE, Fraumeni JF et al. (1983) Tritiated thymidine labeling distribution as a marker for hereditary predisposition to colon cancer. Cancer Res 43:1899–1904
110. Ponz de Leon M, Roncucci L, Di Donato P et al. (1988) Pattern of epithelial cell proliferation in colorectal mucosa of normal subjects and of patients with adenomatous polyps or cancer of the large bowel. Cancer Res 48:4121–4126
111. Anti M, Marra G, Armelao F et al. (1993) Rectal epithelial cell proliferation patterns as predictors of adenomatous colorectal polyps recurrence. Gut 34:525–530
112. Deschner EE, Winawer SJ, Katz S et al. (1983) Proliferative defects in ulcerative colitis patients. Cancer Invest 1:41–47
113. Roncucci L, Ponz de Leon M, Scalmati A et al. (1988) The influence of age on colonic epithelial cell proliferation. Cancer 62:2373–2377
114. Scalmati A, Roncucci L, Ghedini G et al. (1990) Epithelial cell kinetics in the remaining colorectal mucosa after surgery for cancer of the large bowel. Cancer Res 50:7937–7941
115. Cordon-Cardo C, Lloyd KO, Sakamoto J et al. (1986) Immunohistologic expression of blood group antigens in normal human gastrointestinal tract and colonic carcinoma. Int J Cancer 37:667–676
116. Jacoby RF, Llor X, Teng BB et al. (1991) Mutations in the K-ras oncogene induced by 1,2-dimethylhydrazine in preneoplastic and neoplastic rat colonic mucosa. J Clin Invest 87:624–630
117. Melhem MF, Meisler AI, Finley GG et al. (1992) Distribution of cells expressing myc proteins in human colorectal epithelium, polyps, and malignant tumors. Cancer Res 52:5353–5864
118. Friedman E (1981) Differential response of premalignant epithelial cell classes to phorbol ester tumor promoters and to deoxycholic acid. Cancer Res 41:4588–4599
119. Bird RP, McLellan EA, Bruce WR (1989) Aberrant crypts, putative precancerous lesions, in the study of the role of diet in the aetiology of colon cancer. Cancer Surv 8:189–200
120. Roncucci L, Stamp D, Medline A et al. (1991) Identification and quantification of aberrant crypt foci and microadenomas in the human colon. Hum Pathol 22:287–294

121. Roncucci L, Medline A, Bruce WR (1991) Classification of aberrant crypt foci and microadenomas in human colon. Cancer Epidemiol Biomark Prevent 1: 57–60
122. Stopera SA, Bird RR (1993) Effects of all-trans retinoic acid as potential chemopreventive agent on the formation of azoxymethane-induced aberrant crypt foci. Int J Cancer 53:798–804
123. Roncucci L, Pedroni M, Fante R et al. (1993) Cell kinetics evaluation of human colonic aberrant crypts. Cancer Res 53:3726–3729
124. Ponz de Leon M, Sassatelli R, Sacchetti C et al. (1989) Familial aggregation of tumors in the 3-year experience of a population-based colorectal cancer registry. Cancer Res 49:4344–4348
125. Bishop TD, Thomas HJW (1990) The genetics of colorectal cancer. Cancer Surv 9584–9604
126. St John DJB, McDermott FT, Hopper JL et al. (1993) Cancer risk in relatives of patients with common colorectal cancer. Ann Intern Med 118:785–790
127. Woolf CM (1958) A genetic study of carcinoma of the large bowel. Am J Hum Genet 10:42–47
128. Macklin MT (1960) Inheritance of cancer of the stomach and large intestine in man. JNCI 24:551–571
129. Lovett E (1976) Family studies in cancer of the colon and rectum. Br J Surg 63:13–18
130. Duncan JL, Kyle J (1982) Family incidence of carcinoma of the colon and rectum in North-East Scotland. Gut 23:169–171
131. Rozen P, Lynch HT, Figer A et al. (1987) Familial colon cancer in the Tel-Aviv area and the influence of ethnic origin. Cancer 60:2355–2359
132. Bonelli L, Martines H, Conio M et al. (1988) Family history of colorectal cancer as a risk factor for benign and malignant tumours of the large bowel. A case control study. Int J Cancer 41:513–517
133. La Vecchia C, Negri E, Franceschi S et al. (1992) Family history and the risk of stomach and colorectal cancer. Cancer 70:50–55
134. Lynch HT, Kimberling W, Albano WA et al. (1985) Hereditary nonpolyposis colorectal cancer. I. Clinical description and resources. Cancer 56:934–938
135. Burt RW, Bishop TD, Cannon LA et al. (1985) Dominant inheritance of adenomatous colonic polyps and colorectal cancer. N Engl J Med 312:1540–1544
136. Cannon-Albright L, Skolnick MH, Bishop TD et al. (1988) Common inheritance of susceptibility to colonic adenomatous polyps and associated colorectal cancers. N Engl J Med 319:533–537
137. Ponz de Leon M, Scapoli C, Zanghieri G et al. (1992) Genetic transmission of colorectal cancer: exploratory data analysis from a population-based registry. J Med Genet 29:531–538
138. Warthin AS (1913) Heredity with reference to carcinoma. Arch Int Med 12:546–555
139. Hauser IJ, Weller CV (1936) A further report on the cancer family of Warthin. Am J Cancer 26:434–449
140. Lynch HT, Krush AJ (1967) Heredity and adenocarcinoma of the colon. Gastroenterology 53:517–527
141. Lynch HT, Krush AJ (1971) Cancer Family G revisited: 1895–1970. Cancer 27:1505–1511
142. Lynch HT (1986) Frequency of hereditary nonpolyposis colorectal cancer. Gastroenterology 90:486–489
143. Mecklin JP, Jarvinen HJ (1991) Tumor spectrum in cancer family syndrome. Cancer 68:1109–1112

144. Vasen HFA, Mecklin JP, Meera Khan P, Lynch TH (1991) The International Collaborative Study Group on Hereditary Non-polyposis Colorectal Cancer. Dis Colon Rectum 34:424–425
145. Lynch HT, Drouhard TJ, Schuelke GS et al. (1985) Hereditary nonpolyposis colorectal cancer in a Navajo Indian family. Cancer Genet Cytogenet 15: 209–213
146. San Jose BA, Navarro NS, Doble F (1989) Hereditary nonpolyposis colorectal cancer: an awareness. JMMS 25:37–38
147. Lynch HT, Lanspa S, Smyrk T et al. (1991) Hereditary nonpolyposis colorectal cancer. Cancer Genet Cytogenet 53:143–160
148. Jass JR, Stewart SM (1992) Evolution of hereditary nonpolyposis colorectal cancer. Gut 33:783–786
149. Mecklin JP, Jarvinen HJ, Peltokallio P (1986) Cancer family syndrome: genetic analysis of 22 Finnish kindreds. Gastroenterology 90:328–333
150. Mecklin JP (1987) Frequency of hereditary colorectal carcinoma. Gastroenterology 93:1021–1025
151. Westlake PJ, Bryant HE, Huchcroft SA et al. (1991) Frequency of hereditary nonpolyposis colorectal cancer in Southern Alberta. Dig Dis Sci 36:1441–1447
152. Kee F, Collins BJ (1991) How prevalent is cancer family syndrome? Gut 32:509–512
153. Ponz de Leon M, Sassatelli R, Benatti P et al. (1993) Identification of HNPCC in the general population. Cancer 71:3493–3501
154. Benatti P, Sassatelli R, Roncucci L et al. (1993) Tumour spectrum in HNPCC and in suspected HNPCC: a population based study in Northern Italy. Int J Cancer 54:371–377
155. Fitzgibbons RJ, Lynch HT, Stanislav GV et al. (1987) Recognition and treatment of patients with hereditary nonpolyposis colorectal cancer. Ann Surg 206:289–294
156. Vasen HFA, Offerhaus GJA, Jager H et al. (1990) The tumour spectrum in hereditary non-polyposis colorectal cancer: a study of 24 kindreds in the Netherlands. Int J Cancer 46:31–34
157. Mecklin JP, Jarvinen HJ (1986) Clinical features of colorectal carcinoma in cancer family syndrome. Dis Colon Rectum 29:160–164
158. Cristofaro G, Lynch HT, Caruso L et al. (1987) New phenotypic aspects in a family with Lynch syndrome II. Cancer 60:51–58
159. Lynch HT, Kriegler M, Christiansen TA et al. (1988) Laryngeal carcinoma in a Lynch syndrome II kindred. Cancer 62:1007–1013
160. Lynch HT, Richardson JD, Amin M et al. (1991) Variable gastrointestinal and urologic cancers in a Lynch syndrome II kindred. Dis Col Rectum 34:891–895
161. Mecklin JP, Jarvinen HJ, Virolainen M (1992) The association between cholangiocarcinoma and hereditary nonpolyposis colorectal carcinoma. Cancer 69:1112–1114
162. Lynch HT, Smyrk T, Watson P et al. (1991) Hereditary colorectal cancer. Semin Oncol 18:337–366
163. Albano WA, Recabaren JA, Lynch HT et al. (1982) Natural history of hereditary cancer of the breast and colon. Cancer 50:360–363
164. Kee F, Collins BJ, Patterson CC (1991) Prognosis in familial non-polyposis colorectal cancer. Gut 32:513–516
165. Kouri M, Laasonen A, Mecklin JP et al. (1990) Diploid predominance in HNPCC evaluated by flow cytometry. Cancer 65:1825–1829
166. Frei JV (1992) Hereditary nonpolyposis colorectal cancer: diploid malignancies with prolonged survival. Cancer 69:1108–1111

167. Kee F, Patterson CC, Collins BJ et al. (1991) Histologic characteristics and outcome of familial non-polyposis colorectal carcinoma. Scand J Gastroenterol 26:419–424
168. Mecklin JP, Sipponen P, Jarvinen HJ (1986) Histopathology of colorectal carcinoma and adenomas in a cancer family syndrome. Dis Colon Rectum 29:849–853
169. Lanspa SJ, Lynch HT, Smyrk TC et al. (1990) Colorectal adenomas in the Lynch syndromes: results of a colonoscopy screening program. Gastroenterology 98:1117–1122
170. Bailey-Wilson JE, Elston RC, Schuelke GS et al. (1986) Segregation analysis of hereditary nonpolyposis colorectal cancer. Genet Epidemiol 3:27–28
171. Lynch HT, Albano WA, Ruma TA et al. (1983) Surveillance/management of an obligate gene carrier: the cancer family syndrome. Gastroenterology 84: 404–408
172. Mecklin JP, Jarvinen HJ, Aukee S et al. (1987) Screening for colorectal carcinoma in cancer family syndrome kindreds. Scad J Gastroenterol 22:449–453
173. Vasen HFA, Frieda CA, Jager H et al. (1989) Screening for hereditary nonpolyposis colorectal cancer: a study of 22 kindreds in the Netherlands. Am J Med 86:278–281
174. Jass JR, Stewart SM, Schroeder D et al. (1992) Screening for hereditary nonpolyposis colorectal cancer in New Zealand. Eur J Gastroenterol Hepathol 4:523–527
175. Vasen HF, Mecklin JP, Watson P et al. (1993) Surveillance in HNPCC: an international cooperative study of 165 families. Dis Colon Rectum 36:1–4
176. Watson P, Lynch HT (1993) Extracolonic cancer in hereditary nonpolyposis colorectal cancer. Cancer 71:677–685
177. Ponz de Leon M, Benatti P, Pedroni M et al. (1993) Risk of cancer in the follow-up of families with HNPCC. Int J Cancer 55:202–207
178. Vogelstein B, Fearon ER, Hamilton SR et al. (1988) Genetic alterations during colorectal tumor development. N Engl J Med 319:525–532
179. Muleris M, Salmon RJ, Dutrillaux AM et al. (1987) Characteristic chromosomal imbalances in 18 near-diploid colorectal tumors. Cancer Genet Cytogenet 29:289–301
180. Pathak S, Hopwood LV, Hughes JI et al. (1991) Identification of colon cancer-predisposed individuals: a cytogenetic analysis. Am J Gastroenterol 86:679–684
181. Wang L, Li L, Hong Y et al. (1992) t(13q;17p) and del(5q): possibly specific changes in Chinese patients with colorectal cancers. Cancer Genet Cytogenet 62:191–196
182. Remvikos Y, Muleris M, Vielh P et al. (1988) DNA content and genetic evolution of human colorectal adenocarcinoma. A study by flow cytometry and cytogenetic analysis. Int J Cancer 42:539–543
183. Scott N, Quirke P (1993) Molecular biology of colorectal neoplasia. Gut 34: 289–292
184. Forrester K, Almoguera C, Hang K et al. (1987) Detection of high incidence of K-ras oncogenes during human colon tumorigenesis. Nature 327:298–303
185. Finkelstein SD, Sayegh R, Christensen S et al. (1993) Genotypic classification of colorectal adenocarcinoma. Cancer 71:3826–3838
186. Benhattar J, Losi L, Chaubert P et al. (1993) Prognostic significance of K-ras mutations in colorectal carcinoma. Gastroenterology 104:1044–1048
187. Finley GG, Schulz NT, Hill Sa et al. (1989) Expression of the myc gene family in different stages of human colorectal cancer. Oncogene 4:963–971
188. Meltzer SJ, Ahnen DJ, Battifora H et al. (1987) Protooncogene abnormalities in colon cancers and adenomatous polyps. Gastroenterology 92:1174–1180

189. Kinzler KW, Nilbert MC, Su LK et al. (1991) Identification of FAP locus genes from chromosome 5q21. Science 253:661–665
190. Groden J, Thilveris A, Samowitz W et al. (1991) Identification and characterization of the familial adenomatous polyposis coli gene. Cell 66:589–600
191. Powell SM, Zilz N, Beazer-Barclay Y et al. (1992) APC mutations occur early during colorectal tumorigenesis. Nature 359:235–237
192. Kinzler KW, Nilbert MC, Vogelstein B et al. (1991) Identification of a gene located at chromosome 5q21 that is mutated in colorectal cancers. Science 251:1366–1370
193. Miki Y, Nishisho I, Miyoshi Y et al. (1991) Frequent loss of heterozygosity at the MCC locus on chromosome 5q21–22 in sporadic colorectal carcinomas. Jpn J Cancer Res 82:1003–1007
194. D'Amico D, Carbone DP, Johnson BE et al. (1992) Polymorphic sites within the MCC and APC loci reveal very frequent loss of heterozygosity in human small cell lung cancer. Cancer Res 52:1996–1999
195. Boynton RF, Blount PL, Yin J et al. (1992) Loss of heterozygosity involving the APC and MCC genetic loci occurs in the majority of human esophageal cancers. Proc Natl Acad Sci USA 89:3385–3388
196. Fearon ER, Cho KR, Nigro JM et al. (1990) Identification of a chromosome 18q gene that is altered in colorectal cancers. Science 247:49–56
197. Yanoshita R, Konishi M, Fukunari H et al. (1992) Loss of expression of the DCC gene during progression of colorectal carcinomas in familial adenomatous and non-familial adenomatous polyposis patients. Cancer Res 52:3801–3803
198. Hollstein M, Sidransky D, Vogelstein B et al. (1991) p53 mutations in human cancers. Science 253:49–53
199. Van den Broek MH, Renault B, Fodde R et al. (1993) Sites and types of p53 mutations in an unselected series of colorectal cancers in the Netherlands. Anticancer Res 13:587–592
200. Meling GI, Lothe RA, Borresen AL et al. (1993) The TP53 tumour suppressor gene in colorectal carcinoma. Br J Cancer 67:88–92
201. Nigro JM, Baker S, Preisinger AC et al. (1989) Mutations in the p53 gene occur in diverse human tumour types. Nature 342:705–707
202. Baker SJ, Fearon ER, Nigro JM et al. (1989) Chromosome 17 deletions and p53 gene mutations in colorectal carcinomas. Science 244:217–221
203. Scott N, Bell SM, Sagar P et al. (1993) p53 expression and K-ras mutation in colorectal adenomas. Gut 34:621–624
204. Laurent-Puig P, Olschwang S, Delattre O et al. (1992) Survival and acquired genetic alterations in colorectal cancer. Gastroenterology 102:1136–1141
205. Offerhaus GJA, De Feyter EP, Cornelisse CJ et al. (1992) The relationship of DNA aneuploidy to molecular genetic alterations in colorectal carcinoma. Gastroenterology 102:1612–1619
206. Ookawa K, Sakamoto M, Hirohashi S et al. (1993) Concordant p53 and DCC alterations and allelic losses on chromosomes 13q and 14q associated with liver metastases of colorectal carcinoma. Int J Cancer 53:382–387
207. Bardi G, Pandis N, Fenger C et al. (1993) Deletion of 1p36 as a primary chromosomal aberration in intestinal tumorigenesis. Cancer Res 53:1895–1898
208. van der Bosch K, Becker I, Savelyeva L et al. (1992) Deletions in the short arm of chromosome 8 are present in up to 90% of human colorectal cancer cell lines. Genes Chromosomes Cancer 5:91–95
209. Keldysh PL, Dragani TA, Fleischman EW et al. (1993) 11q deletions in human colorectal carcinomas. Genes Chromos Cancer 6:45–50
210. Fujiwara Y, Emi M, Ohata H et al. (1993) Evidence for the presence of two tumor suppressor genes on chromosome 8 for colorectal carcinoma. Cancer Res 53:1172–1174

211. Cunningham C, Dunlop MG, Wyllie AH et al. (1993) Deletion mapping in colorectal cancer of a putative tumour suppressor gene in 8p22–p21.3. Oncogene 8:1391–1396
212. Liu C, Park M, Tsao MS (1992) Overexpression of c-met proto-oncogene but not epidermal growth factor receptor or c-erbB-2 in primary human colorectal carcinomas. Oncogenes 7:181–185
213. Cohn KH, Wang F, DeSoto-Lapaix F et al. (1991) Association of nm23-h1 allelic deletions with distant metastases in colorectal carcinoma. Lancet 338: 722–724
214. Leach FS, Elledge SJ, Sherr CJ et al. (1993) Amplification of cyclin genes in colorectal carcinomas. Cancer Res 53:1986–1989
215. Aaltonen LA, Peltomaki P, Leach FS et al. (1993) Clues to the pathogenesis of familial colorectal cancer. Science 260:812–816
216. Peltomaki P, Sistonen P, Mecklin JP et al. (1991) Evidence supporting exclusion of the DCC gene and a portion of chromosome 18q as the locus for susceptibility to HNPCC in 5 kindreds. Cancer Res 51:4135–4140
217. Peltomaki P, Sistonen P, Mecklin JP et al. (1992) Evidence that the MCC-APC gene region in 5q21 is not the site for susceptibility to HNPCC. Cancer Res 52:4530–4533
218. Bhagirath T, Condie A, Dunlop MG et al. (1993) Exclusion of constitutional p53 mutations as a cause of genetic susceptibility to colorectal cancer. Br J Cancer (in press)
219. Peltomaki P, Aaltonen L, Sistonen P et al. (1993) Genetic mapping of a locus predisposing to human colorectal cancer. Science 260:810–812

Hereditary Gastrointestinal Polyposis Syndromes

> *Hereditary gastrointestinal polyposis syndromes have stimulated the interest of generations of physicians. They provide models for studying the etiology and pathogenesis of intestinal polyps and, in some cases, for investigating the stepwise development of gastrointestinal carcinoma.*
>
> (R.C. Haggitt and B.J. Reid 1986)

Introduction

Familial gastrointestinal polyposis includes various syndromes with common features of numerous adenomatous polyps in the large bowel and a well-defined pattern of genetic transmission. The occurrence of other clinical manifestations will determine the appearance of the specific phenotypes, which have been tentatively classified in Table 1. This, however, is not a simple task, since there is still much debate concerning whether some of these syndromes should be considered separate nosologic entities or part of the spectrum of alterations associated with a single disease. While it is unlikely that further clinical studies will provide new insights into the classification of familial polyposis, this question might be answered in the near future by the biomolecular characterization of the underlying genetic defects.

Familial adenomatous polyposis (FAP or adenomatosis coli) is by far the most common of these polyposis syndromes and the most extensively investigated; moreover, recent studies using sophisticated biomolecular techniques led to the identification of the gene responsible for the disease on the long arm of chromosome 5. The clinical and scientific interest in FAP and related conditions stem from various considerations. Firstly, these syndromes represent "absolute" precancerous lesions, in the sense that in affected individuals who are not treated in due time the development of malignancy can be predicted with almost absolute certainty. Secondly, adenomatosis coli has a clear Mendelian basis (autosomal dominant, usually with a high penetrance); it follows that accurate pedigree analysis, subsequent endoscopic screening of family members at risk, and now linkage and mutation studies of the responsible gene may allow the early identification of affected individuals. Finally, when the disease is diagnosed before the development of cancer, radical surgery may be curative in almost

Table 1. Classification of hereditary polyposis syndromes

	Characteristics (references)
A. Adenomatous polyposis	
1. Adenomatosis coli/ Gardner's syndrome	Colorectal polyps, several other extracolonic manifestations [8, 11, 12]
2. Turcot syndrome	Colorectal adenomas, brain tumors [102, 105]
3. Hereditary flat adenoma syndrome	"Flat" adenomas of the large bowel [94, 95]
4. Zanca syndrome	Polyps of the large bowel, cartilaginous exostosis [46]
B. Hamartomatous polyposis	
1. Peutz-Jeghers syndrome	Polyps of the gastrointestinal tract, pigmented macules of the skin and mucous membranes [108, 109]
2. Juvenile polyposis	Early onset hamartomatous polyps of the gastrointestinal tract [121, 122]
3. Muir-Torre syndrome	Sebaceous tumors, multiple gastrointestinal neoplasms at early onset [130, 131]
4. Cowden's disease	Multiple hamartomas of the skin, oral cavity, and gastrointestinal tract [116, 117]
5. Ruvalcaba-Myrhe-Smith syndrome	Hamartomatous polyps of the large bowel, pigmented macules, macrocephaly, mental deficiency [46, 135]
6. Cronkhite-Canada syndrome	Hamartomatous polyps of the gastrointestinal tract, alopecia, skin hyperpigmentation, nail dystrophy [136, 137]

all cases, although the high frequency of extracolonic manifestations clearly indicates that clinical investigations in these patients should not be limited to the large bowel, and that a surveillance program should be maintained almost indefinitely.

Although not so widely investigated as FAP, and undoubtedly much rarer, virtually all other polyposis syndromes are of some scientific interest and clinical relevance.

Familial Adenomatous Polyposis (Adenomatosis Coli)

Definition and Brief History

Adenomatosis coli is a relatively rare inherited disease characterized by the presence of more than 100 adenomatous polyps scattered throughout the various segments of the large bowel, and by an autosomal dominant type of genetic transmission. In Gardner's syndrome, colorectal adenomas are associated with osteomas of the skull and mandible, epidermoid cysts, soft tissue tumors, and several other neoplastic and nonneoplastic abnormalities. It should be noted that on clinical grounds a sharp distinction between the two syndromes is often impossible; in fact, careful investigations of families with an initial diagnosis of FAP can detect individuals with features of Gardner's syndrome; similarly, various patients in kindreds with this syndrome do not exhibit extracolonic manifestations. Moreover, some patients with FAP may not show overt stigmata of Gardner's syndrome, but these can be found when searched for with more appropriate techniques (for example, osteomas of the mandible and supernumerary teeth are often detected by X-ray examination). The available evidence, therefore, seems to suggest that FAP and Gardner's syndrome are not two different diseases, but that the latter simply represents the full-blown manifestation of a spectrum of clinical features due to the effect of a pleiotropic gene; accordingly, in the rest of this chapter the two clinical conditions will be considered a single nosologic entity. It is likely, however, that the ongoing biomolecular investigations will provide a definitive answer to this debate.

The main advances which have been made in the knowledge of adenomatosis coli are summarized in Table 2. The disease was described independently by various authors at the end of the last century [1–3]. In 1925, a Polyposis Coli Registry was established at St. Mark's Hospital, London [4, 5], and since then most of the progress in our understanding of FAP has been closely related to the activity of this institution and to the efforts of investigators (in particular H.J.R. Bussey) who have been entirely devoted to the study of polyposis and related syndromes. The genetic features of the disease and the main surgical procedures were defined in subsequent years [6, 7], while in 1951 Gardner [8] described the association of colorectal polyps with multiple soft and hard tumors in a large American family. In 1980, a new surgical technique was proposed (i.e., total proctocolectomy with an ileal reservoir and anal anastomosis) which seemed to offer some advantages compared to other precedures [9, 10]. In the same year, several other extracolonic manifestations were described, including polyps in the stomach and small bowel, desmoid tumors, and congenital hypertrophy of the retinal pigment epithelium [11–13]; moreover, a medical treatment of potential benefit (sulindac) in inducing polyp regression was suggested [14]. Finally, between 1986 and 1991 a series of elegant and sophisticated cytogenetic and biomolecular studies led to the mapping of the *FAP* locus on the long arm of chromosome 5, and to the subsequent identification and characterization of the gene responsible for the disease [15–18].

Clinical and Epidemiologic Features

There is a general agreement that at least 100 polyps should be observed in the entire large bowel in order to make the diagnosis of FAP. The number 100 was chosen mainly because all patients with FAP in the St. Mark's

Table 2. Advances in clinical and biological characterization of familial adenomatous polyposis

Authors	Details	Reference
Sklifasowski (1881)	Description of the first patient with FAP	[1]
Cripps (1882)	Description of the first familial aggregate of FAP	[2]
Smith (1887)	Report of colorectal cancer developed in FAP	[3]
Lockhart-Mummery (1925)	Institution of the FAP Registry at St. Mark's Hospital, London	[4]
Cockayne (1927)	Suggestion of an autosomal dominant pattern of inheritance	[6]
Lockhart-Mummery (1934)	Colectomy with ileorectal anastomosis for patients with FAP	[7]
Gardner (1951)	Description of Gardner's syndrome	[8]
Smith (1959)	Description of desmoid tumors in FAP	[12]
Utsunomiya et al. (1974)	Description of gastric polyps in FAP	[12, 48]
Jones et al. (1977)	Description of duodenal lesions in FAP	[13, 53]
Parks et al. (1980)		
Utsunomiya et al. (1980)	Proctocolectomy with ileoanal anastomosis for the treatment of FAP	[9, 10]
Blair et al. (1980)	Congenital hypertrophy of the retinal pigment epithelium (CHRPE)	[40]
Waddel et al. (1983)	Treatment with sulindac	[14]
Herrera et al. (1986)	Interstitial deletion of 5q in a patient with FAP	[15]
Bodmer et al. (1987)	Localization of the *FAP* gene on 5q21–22	[16, 81]
Leppert et al. (1987)	Localization of the *FAP* gene on 5q21–22	
Kinzler et al. (1991)	Identification and sequencing of the *FAP* gene	[17, 18, 82, 83]
Groden et al. (1991)	Identification and sequencing of the *FAP* gene	

registry showed more than 100 polyps, and genetic transmission of polyposis was not observed in patients with less than 100 polyps [5, 11]. However, individuals with multiple polyps in the various large bowel tracts – even if fewer than 100 – should be carefully monitored, since they might be affected patients in whom the full spectrum of the disease did not develop because of variable clinical expressivity; thus, an accurate genealogical tree should be drawn from these patients, and family members at risk should undergo clinical investigation. Moreover, it has been suggested that colonoscopy may underestimate the real number of polyps and, consequently, that all individuals with 50–100 colorectal adenomas should be considered as having suspected FAP [11]. Utsunomiya and Iwama [19] described two types of endoscopic appearance of polyps in Japan – the "dense type" and the "coarse type" – depending on the absolute number and density of adenomas.

At St. Mark's hospital the mean polyp count was in the order of 1000, with a range from 104 to 5000 [5], thus confirming that in the most typical cases the entire large bowel is carpeted with polyps of various dimensions. In other European series [20, 21], polyps were evenly distributed in the various colorectal tracts, but the highest density was observed in the distal colon, where adenomas tended to be larger than in the proximal colon; moreover, rectal polyps were detected in all patients.

The earliest age at which polyps occur and the latest age when the full-blown picture may appear are difficult to determine. In a series of patients who developed FAP while under endoscopic surveillance, the mean age at which polyps were recognized was 22 years (range, 11–53 years), and it is likely that the large majority of individuals carrying the gene will develop polyps (or other manifestations) by the age of 25 years; on the other hand, the risk of polyposis in susceptible individuals becomes small after the age of 35 years [11]. The main symptoms of adenomatosis coli are rectal bleeding, diarrhea, and abdominal discomfort; these usually appear around the age of 30 years, which is not far from the mean age of diagnosis (30–35 years in most clinical series) [11–13, 22]. When the diagnosis of FAP is based on symptom appearance, the probability of having developed a colorectal carcinoma is in the order of 60%–70% [5, 20, 22, 23], while cancer is found in less than 10% of asymptomatic individuals in whom the disease is detected through family screening. These data, therefore, strongly underline the importance of early detection of FAP; however, the extreme variability in the clinical onset of neoplastic lesions in these patients is emphasized by the case report of a woman who had a negative endoscopy at the age of 70 years, but developed polyposis and rectal cancer aged 74 years [11].

Cases of FAP have been described in several countries and races, although the majority of published series concern western Europe, North America, and Japan [20]. Incidence of adenomatosis coli is usually expressed as the frequency at birth of individuals with the *FAP* gene; a reasonably good agreement has been reported between incidence rates in various countries, with values in the order of 1 in 10000–20000 [13, 20, 24]. Recent accurate estimates from the Finnish Cancer Registry indicate that the incidence of FAP in this country is between 1.6 and 2.4/million [23], and that 5–10 new cases of the disease should be expected every year; these figures closely correspond to the incidence rates observed in Denmark [12, 25].

Morphology of Colonic Lesions

The large majority of colorectal polyps in FAP are tubular or tubulovillous adenomas; the density of these lesions varies from 0.15 to 3.0 adenomas/cm^2, and a trend towards increased density from proximal colon to the rectosigmoid region is usually observed [19, 20]. Since the rectum is virtually involved in all patients with FAP, proctosigmoidoscopy should be sufficient for diagnosis, although a careful examination of the entire large bowel is necessary for surveillance of affected individuals before surgery.

The normal appearing colorectal mucosa of patients with adenomatosis coli has been the subject of several investigations. Various types of subtle alterations have been described; these include (a) abnormalities of sialomucin content and properties [26]; (b) expansion of the proliferative region in colonic crypts from the basal zone towards the luminal surface [27–29], and (c) appearance of an increased number of aberrant crypt foci [30], which seem to be precursor lesions for adenomatous polyps and rectal cancer [31] (see chapters on "Biomarkers of Increased Susceptibility to Cancer" and "Hereditary and Familial Colorectal Cancer").

Colorectal cancer is found in more than 60% of probands, but in only 5%–10% of symptom-free patients [12, 20]. In other words, when patients with FAP come to the attention of a physician owing to the appearance of symptoms, the probability of having a malignancy is extremely high. The distribution of carcinomas in FAP is similar to that in sporadic colorectal cancer, i.e., 70%–80% of the lesions are localized in the descending colon and in the rectosigmoid region, while only one-fourth of the tumors develop in the right colon. It is noteworthy that this distribution is different from that of hereditary nonpolyposis colorectal cancer (HNPCC) (see previous chapter), in which the large majority of neoplasms are localized in the proximal colon. Grading, staging, and other morphologic features of carcinomas in FAP do not differ from those of the commonly observed sporadic colorectal cancer [12]. Finally, in Finland the proportion of colorectal carcinomas developing in FAP showed a constant decrease, from 0.53% of all registered colorectal cancers in 1966–1970 to 0.14% in 1986–1990 [23]; the decreasing frequency of this proportion should be attributed to both family screening and increased incidence of sporadic tumors.

Extracolonic Manifestations

After the initial description of Gardner's syndrome [8], several lesions of other organs or tissues have been reported in patients with FAP, and a brief list of these alterations is shown in Table 3. The importance of extracolonic manifestations is twofold; first, they may antedate the appearance or the discovery of colorectal polyps, thus helping in the diagnosis of the underlying intestinal lesions. Second, though most of these changes are benign, some of them may become malignant (duodenal adenomas) or may assume a locally aggressive behavior (desmoid tumors), thus generating additional problems in the follow-up of these patients.

Epidermoid cysts and osteomas are extremely frequent in patients with adenomatosis coli [12, 20, 22]; the former are more often found on the back, the latter especially in the facial skeleton. In various studies [32, 33], panoramic dental radiographs were used to detect occult radiopaque lesions

Table 3. Extracolonic manifestations in adenomatosis coli

Benign	Malignant
Epidermoid cysts	Periampullary carcinoma
Osteomas, odontomas	Thyroid carcinoma
Supernumerary teeth	Hepatoblastoma
Congenital hypertrophy of the retinal pigment epithelium (CHRPE)	Small intestinal carcinoma
Fundic gland polyps	Gastric carcinoma
Gastric adenomas	
Ileal and jejunal adenomas	
Desmoid tumors[a]	

[a] Although considered benign, desmoid tumors are locally invasive neoplasms, and may represent the main clinical problem in FAP patients.

(i.e., osteomas, odontomas, and supernumerary teeth) of the mandible; not surprisingly, abnormalities were detected in the large majority of affected individuals, suggesting that jaw lesions might be a good predictor for polyp development in families with FAP.

Desmoid tumors are locally invasive, nonmetastasizing fibrous neoplasms frequently observed in patients with FAP [11, 13]; these lesions arise in the musculuaponeurotic structures, especially in the anterior abdominal wall at the site of laparotomy wounds. Extremely rare in the general population, these tumors are at least 100 times more common in FAP, and often represent one of the most relevant clinical problems in these patients [34, 35], reaching 20 cm or more in diameter. The frequency of desmoid tumors (which are more often found in women) is in the order of 5%–15% of all patients with FAP [12, 36]. Moreover, intraperitoneal or retroperitoneal fibrous reactions have been reported in these patients [22, 37]; this "fibroproliferative tendency" may involve the intestinal loops, leading to adhesions, fistulas, and obstructions. Treatment of desmoid tumors is basically surgical, with the objective of complete excision of the lesion; surgery, however, is often unsatisfactory, and is accompanied by a high rate of complications and recurrences [36]. Since desmoid neoplasms are usually radioresistant, several medical treatments have been evaluated, including tamoxifen, ascorbic acid, and, more recently, doxorubicin [12, 36, 38, 39]; all these approaches have been of limited value, and the optimal treatment for desmoid tumors has yet to be defined.

Blair et al. [40], and subsequently other investigators [41–45], described patches of congenital hypertrophy of the retinal pigment epithelium (CHRPE) in the majority of patients with adenomatosis coli. At ophthalmoscopy, these lesions are darkly pigmented, usually round or oval shaped, and extremely variable in number (from 1 to 20 or more), dimensions (0.1 to more than 1 optic disk), and distribution (unilateral or bilateral). Histologically, CHRPE consists of a single layer of hypertrophied cells filled with granules of pigment. CHRPE is found in 70%–89% of patients with FAP and in 40%–59% of family members at genetic risk of adenomatosis, while they are extremely rare in the general population (only 6 cases out of 1984 control retinal examinations) [43]. Thus, these lesions, especially when multiple and bilateral, seem to be a rather sensitive and specific biomarker for FAP, although their absence in a family member at risk does not exclude the presence of the disease, and therefore these individuals should regularly be checked according to the usual protocol of surveillance (see later). Since CHRPE has been described in 3- to 12-month-old babies, it is likely that they are congenital lesions.

Gastric adenomas have been considered rare in FAP [11, 12, 46]. In the St. Mark's series [47], 56 out of 102 patients screened prospectively had gastric polyps; however, only 6 of these lesions were adenomatous, whereas in the majority of cases histologic examination showed features of non-adenomatous fundic gland hyperplasia. At variance with the European series, Japanese studies showed the presence of gastric adenomas in approximately half of the patients with FAP [48]; moreover, gastric malignancies have also been described in these patients [48, 49]. It follows that adenomatous lesions of the stomach should be removed at endoscopy, and the patients should be followed up with regular endoscopic controls.

Duodenal polyps represent a much more serious problem; these lesions seem to be present in the majority of patients with FAP and their frequency increases with age; histologic examination almost invariably shows adenomatous changes, which are similar to those of the colon [12]. Moreover, biopsy specimens from apparently normal duodenal mucosa may show early adenomatous changes at histology, thus suggesting that the frequency of these lesions can actually be higher than that usually reported [12, 47, 50]. In keeping with these observations, Spigelman et al. [47] found duodenal adenomatous polyps in 88 out of 102 patients with FAP; adenomas were usually localized in the second and third parts of the duodenum, and were particularly frequent in the periampullary region. Two recent Japanese studies confirmed the high prevalence of adenomatous polyps in FAP [51, 52], and strongly recommended close endoscopic checks (with multiple and repeated biopsies, especially from the periampullary region) for these patients. These conclusions seem warranted by the high prevalence of duodenal and periampullary carcinomas, which occur in adenomatosis coli at a frequency 100 times higher than in the general population [53]. In summary: (a) patients with FAP should be screened at regular intervals for the possible presence of adenomatous lesions in the duodenum; (b) duodenal and periampullary polyps should always undergo endoscopic removal and histologic examination; (c) biopsies from the periampullary area should be taken even when the region appears endoscopically normal; and (d) duodenal carcinomas are frequent in FAP and represent a major cause of death for these patients.

When the entire small bowel could be examined by intraoperative endoscopy, jejunal or ileal adenomatous polyps were found in 20%–40% of patients with FAP [54], although carcinomatous lesions at these anatomic sites are relatively infrequent [55, 56]. Multiple adenomas have been described in the terminal ileum of FAP patients previously treated with total proctocolectomy and ileoanal anastomosis, especially 10 or more years after surgery [57, 58]; moreover, the occurrence of adenocarcinoma of the ileostomy has also been documented [59]. Thus, total colectomy with or without an ileoanal reservoir does not exclude the risk of adenoma or carcinoma development.

There are several reports of thyroid carcinoma (especially of the papillary histologic type) which have developed in patients with FAP, more frequently in the female sex, and it has been estimated that the risk of this type of tumor in a woman with polyposis is more than 100 times the risk in the general population [60, 61]. Bulow et al. [62] suggested that thyroid carcinoma should be included in the list of the extracolonic manifestations which may occur in patients with FAP. Other neoplasms which can be found in these patients include hepatoblastoma [63], carcinoma of the pancreas and biliary tract [64–66], and neoplasms of multiple endocrine organs [67].

Formal Genetics and Counselling

The examination of hundreds of genealogical trees clearly indicates that inheritance in FAP is consistent with an autosomal dominant type of genetic transmission, with a penetrance higher than 90% in most series [12, 13, 68], and a consequent negligible risk of "skipped generations." As already discussed, clinical expressivity may be extremely variable, though in the majority of cases polyps are disseminated throughout the large bowel, thus rendering the diagnosis rather straightforward. In accordance with the type of transmission, the male:female ratio should be close to 1.0, and this has actually been found in most studies; however, it may be of interest that in a large Japanese series of more than 500 cases Utsunomiya et al. [19] found a ratio of 1.7. The authors provided the tentative explanation of the possible existence of an X-linked modifier gene which would influence the expression of polyps [69]. The *FAP* gene does not seem to impair the biological fitness of affected individuals, so that fertility is not reduced in these patients [68].

Age of appearance of colorectal polyps tends to vary both within and between families. After a close endoscopic surveillance of asymptomatic children at risk of FAP, Alm [68] concluded that the most frequent time of appearance of the full-blown picture is in the late teens or early twenties. However, the study also included a 2-year-old girl with a diagnosis of FAP who underwent surgery at the age of 4 years owing to severe symptoms; in addition, development of polyps in infants was reported in various other series [11, 22]. Finally, although cancer occurrence is rare under the age of

20 years, malignant changes have been reported from patients as young as 9 years old [13].

In almost all series, some 30%–40% of all patients with adenomatosis coli are solitary cases, i.e., with only one affected member in a given family [68]; phenotypically, these individuals are indistinguishable from members of families segregating the gene through various generations. Presumably, single cases represent new mutations, although in some patients the gene might have been transmitted through a parent deceased at a very young age, or in whom the disease did not become manifest because of variable expressivity. Recognition of single cases before the appearance of symptoms is obviously difficult (since there are no reasons to suspect a given family) and when this happens it is usually by chance. Since fertility is not reduced, solitary cases can transmit the deleterious gene to their progeny; it follows that in most series, after years of clinical observation, several cases initially labeled as "solitary" eventually became "segregating." Representative pedigrees of solitary and segregating FAP families are shown in Figs. 1 and 2.

Recognition of a family (or a "single" case) of FAP requires accurate counselling of affected individuals and of family members at risk. Physicians should take into account the most recent scientific progress as well as the possible anxiety and, more generally, the psychologic aspects inherent in a genetic neoplastic disease. Detailed information should be provided concerning the hereditary nature of the disease, its natural course, the presence of additional neoplastic activity, various options for surgical treatment, surveillance, and overall prognosis. For asymptomatic family members at risk from the disease (i.e., first-degree relatives of all affected individuals) the most important recommendation is to undergo an initial sigmoidoscopy by the age of 12–16 years. In the case of normal appearing colorectal mucosa, the search for other clinical manifestations of FAP is probably unnecessary, but the patient should be invited back for a repeat endoscopy at regular intervals (3–5 years) until the age of 35–40 years. After this period, the risk of being a carrier of the gene is considered negligible [5, 11], though some sort of endoscopic control remains advisable, owing to the possible late appearance of polyps or nonpenetrance of the gene [70].

Diagnosis, Surgical Treatment, and Prognosis

Since the most distal portions of the large bowel are almost invariably involved, sigmoidoscopy is usually sufficient for the initial diagnosis of FAP; several polyps should be removed for morphologic examination in order to ascertain their adenomatous nature and the degree of differentiation. For subsequent surveillance and diagnostic evaluation, colonoscopy is the technique of choice for exploring the entire large bowel and taking multiple biopsies. Moreover, at the time of diagnosis the patient should also have

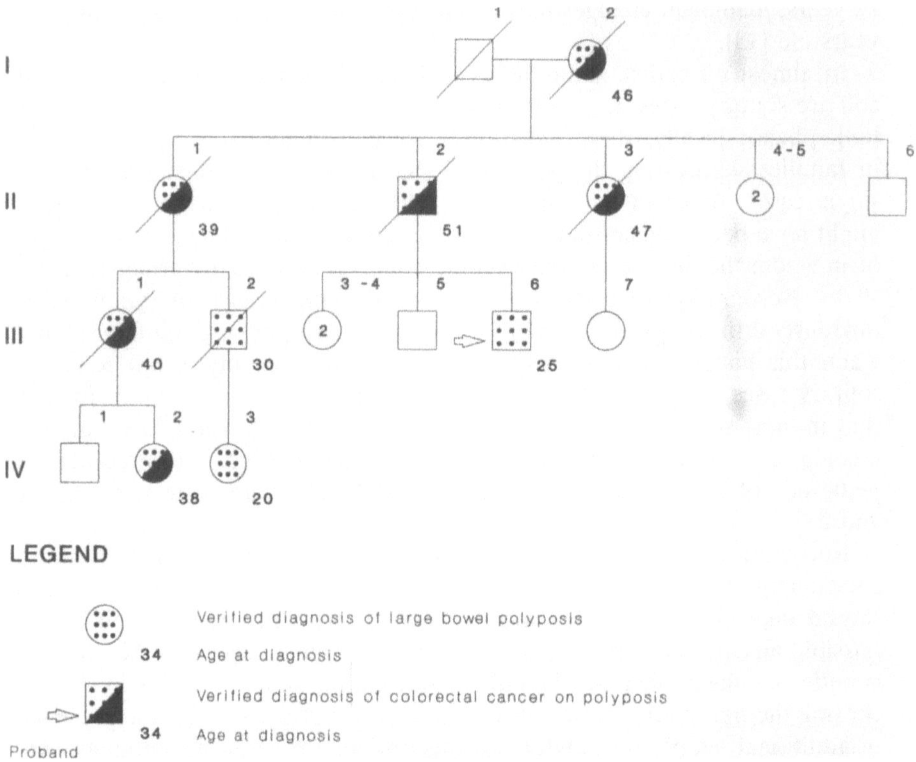

Fig. 1. Representative example of extended family segregating the polyposis trait through several generations. Most affected family members had cancer at the time of diagnosis

an upper endoscopy, in order to verify the possible existence of gastric, duodenal, and especially periampullary lesions [11, 12, 68]. Similarly, at diagnosis or in subsequent years, the presence of other extracolonic manifestations (CHRPE, osteomas, supernumerary teeth, sebaceous cysts, and others) should also be searched for with the appropriate investigations.

After the diagnosis of FAP, time and type of surgery should be taken into consideration. For patients with symptomatic disease, who are usually over the age of 25–30 years, the operation should be carried out as soon as possible; for adolescents and, more generally, for asymptomatic individuals, time of surgery can be individualized, mainly taking into account the endoscopic findings and the fact that it is preferable to carry out the operation after the patient is almost completely physically and sexually mature. As suggested by Bulow [12], the endoscopic findings of large adenomas, rapidly growing polyps, or severe dysplasia all strongly suggest the need for early operation, which is carried out in most series usually when the patient is between the age of 15 and 20 years [11, 68].

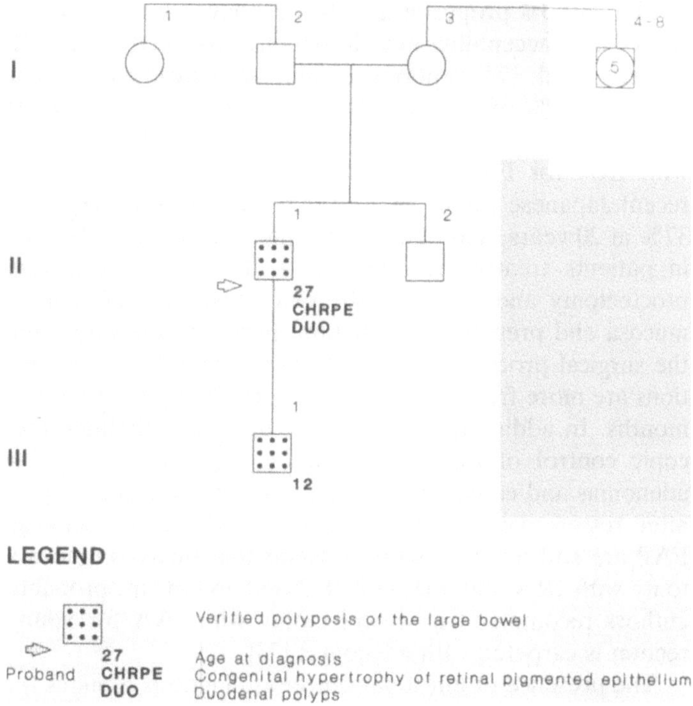

Fig. 2. Pedigree of a small family with FAP. Patient *II-1* was considered to be a "single" case until a full-blown picture of polyposis was diagnosed in his 12-year-old son (*III-1*)

The main surgical procedures for FAP are proctocolectomy with permanent ileostomy, colectomy with ileorectal anastomosis (IRA), and proctocolectomy with ileoanal anastomosis (IAA) [12, 13, 68]. The first of these techniques has virtually been abandoned, or reserved only for patients with carcinoma of the lower rectum. Both the other techniques offer advantages and disadvantages; IRA can be considered if the following conditions are fulfilled: (a) the number of adenomas in the rectum should be limited, in order to be able to remove all of them without damaging the anorectal function; (b) the rectum and the lower sigmoid should not show malignancies; (c) the patient should be aware of the risk of cancer in the remaining rectum, and that in this case a new operation would be required, presumably with a permanent ileostomy; consequently, (d) an endoscopic surveillance program should be undertaken for each individual undergoing this surgical procedure, with removal and histologic examination of all polyps developed in the rectal stump. In the presence of these conditions, most surgeons consider IRA as the method of choice for these patients, mainly because surgery is relatively easy and the functional results in terms of stool frequency and continence are satisfactory.

The authors proposing proctocolectomy with IAA claim that the risk of cancer is unacceptably high in patients operated on by IRA; in particular, Moertel et al. [71] reported a cumulative incidence of cancer in the rectal stump of 59% of patients after 23 years of observation. However, various other studies found a much lower incidence of carcinoma after colectomy with IRA for FAP (10%–15%, after 10–20 years) [72, 73], although a recent Japanese report showed that the risk of cancer in their patients was 37% at 20 years, and that rectal stump was the main factor reducing survival in patients treated with IRA [74]. Total proctocolectomy with mucosal proctectomy and IAA has the two advantages of removing all colorectal mucosa and preserving the natural route of defecation; on the other hand, the surgical procedure is more complex than IRA, postoperative complications are more frequent, and the accommodation period may require several months. In addition, this technique does not eliminate the need for endoscopic control of the pouch and the terminal ileum, since multiple ileal adenomas and carcinoma of the ileostomy have been reported several years after restorative proctocolectomy [57–59]. Thus, surgical approaches for FAP are still under debate; it seems that many surgeons still prefer colectomy with IRA and a close endoscopic follow-up; probably, however, most authors recommend proctocolectomy with IAA for young patients whose rectum is carpeted with adenomas [73].

The presence of intestinal cancer at diagnosis remains the most important determinant of prognosis; in the Danish experience [12], 10-year survival was 41% for FAP patients with cancer as opposed to 87% for those without malignancies. Similarly, in the Finnish experience, life expectancy of individuals diagnosed through family screening was significantly better than that of symptomatic patients [23]. These findings further underscore the importance of recognition and early endoscopic examination of family members at risk. As expected, the main cause of death for patients who underwent prophylactic colectomy was the development of desmoid tumors or periampullary carcinoma [46, 75].

Follow-up and Medical Therapy

After surgery, patients with FAP should continue to be followed at regular intervals virtually for the rest of their life. The main purpose of this close follow-up is the control of additional neoplastic activity in the remaining rectum (after ileorectal anastomosis), in the duodenum, jejunum, terminal ileum, and possibly in other organs such as thyroid and liver. The main guidelines of a tentative surveillance program can be summarized as follows. First, endoscopic examination of the terminal ileum and rectal stump should be carried out at 6-month intervals; newly developed polyps are removed and analyzed for their morphologic features; the appearance of malignant changes usually requires a second operation. Patients treated with proctocolectomy and IAA should also be followed up with endoscopic controls, though at intervals longer than those of patients with residual rectal mucosa. Second, upper gastrointestinal endoscopy should be performed on an annual basis, especially if duodenal polyps are found; other authors proposed that if periampullary adenomas are found in a patient older than 35 years, local excision of the ampulla of Vater might be indicated in order to prevent the development of carcinoma [74]. Moreover, the upper jejunum should also be explored with the help of a jejunoscope or a pediatric colonoscope. Finally, ultrasound examinations of the thyroid gland, the liver, and other abdominal organs are also advisable every 1–2 years.

In recent years, antioxidant vitamins (especially ascorbic acid) and wheat fiber have been tested for possible pharmacologic control of colorectal adenomas in patients with FAP [76, 77], but with rather unsatisfactory overall results. In contrast, regression of rectal adenomas has been reported with the use of sulindac [14, 78], a nonsteroidal antiinflammatory drug which inhibits prostaglandin synthesis. In a controlled crossover study, Labayle et al. [79] confirmed these observations and showed complete or almost complete regression of rectal polyps in five patients with FAP (and previous colectomy with IRA) treated for 4 months with sulindac at the daily dose of 300 mg. More recently, other authors [80] found a significant decrease in the number and size of polyps in 18 unoperated patients with FAP who were treated with sulindac for 9 months; however, complete disappearance of polyps was not observed in any of these patients. Rather interestingly, after interruption of treatment, number and size of polyps tended to increase, but nevertheless after 3 months they still remained below the baseline values. Although the results seem to suggest a possible medical approach to FAP, at present they should be interpreted with caution, and it seems unlikely that in the near future sulindac (or other drugs) may replace surgery as the treatment of choice in these patients.

Molecular Biology

Although the genetic nature of FAP was initially suspected and subsequently confirmed on the basis of simple observation of polyp and cancer occurrence in families, the underlying molecular defect causing the disease has been characterized only in the last few years. The story began in 1986 when Herrera et al. [15] described the clinical case of a 42-year-old man with Gardner's syndrome, mental retardation, and an interstitial deletion removing part of chromosome 5q. The attention of various investigators was therefore focused on probes for the long arm of chromosome 5, and in 1987 two independent research groups [16, 81] localized by linkage analysis the gene responsible for FAP on 5q21–22. Further studies led to the identification of the gene and the detection of constitutional mutations in the coding sequence of patients with adenomatosis coli [17, 18, 82, 83]. Thus, sequencing of the *FAP* gene (also called *APC*, for "adenomatous polyposis coli") revealed an open leading frame of 8535 nucleotides for a predicted sequence of 2843 amino acids coded by 15 exons; rather interestingly, with a length of 6578 nucleotides exon 15 of the *APC* gene is the largest of all known exons [84]. Germline inactivating mutations of *APC* have been found in several patients with FAP but in none of the controls [18, 83–87]; various alterations were detected, including single base substitution leading to amino acid change or stop codons, and small base pair deletions (5–15 bases) leading to frameshift. Most of these mutational events were localized within exon 15 [86], although in about 1/6 of patients mutations were also found in exons 1–14 [18, 84].

The main problem with this kind of biomolecular analysis is that about 50 different mutations of *APC* have been described [16–18, 82–86, 88], so that one should investigate the whole sequence of this 8.5-kb gene in order to identify specific mutations in all individuals at risk. It follows that at present the detection of *APC* mutations is not yet a practical approach for the identification of family members highly susceptible to FAP development, and that the presymptomatic – or even prenatal – diagnosis of adenomatosis coli can be achieved more easily by demonstrating coinheritance of the responsible allele with one or more genetic markers flanking the gene. Several informative markers are available for the diagnosis of FAP through linkage studies [89–91]; however, as the genetic markers are located 1–10 centimorgans from the *APC* gene, some of these seem to be of limited utility for family studies. Recently, Spirio et al. [92] identified a highly polymorphic marker, located only 30–70 kb from the *APC* gene, which should be particularly suitable for linkage studies, thus increasing the accuracy of presymptomatic detection of the disease. Indeed, using this new biomarker the authors were able to determine the carrier status for 20 out of 31 individuals at risk of FAP in 14 investigated families [92]. In conclusion, the increase in the number of available markers and the more precise genetic mapping around the *APC* gene should allow an accurate presymptomatic diagnosis of FAP in high-risk individuals [93].

Other Polyposis Syndromes of the Large Bowel

Hereditary Flat Adenoma Syndrome

Flat adenomas in the large bowel were initially described by Muto et al. [94, 95] as slight elevations of the mucosa with a reddish surface which was dome-shaped but rather flat; histologically, features of tubular adenomas are usually seen [96]. These lesions are difficult to detect in routine endoscopic examinations, mainly because the shape may change with the degree of air insufflation at colonoscopy; nonetheless, recognition of these lesions is important, since the malignant potential of flat adenomas seems to be considerably higher than that of common sessile or pedunculated polyps of the same size [96], thus providing further biological evidence in favor of the adenoma-carcinoma sequence.

Besides the existence of sporadic lesions, a "hereditary flat adenoma syndrome" (HFAS) has recently been described by Lynch and coworkers [46, 97–100]. The main features of this relatively "new" disease include: (a) an autosomal dominant type of genetic transmission; (b) presence of multiple flat adenomas of the large bowel (although more often less than 100); (c) prevalent distribution of adenomas in the proximal colon; (d) high risk of colonic cancer, usually after the age of 50 years; and (e) presence of several extracolonic manifestations, including duodenal adenomas and carcinomas, fundic gland polyps, and adenomas of the stomach. HFAS differs from Lynch syndrome (see previous chapter) mainly because in the latter flat adenomas are rare, and cancer frequently develops below age 45 years. HFAS also shows features of FAP (i.e., presence of polyps and extracolonic changes, high lifetime risk of colorectal cancer); however, in HFAS the endoscopic and pathologic appearance of adenomas is different (they are flat, few in number, and more frequent in the proximal colon), cancer shows a later age of onset and is more often located in the right colon. Management and surveillance of HFAS patients and family members at risk are similar, in general terms, to those already discussed for adenomatosis coli, although a careful endoscopic follow-up with removal and histologic examination of all newly developed polyps may substitute colectomy in many of these patients [46, 99]. Finally, recent biomolecular studies [99, 101], using a series of markers close to the *APC* gene, found a significant linkage of the HFAS trait with the *FAP* locus; besides the possibility of identifying individuals prone to HFAS development by DNA polymorphism analysis, these observations seem to suggest that FAP and HFAS might be due to different mutations of the same gene or, alternatively, to alterations of closely linked genes located in a small region of chromosome 5q. Thus, it is still uncertain whether HFAS represents a clinical variant of FAP (as the biomolecular studies might indicate) or an entirely different nosologic and clinical entity.

Turcot Syndrome

When compared to other polyposis of the large bowel, Turcot syndrome (TS) appears relatively undefined with many controversial aspects. In 1959, Turcot et al. [102] described two siblings with FAP, one of whom developed a medulloblastoma of the spinal cord and the other a glioblastoma of the frontal lobe, while no other member of this family showed intestinal or brain tumors. After this initial observation, several other authors described families, or individuals, with the simultaneous occurrence of multiple adenomatous polyps of the large bowel and tumors of the central nervous system

(CNS) [11, 103], a condition which is now usually referred to as Turcot syndrome. According to some authors [104], colorectal adenomas in TS tend to be larger than in FAP and their number is often less than 100, although they have a strong propensity for malignant transformation. The majority of patients with TS die of tumors of the CNS, which in many cases may develop at a very young age and before the clinical recognition of intestinal adenomas. This also means that affected individuals may not live long enough to have children and to reveal the genetic nature of the disease. Thus, Lewis et al. [105] subdivided patients with TS into three main categories; in type I families, the disease is transmitted in an autosomal recessive mode of inheritance; type II families show features of autosomal dominant transmission, with patients affected by colonic polyps and/or tumors of the CNS in two or more generations. The third type shows no familial history of polyposis or other neoplasms, and should therefore be considered as sporadic.

Kropilak et al. [106] examined 168 kindreds with FAP in the Cleveland Registry and found only 13 patients with tumors of the CNS (mostly medulloblastomas); by reviewing their data and the available literature, the authors concluded that uncertainties concerning inheritance in TS should largely by attributed to the young age of individuals at the appearance of brain tumors, when most of the FAP patients still did not develop the full-blown picture of polyposis. The fact that many of these subjects die before transmitting the disease (and before the clinical appearance of adenomas) may simulate recessive transmission or sporadic cases. The question still remains whether tumors of the CNS should be considered only one of the several extracolonic manifestations of FAP, or whether the association of these neoplasms with diffuse polyposis of the large bowel represents a different clinical entity. The genealogical tree of a family with TS is illustrated in Fig. 3. Finally, recent studies revealed a possible involvement of the *p53* gene in the progression of tumors developed in TS patients [107].

Peutz-Jeghers Syndrome

Peutz-Jeghers syndrome (PJS) [108, 109] is characterized by the presence of hamartomatous polyps of the gastrointestinal tract, melanin spots on the lips and the buccal mucosa, and an autosomal dominant type of genetic transmission [110, 111]. Histologically, hamartomas show a complex branching pattern of smooth muscle supporting normal lamina propria and glands; thus, these polyps are basically composed of normal elements indigenous to the site in which they appear, although their general architecture is markedly abnormal [46]. Hamartomatous polyps are found more frequently in the small bowel, but are usually also present in the colon and stomach and, more rarely, in other mucosal surfaces, such as the upper respiratory and the urinary tracts [112]. Although hamartomatous polyps are commonly not

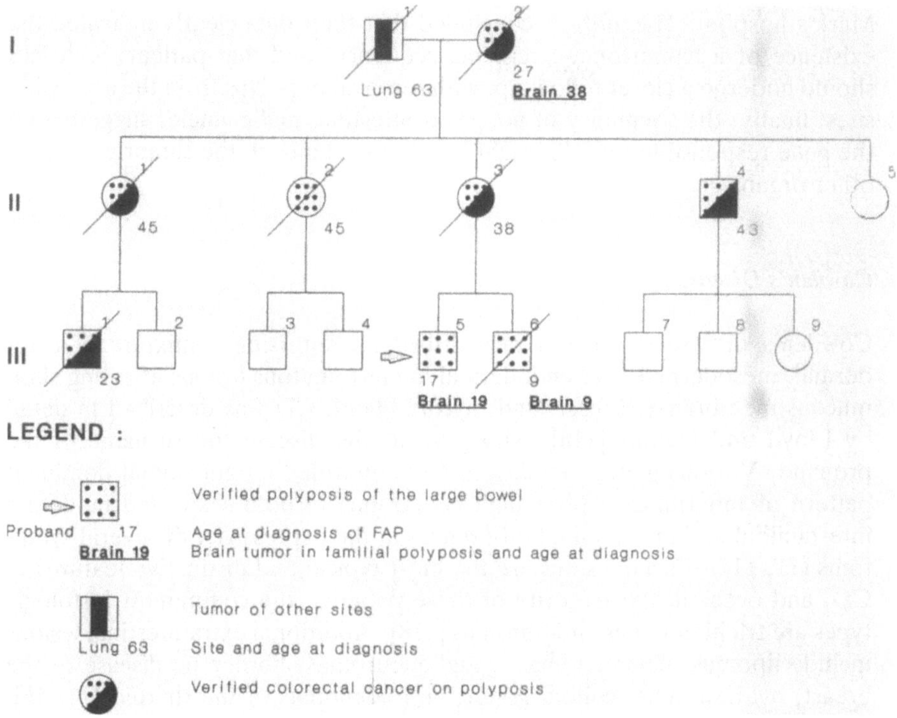

Fig. 3. Representative pedigree of a family with characteristics of Turcot syndrome. Three family members (*I-2*, *III-5*, and *III-6*) were affected by both brain tumors and diffuse intestinal polyposis

considered as precancerous lesions, various studies in the last few years showed the frequent occurrence of gastrointestinal malignancies in PJS; even more interestingly, these patients seem to be prone to the development of tumors of other organs. Thus, Giardiello et al. [113] reported the occurrence of cancer in 15 out of 31 patients with PJS after an average interval of 25 years from the diagnosis. Only four of these tumors were localized in the gastrointestinal tract, whereas the others occurred in various organs, including pancreas, breast, lung, and ovary. According to these findings, the relative risk of cancer in PJS patients was 18 times higher than that of the general population. Similarly, Foley et al. [111] found two gastrointestinal malignancies in the follow-up of the first family with PJS described in the United States (the "Harrisburg family") [114]; in addition, the authors documented the presence of adenomatous and carcinomatous changes in a duodenal hamartomatous polyp, thus suggesting the possible existence of a hamartoma-adenoma-carcinoma sequence in gastrointestinal tumorigenesis. A similar excess of gastrointestinal and nongastrointestinal malignancies was reported by Spiegelman et al. [115] in 72 patients with PJS studied at St.

Mark's hospital. The authors concluded that their data clearly indicated the existence of a hamartoma-carcinoma sequence, and that patients with PJS should undergo a closer follow-up, with removal of polyps from the accessible sites; finally, the frequency of nongastrointestinal malignancies suggests that the gene responsible for PJS might be of importance in the tumorigenesis of other organs.

Cowden's Disease

Cowden's disease (CD) is a rare disorder comprising a mixture of ectodermal, mesodermal, and endodermal hamartomatous lesions affecting skin, mucous membranes, breast, and thyroid gland. CD was described in detail by Lloyd and Dennis [116], who gave to the disease the surname of the proband. Various genetic studies in CD confirmed an autosomal dominant pattern of inheritance with a high penetrance in both sexes and moderate interfamilial and intrafamilial differences in the expressivity of several symptoms [11, 117]. Facial lesions are the most typical and distinctive features of CD, and occur in the majority of these patients; the commonest histologic types are trichilemomas and fibromas [118]. Additional extraintestinal lesions include lipomas, hemangiomas, ganglioneuromas, fibrocystic disease of the breast, ovarian cysts, colloid goiter, and adenomas of the thyroid [11, 46]; moreover, other congenital abnormalities – such as craniomegaly, arched palate, and adenoid facies – have been described in these families [11, 117]. In CD, polyps can be seen in various gastrointestinal tracts, from the esophagus to the rectum, and their frequency is in the order of 30%–60% of all cases [46, 117]; the morphologic aspect of these lesions, however, is rather peculiar, being characterized by fibrosis of the lamina propria, cystic dilatations of glands, extension of the muscularis mucosae into the lamina propria, accumulation of adipose tissue, and frequent lymphoid follicles [11, 119]. Although there is no evidence that these gastrointestinal polyps may progress to frank malignancy, patients with CD are at high risk of other cancers, in particular breast and thyroid carcinoma; indeed, the risk of breast cancer is so high for these patients that some authors [120] recommend prophylactic bilateral total mastectomy by their 3rd decade. Cytogenetic investigations, DNA repair studies, and, more recently, analysis of the amplification or rearrangements of genes (*ras* and c-*erbB-2*) presumably involved in the pathogenesis of various tumors did not reveal appreciable abnormalities in CD, so that the genetic cause of the syndrome remains unknown [117, 120].

Familial Juvenile Polyposis

Familial juvenile polyposis (FJP) is another hamartomatous polyposis syndrome characterized by an autosomal dominant type of inheritance and an excess of gastrointestinal malignancies. Polyps usually number more than 10, but less than 200, and can be found in the large bowel (where they are most common), in the stomach, and in the small bowel. The average diameter of these lesions is 1–2 cm; histologic examination shows dilated and elongated glands with slightly irregular contours set in an abundant stromal tissue [121]; the glands are lined by normal colonic epithelial cells, and the stroma is often inflamed and edematous. Mixed polyps can be found in which adenomatous areas can be recognized in the context of a hamartomatous lesion, and this may explain the frequency of malignant changes reported by various authors [11, 46, 121]. The first description of FJP represents a further contribution of St. Mark's hospital to our understanding of hereditary polyposis [122]. The St. Mark's registry includes 36 families with FJP, although only 9 of these are clearly genetically transmitted [123]. Nonfamilial cases might simply be phenocopies or can be due to new mutation of the putative gene responsible for the disease. It is interesting to note that birth defects (craniomegaly, intellectual handicap, cryptorchidism, malrotation of the bowel, cardiac lesions, and others) are relatively frequent in nonfamilial juvenile polyposis, but rare in FJP [11, 124].

Several authors reported the development of gastrointestinal carcinoma in patients with FJP or in their family members [125–127]. By reviewing this topic, Jarvinen and Franssila [128] found 9 cases of colorectal cancer out of 102 patients with FJP, and a positive family history for this tumor (usually at an early onset) in the majority of these kindreds. Moreover, a recent report from the St. Mark's registry showed that 18 out of 87 patients with juvenile polyposis developed cancer of the large bowel in the follow-up [121]. The high risk for cancer in these patients seems to be limited to the colorectal tract; it is likely that some hamartomatous lesions evolve into adenomas of various degrees of dysplasia and then undergo carcinomatous changes. Because of this risk, various authors advocated subtotal colectomy with ileorectal anastomosis as a prophylaxis of large bowel cancer, especially in FJP patients with numerous polyps [20, 128]; alternatively, lifetime endoscopic surveillance of the gastrointestinal tract is strongly recommended [129].

Muir-Torre Syndrome and Other Rare Polyposis

Several other syndromes basically characterized by multiple polyps of the large bowel associated with various extraintestinal manifestations have been described. These can be summarized as follows. Muir-Torre syndrome was described independently by the two authors in 1967 [130, 131]; the main feature of this disease is the association of multiple tumors of sebaceous glands with adenomas and carcinomas of the gastrointestinal tract; in addition, several other neoplasms can be seen in these families, including endometrial and breast cancer, urinary tract and prostate tumors, leukemia, and brain tumors [132]. Owing to the preponderance of early onset cancer of the large bowel in these kindreds, some authors suggested that Muir-Torre syndrome represents a different phenotypic expression of hereditary nonpolyposis colorectal cancer (see previous chapter) [133–134].

Ruvalcaba-Myrhe-Smith syndrome (RMSS) [46, 135] is characterized by hamartomatous polyps of the large bowel associated with mental retardation, unusual craniofacial appearance, and pigmented macules on the penis; although only few patients have been described, the disease seems to be transmitted through an autosomal dominant type of inheritance. The close histologic similarity of hamartomatous lesions in this syndrome and in FJP, and the frequency of congenital abnormalities in patients with juvenile polyps, suggest that RMSS might be a variant of FJP [11].

In Cronkhite-Canada syndrome (CCS) [136, 137], hamartomatous polyps of the gastrointestinal tract usually appear in adults, and are histologically similar to those seen in juvenile polyposis. CCS does not seem to be genetically transmitted, while it is frequently associated with the development of colorectal cancer [138]; additional clinical features of CCS include alopecia, skin hyperpigmentation, nail dystrophy, and protein-losing enteropathy [46]. Finally, in Zanca's syndrome [46], diffuse polyposis of the large bowel is associated with cartilaginous exostoses; it is likely that the disease represents a variant of adenomatosis coli characterized by a rather characteristic extracolonic manifestation.

References

1. Sklifasowski NW (1881) Polyadenoma tractus intestinalis. Vrac 4:55–57
2. Cripps WH (1882) Two cases of disseminated polypus of the rectum. Trans Pathol Soc Lond 33:165–168
3. Smith T (1887) Three cases of multiple polypi of the large bowel occurring in one family. S Barth Hosp Rep 23:225–229
4. Lockhart-Mummery P (1925) Cancer and heredity. Lancet 1:427–429
5. Bussey HJR (1975) Familial polyposis coli. John Hopkins University Press, New York
6. Cockayne EA (1927) Heredity in relation to cancer. Cancer Rev 2:337–347
7. Lockhart-Mummery JP (1934) The causation and treatment of multiple adenomatosis of the colon. Ann Surg 99:178–184
8. Gardner EJ (1951) A genetic and clinical study of intestinal polyposis, a predisposing factor to carcinoma of the colon and rectum. Am J Hum Genet 3:167–176
9. Parks AG, Nicholls RJ, Beliveau P et al. (1980) Proctocolectomy with ileal reservoir and anal anastomosis. Br J Surg 67:533–538
10. Utsunomiya J, Iwama T, Imajo M et al. (1980) Total colectomy, mucosal proctectomy and ileal anastomosis. Dis Colon Rectum 23:459–466
11. Haggitt RC, Reid BJ (1986) Hereditary gastrointestinal polyposis syndromes. Am J Surg Pathol 10(12):871–887
12. Bulow S (1989) Familial adenomatous polyposis. Ann Med 21:299–307
13. Naylor EW, Lebenthal E (1980) Gardner's syndrome: recent developments in research and management. Dig Dis Sci 25:945–959
14. Waddell WR, Longhry RW (1983) Sulindac for polyposis of the colon. J Surg Oncol 24:83–87

15. Herrera L, Kakati S, Gibas L et al. (1986) Gardner syndrome in a man with an interstitial deletion of 5q. Am J Med Genet 25:473–476
16. Bodmer WF, Bailey CJ, Bodmer J et al. (1987) Localization of the gene for FAP on chromosome 5. Nature 328:614–619
17. Kinzler KW, Nilbert MC, Su LK et al. (1991) Identification of FAP locus from chromosome 5q21. Science 253:661–665
18. Groden J, Thliveris A, Samowitz W et al. (1991) Identification and characterization of the familial adenomatous polyposis gene. Cell 66:589–600
19. Utsunomiya J, Iwama T (1980) Adenomatosis coli in Japan. In: Winawer S, Schottenfeld D, Sherlock P (eds) Colorectal cancer: prevention, epidemiology and screening. Raven, New York, pp 83–95
20. Alm T (1985) Hereditary adenomatosis of the colon and the rectum. In: Lynch HT, Lynch PM (eds) Colon cancer genetics. Von Nostrand Reinhold, New York, pp 30–51
21. Alm T, Lieznerski G (1973) The intestine polyposis. Clin Gastroenterol 2: 577–602
22. Ponz de Leon M, Sassatelli R, Zanghieri G et al. (1989) Hereditary adenomatosis of the colon and rectum: clinical features of 8 families from Northern Italy. Am J Gastroenterol 84:906–916
23. Jarvinen HJ (1992) Epidemiology of familial adenomatous polyposis in Finland: impact of family screening on the colorectal cancer rate and survival. Gut 33:357–360
24. Lipkin M, Winawer SJ, Sherlock P (1981) Early identification of individuals at increased risk for cancer of the large intestine. Clin Bull 11:13–21
25. Bulow S, Holm NV, Hauge M (1986) The incidence and prevalence of familial polyposis in Denmark. Scand J Soc Med 14:67–74
26. Muto T, Kamiya J, Sawada T et al. (1985) Mucin abnormality of colonic mucosa in patients with FAP. Dis Colon Rectum 28:147–148
27. Deschner E, Lipkin M (1975) Proliferative pattern in colonic mucosa in familial polyposis. Cancer 35:413–418
28. Lipkin M, Blattner WE, Fraumeni JF et al. (1983) Tritiated thymidine labeling distribution as a marker for hereditary predisposition to colon cancer. Cancer Res 43:1899–1904
29. Farmer KCR, Phillips RKS (1993) Colectomy with ileorectal anastomosis lowers rectal mucosal cell proliferation in FAP. Dis Colon Rectum 36:167–171
30. Roncucci L, Stamp D, Medline A et al. (1991) Identification and quantification of aberrant crypt foci and microadenomas in the human colon. Hum Pathol 22:287–294
31. Stopera SA, Bird RR (1993) Effects of all-trans retinoic acid as potential chemopreventive agent on the formation of azoxymethane-induced aberrant crypt foci. Int J Cancer 53:798–804
32. Utsunomiya J, Nakamura T (1975) The occult osteomatous changes in the mandible in patients with familial polyposis coli. Br J Cancer 62:45–51
33. Offerhaus GJA, Levin LS, Giardiello FM et al. (1987) Occult radiopaque jaw lesions in FAP and hereditary nonpolyposis colorectal cancer. Gastroenterology 93:490–497
34. Naylor EW, Gardner EJ, Richards R (1979) Desmoid tumors and mesenteric fibromatosis in Gardner syndrome. Arch Surg 114:1161–1185
35. Erbe RW (1976) Current concepts in genetics: inherited gastrointestinal polyposis syndromes. N Engl J Med 294:1101–1104
36. Jones IT, Fazio VW, Weakley FL et al. (1986) Desmoid tumors in familial polyposis coli. Ann Surg 204:94–97
37. Watne AL, Core SK, Carrier JM (1975) Gardner's syndrome. SGO 141:53–56

38. Itoh H, Ikeda S, Oohata Y et al. (1988) Treatment of desmoid tumors in Gardner's syndrome. Dis Colon Rectum 31:459–461
39. Seiter K, Kemeny N (1993) Successful treatment of a desmoid tumor with doxorubicin. Cancer 71:2242–2244
40. Blair NP, Trempe CL (1980) Hypertrophy of the retinal pigment epithelium associated with Gardner's syndrome. Am J Ophthalmol 90:661–667
41. Traboulsi EI, Krush AJ, Gardner EJ et al. (1987) Prevalence and importance of pigmented ocular fundus lesions in Gardner's syndrome. N Engl J Med 316:661–668
42. Baker RH, Heinemann MH, Miller HH et al. (1988) Hyperpigmented lesions of the retinal pigment epithelium in familial adenomatous polyposis. Am J Med Genet 31:427–435
43. Baba S, Tsuchiya M, Watanabe I et al. (1990) Importance of retinal pigmentation as a subclinical marker in familial adenomatous polyposis. Dis Colon Rectum 33:660–665
44. Heyen F, Jagelman DG, Romania A et al. (1990) Predictive value of CHRPE as a clinical marker for familial adenomatous polyposis. Dis Colon Rectum 33:1003–1008
45. Lyons LA, Lewis RA, Strong LC et al. (1988) A genetic study of Gardner syndrome and congenital hypertrophy of the retinal pigment epithelium. Am J Hum Genet 42:290–296
46. Lynch HT, Smyrk T, Watson P et al. (1991) Hereditary colorectal cancer. Semin Oncol 18:337–366
47. Spigelman AD, Williams GB, Talbot IC et al. (1989) Upper gastrointestinal cancer in patients with familial adenomatous polyposis. Lancet 2:783–785
48. Ida M, Tsuneyoshi Y, Itoh H et al. (1988) Natural history of gastric adenomas in patients with familial adenomatosis coli/Gardner's syndrome. Cancer 61: 605–611
49. Goodman AJ, Dundas SAC, Scholefield JH et al. (1988) Gastric carcinoma and FAP. Int J Colorectal Dis 3:201–203
50. Watanabe H, Enjoji M, Yao T et al. (1978) Gastric lesions in familial adenomatosis coli. Hum Pathol 9:269–283
51. Iida M, Yao T, Itoh H et al. (1989) Natural history of duodenal lesions in Japanese patients with familial adenomatosis coli. Gastroenterology 96: 1301–1306
52. Noda Y, Watanabe H, Iida M et al. (1992) Histologic follow-up of ampullary adenomas in patients with familial adenomatosis coli. Cancer 70:1847–1856
53. Jagelman DG, DeCosse JJ, Bussey HJR et al. (1988) Upper gastrointestinal cancer in familial adenomatous polyposis. Lancet 1:1149–1151
54. Iida M, Ohsato K, Itoh H et al. (1989) Diagnostic value of intraoperative fiberoscopy for small intestinal polyps in familial adenomatosis coli. Endoscopy 12:161–165
55. Philips LG (1981) Polyposis and carcinoma of the small bowel and familial colonic polyposis. Dis Colon Rectum 24:478–481
56. Ross JE, Mara JE (1974) Small bowel polyps and carcinoma in multiple intestinal polyposis. Arch Surg 108:736–738
57. Myrhoj T, Bulow S, Mogensen AM (1989) Multiple adenomas in terminal ileum 25 years after restorative proctocolectomy for FAP. Dis Colon Rectum 32:618–620
58. Iida M, Itoh H, Matsui T (1989) Ileal adenomas in postcolectomy patients with familial adenomatosis coli/Gardner's syndrome. Dis Colon Rectum 32: 1034–1038

59. Gilson TP, Sollenberger LL (1992) Adenocarcinoma of an ileostomy in a patient with FAP. Dis Colon Rectum 35:261–265
60. Thompson JS, Harned RK, Anderson JC et al. (1983) Papillary carcinoma of the thyroid and FAP. Dis Colon Rectum 26:583–585
61. Plail RO, Bussey HJR, Glazer G et al. (1987) Adenomatous polyposis: an association with carcinoma of the thyroid. Br J Surg 74:377–380
62. Bulow S, Holm NV, Mellemgaard A (1988) Papillary thyroid carcinoma in Danish patients with FAP. Int J Colorectal Dis 3:29–31
63. Bernstein IT, Bulow F, Mauritzen K (1992) Hepatoblastoma in two cousins in a family with adenomatous polyps. Dis Colon Rectum 35:373–374
64. Komorowski RA, Tresp MG, Wilson SD (1986) Biliary neoplasia in Gardner's syndrome. Dis Colon Rectum 29:55–58
65. Jarvinen H, Nyberg M, Peltokallio P (1983) Biliary involvement in familial adenomatosis coli. Dis Colon Rectum 26:525–528
66. Giardiello FM, Offerhaus GJA, Lee DH et al. (1993) Increased risk of thyroid and pancreatic carcinoma in familial adenomatous polyposis. Gut 34:1394–1396
67. Painter TA, Jagelman DG (1985) Adrenal adenomas and adrenal carcinomas in association with hereditary adenomatosis of the colon and rectum. Cancer 55:2001–2004
68. Bussey HJR, Morson BC (1978) Familial polyposis coli. In: Lipkin M, Good RA (eds) Gastrointestinal tract cancer. Plenum Medical, New York, pp 275–294
69. Utsunomiya J, Murata M, Tanimura M et al. (1980) An analysis of the age distribution of colon cancer in adenomatosis coli. Cancer 45:198–205
70. Evans DGR, Guy SP, Thakker N et al. (1993) Non-penetrance and late appearance of polyps in families with FAP. Gut 34:1389–1393
71. Moertel CG, Hill JR, Adson M (1970) Surgical management of multiple polyposis. Arch Surg 100:521–525
72. Bussey HJR, Eyers AA, Ritchie SM et al. (1985) The rectum in adenomatous polyposis. Br J Surg 72[Suppl]:29–31
73. Berk T, Bulow S, Cohen Z et al. (1988) Symposium: surgical aspects of FAP. Int J Colorectal Dis 3:1–16
74. Iwama T, Mishima Y, Utsunomiya J (1993) The impact of FAP on the tumorigenesis and mortality at several organs. Ann Surg 217:101–108
75. Arvanitis ML, Jagelman DG, Fazio VW et al. (1990) Mortality in patients with FAP. Dis Colon Rectum 33:639–642
76. Bussey HJR, DeCosse JJ, Deschner EE et al. (1982) A randomized trial of ascorbic acid in polyposis coli. Cancer 50:1434–1439
77. DeCosse JJ, Miller HH, Lesser ML (1989) Effect of wheat fiber and vitamins C and E on rectal polyps in patients with FAP. JNCI 81:1290–1297
78. Waddell WR, Ganser GF, Cerise EJ et al. (1989) Sulindac for polyposis of the colon. Am J Surg 157:175–179
79. Labayle D, Fisher D, Vielh P et al. (1991) Sulindac causes regression of rectal polyps in FAP. Gastroenterology 101:635–639
80. Giardiello FM, Hamilton SR, Krush AJ et al. (1993) Treatment of colonic and rectal adenomas with sulindac in FAP. N Engl J Med 328:1313–1316
81. Leppert M, Dobbs M, Scambler P et al. (1987) The gene for familial polyposis coli maps to the long arm of chromosome 5. Science 238:1411–1413
82. Joslyn G, Carlson M, Thliveris A et al. (1991) Identification and deletion mutations and three new genes at the familial polyposis locus. Cell 66:601–613
83. Nishisho I, Nakamura Y, Miyoshi Y et al. (1991) Mutations of chromosome 5q21 genes in FAP and colorectal cancer patients. Science 253:665–669

84. Olschwang S, Laurant-Puig P, Groden J et al. (1993) Germ-line mutations in the first 14 exons of the APC gene. Am J Hum Genet 52:273–279
85. Groden J, Gelbert L, Thliveris A et al. (1993) Mutational analysis of patients with adenomatous polyposis: identical inactivating mutations in unrelated individuals. Am J Hum Genet 52:263–272
86. Varesco L, Gismondi V, Jamer R et al. (1993) Identification of APC gene mutations in Italian adenomatous polyposis coli patients by PCR-SSCP analysis. Am J Hum Genet 52:280–285
87. Su LK, Johnson KA, Smith KJ et al. (1993) Association between wild type and mutant APC gene products. Cancer Res 53:2728–2731
88. Ando H, Miyoshi Y, Nagase H et al. (1993) Detection of 12 germ-line mutations in the adenomatous polyposis gene by polymerase chain reaction. Gastroenterology 104:989–993
89. Tops CMJ, Wijnen JT, Griffioen G et al. (1989) Presymptomatic diagnosis of FAP by bridging DNA markers. Lancet 2:1361–1363
90. Paul P, Jagelman DG, Fazio VW et al. (1990) Evaluation of polymorphic genetic markers for linkage to the FAP locus on chromosome 5. Dis Colon Rectum 33:740–744
91. Olschwang S, Weiffenbach B, Laurent-Puig P et al. (1991) Genetic characterization of the APC locus involved in FAP. Gastroenterology 101:154–160
92. Spirio L, Nelson L, Ward K et al. (1993) A CA-repeat polymorphism close to the APC gene offers improved diagnostic testing for familial APC. Am J Hum Genet 52:286–296
93. Burt RW, Groden J (1993) The genetic and molecular diagnosis of FAP. Gastroenterology 104:1211–1214
94. Muto T, Kamiya J, Sawada T et al. (1983) Morphogenesis of human colonic cancer. Dis Colon Rectum 26:257–262
95. Muto T, Kamiya J, Sawada T et al. (1985) Small flat adenoma of the large bowel with special reference to its clinicopathologic features. Dis Colon Rectum 28:847–851
96. Adachi M, Muto T, Okinaga K et al. (1991) Clinicopathologic features of flat adenoma. Dis Colon Rectum 34:981–986
97. Lynch HT, Smyrk T, Lanspa SJ et al. (1988) Flat adenomas in a colon cancer-prone kindred. JNCI 80:278–282
98. Lynch HT, Smyrk TC, Lanspa SJ et al. (1990) Phenotypic variation in colorectal adenoma/cancer expression in 2 families: hereditary flat adenoma syndrome. Cancer 66:909–915
99. Lynch HT, Smyrk TC, Watson P et al. (1992) Hereditary flat adenoma syndrome: a variant of FAP? Dis Colon Rectum 35:411–421
100. Lynch HT, Smyrk TC, Lanspa SJ et al. (1993) Upper gastrointestinal manifestations in families with hereditary flat adenoma syndrome. Cancer 71:2709–2714
101. Spirio L, Otterud B, Stauffer D et al. (1992) Linkage of variant or attenuated form of adenomatous polyposis coli to the APC locus. Am J Hum Genet 51:92–100
102. Turcot J, Despres JP, St Pierre F (1959) Malignant tumors of the central nervous system associated with familial polyposis of the colon: report of two cases. Dis Colon Rectum 2:465–468
103. Newton HB, Rosenblum MK, Malkin MG (1991) Turcot's syndrome: flow cytometric analysis. Cancer 68:1633–1639
104. Itoh H, Ohsato M, Yao T et al. (1979) Turcot's syndrome and its mode of inheritance. Gut 20:414–419
105. Lewis JH, Ginsberg AL, Toomey KE (1983) Turcot's syndrome: evidence for autosomal dominant inheritance. Cancer 51:524–528

106. Kropilak M, Jagelman MD, Fazio VW et al. (1989) Brain tumors in familial adenomatous polyposis. Dis Colon Rectum 32:778–782
107. Kikuchi T, Rempel SA, Rutz HP et al. (1993) Turcot's syndrome of glioma and polyposis occurs in the absence of germ line mutations of exons 5 to 9 of p53. Cancer Res 53:957–961
108. Peutz JLA (1921) Very remarkable case of familial polyposis of mucous membranes of intestinal tract and nasopharynx accompanied by peculiar pigmentations of the skin and mucous membranes. Ned Maand Geneeskd 10:134–146
109. Jeghers H, McKusick VA, Katz KH (1949) Generalized intestinal polyposis and melanin spots of oral mucosa, lips and digits: a syndrome of diagnostic significance. N Engl J Med 241:993–1005
110. Burdick D, Prior JT, Scanlon GT (1963) Peutz-Jeghers syndrome: a clinical-pathological study of a large family with a ten-year follow-up. Cancer 16: 854–867
111. Foley TR, McGarrity TJ, Abt AB (1988) Peutz-Jeghers syndrome: a clinicopathologic survey of the "Harrisburg Family" with a 49-year follow-up. Gastroenterology 95:1535–1540
112. Sommerhaug RG, Mason T (1970) Peutz-Jeghers syndrome and ureteral polyposis. JAMA 211:120–122
113. Giardiello F, Welsh SB, Hamilton SR et al. (1987) Increased risk of cancer in the Peutz-Jeghers syndrome. N Engl J Med 316:1511–1514
114. Bartholomew LG, Moore CE, Dahlin DC et al. (1962) Intestinal polyposis associated with mucocutaneous pigmentation. Surg Gynecol Obstet 115:1–11
115. Sligelman AD, Murday V, Phillips RKS (1989) Cancer and the Peutz-Jeghers syndrome. Gut 30:1588–1590
116. Salem OS, Steck WD (1983) Cowden's disease (multiple hamartoma and neoplasia syndrome). J Am Acad Dermatol 8:686–696
117. Starink TM, van der Veen JPW, Arwert F et al. (1986) The Cowden syndrome: a clinical and genetic study in 21 patients. Clin Genet 29:222–233
118. Brownstein MH, Mehregan AM, Bikowski JB et al. (1979) The dermatopathology of Cowden's syndrome. Br J Dermatol 100:667–673
119. Weary PE, Gorlin RJ, Gentry WC et al. (1972) Multiple hamartoma syndrome (Cowden's disease). Arch Dermatol 106:682–690
120. Williard W, Borgen P, Bol R et al. (1992) Cowden's disease: a case report with analysis at the molecular level. Cancer 69:2969–2974
121. Jass JR, Williams CB, Bussey HJR (1988) Juvenile polyposis – a precancerous condition. Histopathology 13:619–630
122. McColl I, Bussey HJR, Veale AMO et al. (1964) Juvenile polyposis coli. Proc R Soc Med 57:896–897
123. Bussey HJR, Veale AMO, Morson BC (1978) Genetics of gastrointestinal polyposis. Gastroenterology 74:1325–1330
124. Walpole IR, Cullity G (1989) Juvenile polyposis: a case with early presentation and death attributable to adenocarcinoma of the pancreas. Am J Med Genet 32:1–8
125. Grotsky HW, Rickert RR, Smith WD et al. (1982) Familial juvenile polyposis coli: a clinical and pathological study of a large kindred. Gastroenterology 82:494–501
126. Mills SE, Fechner RE (1982) Unusual adenomatous polyps in juvenile polyposis coli. Am J Surg Pathol 6:177–183
127. Longo WE, Touloukian RJ, West AB et al. (1990) Malignant potential of juvenile polyposis coli. Dis Colon Rectum 33:980–984
128. Jarvinen H, Franssila KO (1984) Familial juvenile polyposis coli: increased risk of colorectal cancer. Gut 25:792–800

129. Saul SH, Raffensperger E (1988) Juvenile polyposis: intramucosal signet-cell adenocarcinoma arising in a polyp at a gastro-jejunostomy site. Surg Pathol 1:159–164
130. Torre D (1968) Multiple sebaceous tumors. Arch Dermatol 98:549–551
131. Muir EG, Belly AJY, Barlow KA (1967) Multiple primary carcinomata of the colon, duodenum and larynx associated with kerato-acanthomata of the face. Br J Surg 54:191–195
132. Alessi E, Brambilla L, Luporini G et al. (1985) Multiple sebaceous tumors and carcinomas of the colon: Torre syndrome. Cancer 55:2566–2574
133. Lynch HT, Lynch PM, Pester J et al. (1981) The cancer family syndrome: rare cutaneous phenotypic linkage of Torre's syndrome. Arch Intern Med 141:607–611
134. Anderson DE (1980) An inherited form of large bowel cancer: Muir's syndrome. Cancer 45:1103–1107
135. Ruvalcaba RHA, Myhre S, Smith DW (1980) Sotos syndrome with intestinal polyposis and pigmentary changes of the genitalia. Clin Genet 18:413–416
136. Daniel ES, Ludwig SL, Lewin KS et al. (1974) The Cronkhite-Canada syndrome: an analysis of clinical and pathologic features and therapy in 55 patients. Medicine 61:293–308
137. Burke AP, Sobin LH (1989) The pathology of Cronkhite-Canada polyps: a comparison to juvenile polyposis. Surg Pathol 13:940–946
138. Rappaport LB, Sperling HV, Stavrides A (1986) Colon cancer in the Cronkhite-Canada syndrome. J Clin Gastroenterol 8:199–202

Familial Aspects in Carcinoma of the Pancreas

> *Treatment of adenocarcinoma of the pancreas gives rise to little ground for optimism. Progress in understanding of the causes of this appalling disease remains disappointingly slow, and despite major improvements in our ability to detect its presence, diagnosis is almost invariably delayed until the disease has spread beyond the reach of surgical cure.*
>
> (D.C. CARTER 1990)

Introduction

Cancer of the exocrine pancreas is a rapidly progressive disease whose etiology remains largely obscure. This neoplasm is relatively frequent throughout the Western world, where it represents the fifth commonest cause of cancer-related mortality, accounting for approximately 25 000 annual deaths in the United States and 4000–6000 in countries such as Italy and the United Kingdom. The main features of pancreatic carcinoma are the almost absolute lack of pathogenetic hypotheses – either from animal experimentation or epidemiologic investigations – and the extremely poor prognosis; it follows that the diagnosis of this enigmatic disease represents a virtual death sentence for the patient.

At variance with endocrine pancreatic tumors, whose genetic basis has been well characterized within the multiple endocrine neoplasia syndromes, until recently there were only few anecdotal reports on the familial occurrence of pancreatic adenocarcinoma. However, more recent studies suggest that familial clustering of the disease is not rare, and that about 5% of patients with this tumor may show a family history of pancreatic cancer. Moreover, the possible role of oncogene and/or tumor suppressor gene alterations in the development of pancreatic carcinoma has recently become the object of intense investigation, thus leading to the formulation of some promising pathogenetic hypotheses.

General Aspects

Clinical and Epidemiologic Features

In the last 2 decades the incidence of pancreatic carcinoma in Western countries has shown only slight fluctuations; at present, it is estimated to be in the order of 10–15 new cases/100 000 inhabitants per year, with a male to female ratio of 1.3–1.5 [1, 2]. Lower rates are usually seen in Eastern countries, though in Japan the incidence rose consistently during the last 30 years [3].

Of the various risk factors, cigarette smoking seems to be the most important determinant of pancreatic cancer, with relative risks higher than 2.0 for individuals smoking more than 1 pack of cigarettes per day [4, 5]. Although the pathogenetic link between smoking habit and tumor development remains unknown, it is of interest that in rats pancreatic tumors can be induced by the administration of nitrosamines contained in tobacco smoke [6, 7]. As for many other human tumors, a diet rich in animal fat and meat might enhance the risk of pancreatic cancer, while diets rich in fruits or vegetables seem to show a protective effect [8]. In contrast, no association could be found between risk of the disease and consumption of tea, beer, or alcoholic beverages [5]. In 1981, McMahon et al. [9] gathered epidemiologic evidence of a possible link between coffee consumption and increased risk of pancreatic cancer; these results, however, were not confirmed by subsequent prospective investigations [10]. An increased risk of pancreatic carcinoma has also been associated with a history of subtotal gastrectomy [5], diabetes mellitus [11], and chronic pancreatitis [12], and with some working activities [13].

In most patients the diagnosis of pancreatic tumor is still based on the presence of symptoms. Epigastric pain, jaundice, and weight loss represent the typical manifestations of tumors localized in the head or the body of the gland. Cancers of the tail do not compress the bile duct and may remain painless for a longer time; in this case, therefore, the appearance of jaundice or pain usually indicates liver metastasis. All these symptoms are virtually of no clinical value, since by their appearance the disease is almost invariably in an advanced stage, with little or no prospect of cure. On the other hand, it is extremely difficult to diagnose pancreatic carcinoma at an early stage, before obstruction of the bile duct or infiltration of the duodenum or other organs; even the availability of tumor markers, i.e., CA-19.9, carcinoembryonic antigen (CEA), appears to be of little help, since the levels are frequently normal in the early stages of the disease [14].

The large majority of histologically verified tumors are adenocarcinomas originating from the ductular or ductal epithelium; other common histologic types include giant cell carcinoma, mucinous carcinoma, cystoadenocarcinoma (which carries a relatively good prognosis), and microadenocarcinoma [15]. Acinar cell tumors constitute 5% of the total. At diagnosis, almost 90% of pancreatic tumors are no longer confined to the gland; early metastatic spread to adjacent or distal lymph nodes and perineural invasion within and beyond the organ are extremely frequent, whereas liver, peritoneum, and lung represent the commonest sites of extranodal metastasis [16]. Pancreatic carcinomas are usually staged into four main categories. In stage I, the malignant tissue is limited to the pancreas with no direct extension beyond the gland; stage II tumors extend into the surrounding tissues but without lymph node involvement; in stage III, the neoplasms spread to regional lymph nodes, and in stage IV distant metastases are present.

Besides clinical symptoms, the diagnosis of pancreatic cancer is based on the careful evaluation of recent imaging techniques, in particular abdominal ultrasounds, computed tomography, and magnetic resonance imaging. Endoscopic retrograde cholangiopancreatography and angiography are also of value for diagnosing neoplasms of the pancreatobiliary junction and for a proper assessment of the major vascular involvement. Since some benign conditions (including bile duct stones and chronic pancreatitis) may induce clinical manifestations similar to those of pancreatic carcinoma, cytologic or histologic confirmation of the diagnosis should be obtained. Percutaneous fine-needle aspiration cytology and tru-cut biopsy are the techniques of choice for morphologic diagnosis, though these maneuvers may expose the patient to the risk of seeding neoplastic cells along the needle tract [17, 18]. Once a diagnosis has been made, a critical evaluation of the various procedures may allow an accurate preneoplastic staging, with the objective of identifying tumors that can be removed with some chance of cure, those for which resection appears more difficult, and cases in which surgery is not feasible [19]. Besides ultrasonography and computed tomography, laparoscopy is particularly helpful in staging the disease, since it can visualize small liver, peritoneal, and omental metastases which are usually undetectable by imaging techniques [20]. Somewhat intuitively, it can be said that curative surgery is virtually limited to stage I patients, and these unfortunately represent only a small proportion of the total.

Management and Prognosis

Although there is little doubt that radical surgical resection offers the only hope of cure for patients with pancreatic cancer, this objective is much more utopian than real, for the following reasons. First of all, only a minority of patients – 5%–20%, according to the published series [21, 22] – have resectable disease, whereas the remaining affected individuals require only palliation for symptom relief. Secondly, the two standard surgical procedures for pancreatic cancer are pancreatoduodenectomy (or Whipple's operation) and total pancreatectomy, both complex operations which can be followed by serious postoperative problems, including fistulas at the anastomotic site and insulin-dependent diabetes. Thirdly, besides staging at diagnosis no biological marker indicative of the clinical outcome has been detected, though preliminary observations in a small number of patients seem to suggest that aneuploid tumors are associated with a more severe prognosis [23–25]. Finally, Gudjonsson recently reviewed the results of surgical treatment of pancreatic cancer over the 50 years which have elapsed from the first pancreatoduodenal resection [26]; of the 37300 patients considered, 4100 underwent surgical resection, and only 157 survived 5 years (3.5% of the operated, 0.4% of the total). It is noteworthy that 12 out of the 157 long-term survivors had not been operated upon. Moreover, operative mortality tended to improve gradually with time, though in 1980 it was still around 15%. The author was led to the conclusion that surgery had such a small effect on survival that this kind of operation, with the purpose of cure, should be abandoned. After this comprehensive report, new studies indicated a slightly more favorable outcome, with 5-year survival in the order of 15%–25% of total patients who underwent resection [27, 28]; there is no doubt, however, that early diagnosis and cure remain rare events for patients with pancreatic cancer. The use of adjuvant chemotherapy (fluorouracil alone, or in combination with mitomycin, streptozocin, and ifosfamide) or radiotherapy are of very little help in the management of these patients, although intraoperative radiation may be of some help for the relief of pain in many cases [29–31].

Familial Pancreatic Cancer

Despite its relative frequency, cancer of the exocrine pancreas has only rarely been reported in families, and consequently is not regarded as a familial tumor. However, during the last 20 years several anecdotal reports showed familial clustering of this disease; moreover, recent population-based case-control studies showed a significant excess of pancreatic cancer among close relatives of affected patients and, in addition, these tumors are not infrequent in the neoplastic spectrum of Lynch syndrome II (see chapter on "Hereditary and Familial Colorectal Cancer") [32, 33].

Reiner et al. [34] reported the occurrence of pancreatic carcinoma in a father and son who had both prior exposure to toxic chemicals, thus suggesting a possible interaction between environmental factors and genetic susceptibility. Interestingly, in the son cancer developed at the age of 39 years, a very early occurrence for this type of tumor. In 1973, MacDermott and Kramer described a remarkable family in which three brothers and a sister were affected by pancreatic cancer between the ages of 59 and 72 years [35]. A few years later a similar family was reported in which four brothers developed adenocarcinoma of the pancreas in the 7th or 8th decade of life [36]. This family also included cases of colorectal tumors, prostate cancer, and a carcinoma "in situ" of the cervix uteri; however, despite the striking aggregation of neoplasms and the absence of vertical transmission, the rarity of multiple and of early onset tumors does not allow this kindred to be defined as a Lynch syndrome II. In contrast, apparent vertical transmission was observed by Ehrenthal et al. [37] in a family in which pancreatic carcinoma developed in three women of consecutive generations who died of the disease at progressively younger ages. Although two of these patients were smokers, the early age of onset of cancer in the second and third generations (42 and 29 years, respectively) makes it unlikely that tumors developed only as a pure coincidence in these individuals, but rather suggests the existence of a genetic predisposition to the disease.

In a hospital-based case-control study, Falk et al. [38] evaluated family history of pancreatic carcinoma as part of a comprehensive study of this disease in Louisiana (United States). The study included 363 cases of pancreatic tumor diagnosed between 1979 and 1983, and 1234 controls from the same geographic area. The authors found a significant excess of either cancers of all sites or of the pancreas among case relatives (odds ratio, 1.86 and 5.2; CI, 1.4–2.4 and 2.0–13.2, respectively), and suggested that in their series there was a certain familial tendency for pancreatic carcinoma, although environmental factors were also implicated in the study (i.e., cigarette smoking and dietary habits) in the pathogenesis of these tumors. Similar results were reported in a recent Canadian study; Ghadirian et al. [39] carried out a population-based case-control study involving 150 patients with documented pancreatic cancer and 150 matched controls. Ten out of 150 cases (6.7%) had a positive family history for pancreatic carcinoma, often with more than one case of cancer besides the proband; in contrast, only one individual in the control group reported a family history of the disease. The authors interpreted their data as indicative of some familial predisposition to pancreatic tumors in approximately 6%–7% of the affected patients.

A detailed description of the main clinical and pathologic characteristics of familial pancreatic cancer has recently been provided by Lynch and colleagues [40] in a large series of 18 nuclear families. The main features of the study can be summarized as follows. First, the families were identified by the occurrence of pancreatic cancer in two or more first-degree relatives; a total of 48 individuals from these families reported a diagnosis of the disease, and in 39 of them (81.2%) medical charts or death certificates were available. Second, the histologic type was known for 28 patients; all tumors were ductal adenocarcinomas, with the exception of a malignant islet cell neoplasm. Third, early appearance of pancreatic cancer was rare in these families, with a median age at diagnosis of 70 years, and a range from 46 to 94 years; survival (22% at 1 year, and 3% at 2 years) in this series did not differ from that of the sporadic counterpart. Fourth, many members of the investigated families reported cancers of other sites; these included 17 breast carcinomas, 11 colorectal cancers, and 5 lung cancers, whereas melanomas, prostate, and other tumors were seen more rarely. Unfortunately the investigation was not population based, and this does not allow the definition of a precise estimate of the frequency of familial pancreatic cancer in the general population. A further problem might be the inclusion in the sample of families with Lynch syndrome II, which besides colonic, endometrial, and gastric carcinomas may also include – although more rarely – pancreatic neoplasms (see chapter on "Hereditary and Familial Colorectal Cancer"). However, other features of Lynch syndrome II (i.e., early age of onset and multiple tumors) were virtually absent in this series of investigated families.

Molecular Biology

Progress in understanding the biomolecular events of pancreatic tumorigenesis has been hindered by the limited availability of tumor material in comparison with other more accessible human neoplasms. Despite this, several abnormalities in oncogenes, tumor suppressor genes, and growth factors have been detected, although the observed findings do not allow the outline of an ordered sequence of genetic changes in pancreatic cancer development.

Overexpression of the epidermal growth factor receptor and of transforming growth factor alpha have been reported in several human pancreatic tumor cell lines [41–43]; in addition, Hall et al. reported abnormalities in the c-*erbB-2* oncogene expression in about 20% of pancreatic carcinomas [44]. However, the most interesting molecular feature of these tumors is mutations of the K-*ras* oncogene at codon 12, which have been found in more than 90% of the neoplasms and that might represent an early event in pancreatic tumorigenesis. Thus, Almoguera et al. found K-*ras* mutations in 21 out of 22 cases of pancreatic cancer, Smith et al. in 28 of 30 cases, and Toda and colleagues in all 18 patients investigated with the disease [45–47]. Similarly, Shibata et al. [48] used polymerase chain reaction and the RNAase A mismatch cleavage assay to investigate K-*ras* mutations in fine-needle aspirates of human pancreatic carcinoma; among the investigated patients, mutant K-*ras* oncogenes were found in 18 of 25 (72%) with malignant cells at histology, but in none of the benign aspiration cytologies, thus confirming the specificity of this genetic alteration. Moreover, in the study by Tada et al. [47], while all pancreatic carcinomas showed mutation of the K-*ras* gene at codon 12, no mutation was found in insulinomas (*n*, 2), gallbladder carcinomas (*n*, 11), chronic pancreatitis (*n*, 6), or normal pancreas (*n*, 16). Since the diagnosis of pancreatic carcinoma is often difficult, these findings might have a clinical application; in fact, this biomolecular procedure can be used either to differentiate pancreatic cancer, or to complement morphologic diagnosis. It is likely, therefore, that K-*ras* mutations will become a useful biological marker of pancreatic cancer [49].

Tumor suppressor gene abnormalities have also been implicated in the pathogenesis of pancreatic cancer. Alterations of the *p53* antioncogene are of particular interest, since germline mutations of this gene have recently been reported in Li-Fraumeni syndrome (see next chapter), which may occasionally include pancreatic carcinomas [50]. Ruggeri et al. [51], by sequence analysis, found point mutations in the conserved region of the gene (exons 5–8) in all seven human pancreatic carcinoma cell lines and in 40% of primary pancreatic tumors. Of the ten mutations detected, nine were transitions causing various amino acid changes (the most common being arginine to histidine), and 40% were in a "hot-spot" at codon 273; moreover, alterations of the retinoblastoma (*Rb*) gene were found in two of the seven cell lines, and in two of ten pancreatic carcinomas. The authors concluded that inactivation of the two tumor suppressor genes *p53* and *Rb* might play a role in the development of pancreatic cancer, though this does not exclude the possible involvement of other antioncogenes located on chromosomes 5q, 8p, or others [51–54].

Finally, Hohne et al. [55] studied, by Southern blot analysis, the expression of the *DCC* gene in pancreatic carcinoma. The gene, located on chromosome 18q21.3, has frequently been found deleted in colorectal carcinoma, and this is consistent with a putative tumor suppressor function of its product (*DCC* is for "deleted in colorectal carcinoma", see chapter on "Hereditary and Familial Colorectal Cancer") [56]. The authors found a greatly reduced or even extinct expression of *DCC* in the majority of the investigated pancreatic tumor cell lines and in 50% of primary cancers, thus suggesting a certain role of this gene in pancreatic tumorigenesis [55]. These findings might be of interest for at least two reasons. First, changes in the *DCC* gene do not seem to be limited to colorectal carcinoma, but it is likely that they represent a frequent event and, perhaps, a common pathogenetic step for several tumors of the digestive organs. Second, the *DCC* gene product shows similarities with the neural cell adhesion molecule [56]; since pancreatic cancer shows a marked tendency toward perineural metastatic diffusion, it is possible that this propensity reflects an altered expression of cell surface molecules which control the interaction between tumor cells and intercellular matrix. Thus, on theoretical grounds, loss or alterations of the *DCC* gene product might represent a major determinant of the characteristic invasiveness and poor prognosis of pancreatic cancer.

References

1. Gordis L, Gold LB (1984) Epidemiology of pancreatic cancer. World J Surg 8:808–821
2. Swedish Cancer Registry (1991) Cancer incidence in Sweden, 1988. National Board of Health and Welfare, Stockholm
3. Hirayama T (1989) Epidemiology of pancreatic cancer in Japan. Jpn J Clin Oncol 19:208–215
4. MacMahon B (1982) Risk factors for cancer of the pancreas. Cancer 50:2676–2680

5. Mack TM, Yu MC, Hanisch R et al. (1986) Pancreas cancer and smoking, beverage consumption, and past medical history. JNCI 76:49–60
6. Rivenson A, Hoffman D, Prokopczyk B et al. (1987) Induction of lung and exocrine pancreas tumors in F344 rats by tobacco-specific N-nitrosamines. Cancer Res 48:6912–6917
7. Rao MS (1987) Animal models of exocrine pancreatic carcinogenesis. Cancer Metastasis Rev 6:665–676
8. Norell SE, Ahlbom A, Erwald R et al. (1986) Diet and pancreatic cancer: a case-control study. Am J Epidemiol 124:894–902
9. MacMahon B, Yen S, Trichopoulos D et al. (1981) Coffee and cancer of the pancreas. N Engl J Med 304:630–633
10. Gordis L (1990) Consumption of methylxanthine-containing beverages and risk of pancreatic cancer. Cancer Lett 52:1–12
11. Cuzick J, Babiker AG (1989) Pancreatic cancer, alcohol, diabetes mellitus and gallbladder disease. Int J Cancer 43:415–421
12. Lowenfels AB, Maisonneuve P, Cavallini G et al. (1993) Pancreatitis and the risk of pancreatic cancer. N Engl J Med 328:1433–1437
13. Mancuso TF, El-Attar AA (1967) Cohort study of workers exposed to betanaphthylamine and benzidine. J Occup Med 9:277–285
14. Frebourg T, Bercoff E, Manchon N et al. (1988) The evaluation of CA 19.9 antigen level in the early detection of pancreatic cancer. Cancer 62:2287–2290
15. Morohoshi T, Held G, Kloppel G (1983) Exocrine pancreatic tumors and their histological classification. Histopathology 7:645–661
16. Nagai H, Kuroda A, Morioka Y (1986) Lymphatic and local spread of T1 and T2 pancreatic cancer. Ann Surg 204:65–71
17. Ferrucci JT, Wittenberg J, Margolies MN et al. (1979) Malignant seeding of the tract after thin needle aspiration biopsy. Radiology 130:345–346
18. Weiss SM, Skibber JM, Mohiuddin M et al. (1985) Rapid intra-abdominal spread of pancreatic cancer. Arch Surg 120:415–416
19. Warshaw AL, Fernandez del Castillo C (1992) Pancreatic carcinoma. N Engl J Med 326:455–465
20. Warshow AL, Tepper JE, Shipley WU (1986) Laparoscopy in the staging and planning of therapy for pancreatic cancer. Am J Surg 151:76–80
21. Rosenberg JM, Welch JP, Macaulay WP (1985) Cancer of the head of the pancreas: an institutional review with emphasis on surgical therapy. J Surg Oncol 28:217–221
22. Connolly MM, Dawson PJ, Michelassi F et al. (1987) Survival in 1001 patients with carcinoma of the pancreas. Ann Surg 206:366–373
23. Weger AR, Glaser KS, Schwab G et al. (1991) Quantitative nuclear DNA content in fine needle aspirates of pancreatic cancer. Gut 32:325–328
24. Allison DC, Bose KK, Hruban RH et al. (1991) Pancreatic cancer cell DNA content correlates with long term survival after pancreatoduodenectomy. Ann Surg 214:648–656
25. Porschen R, Remy U, Bevers G et al. (1993) Prognostic significance of DNA ploidy in adenocarcinoma of the pancreas. Cancer 71:3846–3850
26. Gudjonsson B (1987) Cancer of the pancreas: 50 years of surgery. Cancer 60:2284–2303
27. Trede M, Schwall G, Saeger HD (1990) Survival after pancreatoduodenectomy. Ann Surg 211:447–458
28. Cameron JL, Crist DW, Sitzmann JV et al. (1991) Factors influencing survival after pancreaticoduodenectomy for pancreatic cancer. Am J Surg 161:120–125
29. Moertel CG, Frytak S, Hahn RG et al. (1981) Therapy of locally unresectable pancreatic carcinoma. Cancer 48:1705–1710

30. Dobelbower RR Jr, Konski AA, Merrick HW III et al. (1991) Intraoperative electron beam radiation therapy for carcinoma of the exocrine pancreas. Int J Radiat Oncol Biol Phys 20:113–119
31. Wils JA (1990) Current status of chemotherapy in metastatic pancreatic cancer. Anticancer Res 9:1027–1032
32. Watson P, Lynch HT (1993) Extracolonic cancer in HNPCC. Cancer 71:677–685
33. Lynch HT, Smyrk TC, Watson P et al. (1993) Genetics, natural history, tumor spectrum, and pathology of HNPCC. Gastroenterology 104:1535–1549
34. Raimer RR, Fraumeni JF, Ozols RF et al. (1977) Pancreatic cancer in father and son. Lancet 1:911–912
35. MacDermott RP, Kramer P (1973) Adenocarcinoma of the pancreas in four siblings. Gastroenterology 65:137–139
36. Friedman JM, Fialkow PJ (1976) Familial carcinoma of the pancreas. Clin Genet 9:463–469
37. Ehrenthal D, Haeger L, Griffin T et al. (1987) Familial pancreatic adenocarcinoma in 3 generations. Cancer 59:1661–1664
38. Falk RT, Pickle LW, Fontham ET et al. (1988) Life-style risk factors for pancreatic cancer in Louisiana: a case-control study. Am J Epidemiol 128:324–336
39. Ghadirian P, Simard A, Baillargeon J (1988) Family aggregation of pancreatic cancer: a population-based case-control study. Proc Am Assoc Cancer Res 29:257
40. Lynch HT, Fitzsimmonds RN, Smyrk TC et al. (1990) Familial pancreatic cancer: clinicopathologic study of 18 nuclear families. Am J Gastroenterol 85:54–60
41. Korc M, Meltzer P, Trent J (1986) Enhanced expression of epidermal growth factor receptor correlates with alterations of chromosome 7 in human pancreatic cancer. Proc Natl Acad Sci USA 83:5141–5144
42. Poston GJ, Gillespie J, Guillou PJ (1991) Biology of pancreatic cancer. Gut 32:800–812
43. Davies N, Kapur K, Gillespie J et al. (1993) Transforming growth factor alpha is trophic to pancreatic cancer in vivo. Gut 34:1097–1098
44. Hall PA, Hughes CM, Staddon SL et al. (1990) The c-erbB-2 proto-oncogene in human pancreatic cancer. J Pathol 161:195–200
45. Almoguera C, Shibata D, Forrester K et al. (1988) Most human carcinomas of the exocrine pancreas contain mutant c-K-ras genes. Cell 53:549–554
46. Smit VTHBM, Boot AJM, Smits AMM et al. (1988) K-ras codon 12 mutations occur very frequently in pancreas adenocarcinomas. Nucleic Acids Res 16:7773–7782
47. Tada M, Omata M, Otho M (1991) Clinical applications of ras gene mutation for diagnosis of pancreatic adenocarcinoma. Gastroenterology 100:233–238
48. Shibata D, Almoguera C, Forrester K et al. (1990) Detection of c-K-ras mutations in fine needle aspirates from human pancreatic adenocarcinoma. Cancer Res 50:1279–1283
49. Motojima K, Urano T, Nagata Y et al. (1993) Detection of point mutations in the K-ras oncogene provides evidence for the multicentricity of pancreatic carcinoma. Ann Surg 217:138–143
50. Malkin D, Li FP, Strong LC et al. (1990) Germ line p53 mutations in a familial syndrome of breast cancer, sarcomas, and other neoplasms. Science 250:1233–1238
51. Ruggeri B, Zhang SY, Caamano J et al. (1992) Human pancreatic carcinomas and cell lines reveal frequent and multiple alterations in the p53 and Rb-1 tumor-suppressor genes. Oncogenes 7:1503–1511

52. Michelassi F, Erroi F, Angriman I et al. (1989) Loss of heterozygosity on chromosome 5q in gastric, colorectal and pancreatic cancer. Ital J Surg Sci 19:341–344
53. Wasylyshyn ML, Neuman WL, Angriman I et al. (1990) Evidence for a new tumor suppressor gene involved in gastrointestinal malignancies. Surgery 110: 265–269
54. Horii A, Nakatsuru S, Miyoshi Y et al. (1992) Frequent somatic mutations of the APC gene in human pancreatic cancer. Cancer Res 52:6696–6698
55. Hohne MW, Halatsch ME, Khal GF et al. (1992) Frequent loss of expression of the potential tumor suppressor gene DCC in ductal pancreatic adenocarcinoma. Cancer Res 52:2616–2619
56. Fearon ER, Cho KR, Nigro JM et al. (1990) Identification of a chromosome 18q gene that is altered in colorectal carcinoma. Science 247:49–56

Li-Fraumeni Syndrome

Families with Li-Fraumeni syndrome are rare, but nevertheless recognition of such families is important in identifying individuals at risk, who may benefit from genetic counselling and screening. Of wider importance, such families provide a model of cancer susceptibility, not only to rare cancer, such as soft tissue sarcomas and adrenocortical tumours, but also to very common malignancies.

(J.M. BIRCH 1990)

Introduction

Li-Fraumeni syndrome (LFS) is a rare inherited disease characterized by soft tissue sarcomas in children and young adults, early onset breast cancer in their close relatives, and frequent occurrence of adrenocortical and brain tumors, osteosarcomas, leukemia, and other neoplasms. Despite its rarity, the disease is of considerable clinical and biological interest for several reasons. First of all, LFS was one of the first cancer family syndromes in which an autosomal dominant type of genetic transmission was documented, initially on the basis of clinical reports on clustering of neoplasms in families, subsequently with segregation analysis, and finally with the observation of a continued excess of cancers in the follow-up. Second, germline mutations of the *p53* tumor suppressor gene have been detected in several families with LFS; although the paradigm that "not all investigated families showed germline *p53* mutations, and these were found not only in LFS" holds true, there is nevertheless no doubt that these observations represent a major advance towards the understanding of the molecular biology of inherited tumors. Third, if germline *p53* mutations can be considered a biological marker of increased susceptibility to the tumor spectrum of LFS, then it is possible to identify asymptomatic individuals who are at risk of the disease, and to develop a long-term program of screening and follow-up. Finally, the "molecular definition" of increased susceptibility to cancer in LFS (i.e., *p53* mutations) raises several clinical and ethical questions. For example, since tumor spectrum and age of onset of neoplasms in LFS are very wide, to devise an effective screening program for early detection of cancer in family members at risk might be extremely complex. Moreover, the benefit of reassuring a high-risk individual with a negative test (i.e., no *p53* mutation) should be balanced by the unavoidable anxiety and possible social discrimination of asymptomatic subjects who may show *p53* mutations.

Clinical, Epidemiologic, and Morphologic Features

Table 1 summarizes the main historical highlights in the identification and biological characterization of Li-Fraumeni syndrome. In 1968, Bottomley and colleagues [1] described a large family with a striking aggregation of cancers (early onset sarcomas, brain tumors, breast cancer, leukemia, and adrenal cortical carcinoma) over three generations; after a few years, in a second report [2], the pedigree of this family was extended to 5 generations including more than 400 members. The authors suggested that tumor aggregation and the apparent vertical transmission were consistent with an autosomal dominant type of inheritance. In 1969, Li and Fraumeni, by reviewing the clinical records of 648 children with rhabdomyosarcoma, found four families in which close relatives of the proband had childhood sarcomas; moreover, breast cancer, brain tumors, and other neoplasms were frequently detected among family members, thus suggesting the possible existence of a new cancer family syndrome [3–5]. Several years later, Lynch and collaborators [6, 7] reported a similar association of tumors in families

Table 1. Advances in the clinical and biological characterization of Li-Fraumeni syndrome and related conditions

Authors	Highlights	Reference
Bottomley et al. (1967)	Clinical report of the first family	[1]
Li and Fraumeni (1969)	Description of four families with the clinical features of LFS	[3]
Lynch et al. (1973)	Report of LFS ascertained through familial breast cancer	[6]
Li et al. (1988)	Updated report of 24 families with LFS	[11]
Malkin et al. (1990)	First report of germline mutations of *p53* in LFS	[21]
Srivastava et al. (1990)	First report of germline mutations of *p53* in LFS	
Santibanez-Koref et al. (1991)	Point mutations of *p53* present only in part of the families with LFS	[24]
Malkin et al. (1992)	*p53* mutations in children with multiple tumors	[31]
Toguchida et al. (1992)	*p53* mutations in patients with sarcoma	[32]
Prosser et al. (1992)	*p53* mutations in a breast/ovary cancer family	[35]

discovered through familial breast cancer; in accordance with the observed tumor spectrum, the authors proposed the acronym SBLA to designate this new syndrome ("S" for sarcoma; "B" for breast and brain tumors; "L" for leukemia, lung and laryngeal carcinoma; "A" for adrenal cortical cancer). Thus, virtually within the same period, at least three different research groups described families with almost identical clinical features, which were therefore highly suggestive of a new form of hereditary cancer which is now usually referred to as "Li-Fraumeni syndrome" (for the continued efforts of these investigators to update the family trees, and to define the main biological features of the disease).

The clinical diagnosis of LFS is mainly based on an accurate evaluation of extended family trees. In recent years, follow-up studies have broadened the tumor spectrum which features the syndrome, so that it may be difficult to distinguish tumors occurring by chance in large families over many years (phenocopies) from tumors that develop owing to a genetic predisposition. As already discussed for other hereditary tumors, the small size of modern families, especially in Western countries, renders the identification of LFS even more complex. In a recent survey of 24 families with LFS, Li et al. [8] reported a total of 151 verified malignancies, the large majority being diagnosed before the age of 45 years; the number of affected patients per family ranged between 3 and 17. Sarcomas (of soft tissues or bones) were diagnosed in about one-third of the patients (55 cases), and were more frequent in the age groups 0–14 and 15–29 years. Brain tumors, leukemia, and adrenocortical carcinoma were also seen almost exclusively in younger individuals, while breast cancer and several other carcinomas (including lung tumors, pancreatic, colorectal and prostate cancer) were more often diagnosed after the age of 30 years. Moreover, these tumors accounted for the large majority (73%) of the multiple primaries which developed in 15 family members. Finally, the authors provided a "tentative definition" of the syndrome according to the following minimum criteria: (a) The family should include one individual, designated as the proband, with a diagnosis of sarcoma before the age of 45 years; (b) a first-degree relative should be affected by cancer developed in the same age interval; and (c) another first- or second-degree relative in the lineage should have cancer in this age interval or sarcoma at any age. By using these criteria, Birch et al. [9, 10] identified 5 families with LFS in a population-based series of 177 children with soft tissue sarcoma diagnosed below the age of 15 years.

Little is known of the main epidemiologic features of LFS. Most of the published series concern American families [1–8], but the disease has also been described in the United Kingdom [9] and in Japan [11]; rather interestingly, two of the families reported by Li et al. [8] are black, and one is American Indian [12]. It is likely, therefore, that the disease is present in all races and continents, and that the lack of reports from other countries should be attributed to the difficulty of its identification. Accurate estimates of incidence and prevalence rates of LFS are lacking. Sarcomas, breast carcinoma, and other tumors occurring in LFS do not seem to show any characteristic location or histologic type which might allow the differentiation of these genetically determined neoplasms from the sporadic cases. However, Lynch and coworkers [7] reported the frequent occurrence, in their families, of some pathologic features, including multinucleate giant cells, intravacuolar inclusion within nucleoli, intranuclear inclusion of invaginated cytoplasm, erythrophagocytosis by tumor cells, and intracytoplasmic acidophilic inclusions. The clinical and diagnostic significance of these morphologic changes remains undefined. Finally, Hartley et al. [13] reported the occurrence of germ cell tumors (of the testis or ovary) among relatives of children with soft tissue or bone sarcoma, and suggested that this type of tumor might represent an uncommon clinical manifestation of LFS.

Genetic Transmission

Since the lifetime risk of cancer is in the order of 25%–30% in most Western countries, familial aggregates of tumors might simply be due to casual association. However, despite this theoretical possibility, the genetic nature of LFS has always been suspected; in fact, several lines of evidence support the autosomal dominant model of transmission and render unlikely any cluster of cancers due to random distribution. First, the simple observation of the published family trees [7, 8] reveals, in almost all cases, the features of autosomal dominant inheritance (i.e., verticality, no "skipped generation," segregation ratio around 50%) which have been discussed in the chapter on "Genetic Aspects of Disease: Categories of Genetic Disorders". Second, cancer aggregates unrelated to genetic factors, but presumably due to commonly shared environmental agents, are usually seen in older individuals, and concern neoplasms of frequent occurrence; in contrast, the large majority of tumors in LFS develop before the age of 45 years, and some of them (i.e., adrenocortical carcinoma) are extremely rare in the general population. Moreover, multiple tumors – again a constant feature of hereditary cancer (see chapters on "Hereditary and Familial Breast Cancer" and "Hereditary and Familial Colorectal Cancer") – are common in LFS [8]. Third, various studies showed a significant excess of neoplasms among close relatives of children with soft tissue sarcoma [9, 14, 15]; the large majority of these tumors were early onset breast carcinoma and pediatric malignancies (often sarcoma of the bones or soft tissue), thus indicating a possible genetic basis for many sarcomas of childhood. Finally, clinical follow-up of individuals at risk of tumors in LFS kindreds was consistent with the proposed model of transmission; in fact, during a follow-up period of almost 20 years, neoplasms continued to occur more frequently than expected in the entire cohort [16, 17]. The risk of cancer was particularly high in the age group 0–18 years (relative risk, RR, 21.1; confidence intervals, CI, 7.7–46) whereas it tended to decline with increasing age (after the age of 60 years, RR = 1); moreover, the excess of cancers was virtually limited to those neoplasms seen in the syndrome, while altogether other tumors did not occur more often than in the general population. Of individuals younger than 45 years, nearly 90% of cancers developed in subjects at risk of being carriers of the gene. Taken together, these observations strongly support the expression of an autosomal dominant gene among family members of LFS.

Segregation analyses were also of help in elucidating the genetic basis of LFS. Lynch et al. [7] studied six pedigrees with features of LFS including a total of 84 cases of cancer; the estimated "segregation parameter" was 45.6% ± 11%, which is close to the theoretical 50% expected for a fully penetrant autosomal dominant trait. Similarly, Williams and Strong [18] defined an autosomal dominant mode of transmission in nine families of children with bone or soft tissue sarcoma; according to this analysis, cancer occurred in one-half of high-risk family members by the age 30 years.

In summary, there is a general consensus that in LFS primary genetic factors are the major determinant of the susceptibilty to the development of a few specific neoplasms; as will be discussed in the next section, the molecular basis of this predisposition has partially been defined with the discovery of *p53* mutations in germline cells of many affected individuals. Although these findings do not exclude the possible role of environmental factors in the pathogenesis of LFS, our present knowledge of these hypothetical agents remains elusive.

Molecular Genetics

Germline Mutations of p53

As already discussed (see chapters on "Oncogenes and Tumor Suppressor Genes," "Genetic Factors in Solid Tumors of Childhood," and "Retinoblastoma"), tumor suppressor genes seem to be strongly associated with familial cancer. Of these genes, *p53*, located on chromosome 17p13, appeared of considerable biological interest in LFS because of the frequent inactivating mutations in tumors which characterize the syndrome [19, 20]. It is not surprising, therefore, that several investigators were attracted by the possibility that mutations of this gene might underlie cancer predisposition in LFS, and in 1990, almost simultaneously, two research groups reported germline *p53* mutations in families with a tumor spectrum consistent with LFS. Malkin et al. [21] studied skin fibroblasts and peripheral lymphocytes from both affected and unaffected members of five LFS families; after sequencing the entire genomic region of *p53* on both strands, C to T or G to A mutations were found at codons 245, 248, 252, or 258 in seven affected individuals and in two gene carriers, while no mutations were found in noncarriers. Similarly, Srivastava et al. [22] analyzed the *p53* gene in a large family with LFS; DNA sequence analysis from normal skin fibroblasts showed G to A mutations at codon 245 in four affected individuals spanning two different generations. The mutation led to change of aspartic acid for glycine in one of the "hot-spot" regions of the gene. Point mutations were not observed in the DNA of another affected family member (possible phenocopy?); more importantly, molecular analysis showed a normal *p53* sequence in various unaffected individuals. The authors of both research groups concluded that changes in the *p53* gene occur not only as somatic events in human neoplasia, but also as germline mutations in rare cancer family syndromes, and that these inherited mutations might render family members highly susceptible to cancer development [23].

Subsequent reports extended our knowledge of *p53* mutations in LFS and, as usual, rendered the issue more complex. Thus, in 1991, Santibanez-Koref et al. [24] carried out *p53* sequence studies in eight British families fulfilling the clinical criteria of LFS [8]; since previous investigators [21, 22] indicated a hot-spot region for mutation between codon 245 and 258, sequence of the gene was limited to exon 7. Germline mutations at codon 248 (one G to A and one C to T, causing changes of arginine to glycine or tryptophan respectively) were found in four affected members of two families only, whereas the investigated individuals (*n*. 8) of the remaining six families all showed the wild-type gene sequence. The authors concluded that *p53* might be the primary lesion in some but not all families with LFS, and suggested that genetic counselling in these families or attribution of risk for cancer on the basis of *p53* status should be done with caution. However, from this study the possibility of *p53* mutations in other regions of the gene could not be excluded; indeed, Low et al. [25] recently reported a specific germline mutation of *p53* at codon 133 (exon 5) in nine affected or high-risk individuals of a large LFS family. This study indicates that *p53* alterations are not restricted to a well-defined region of the gene, and that germline

Table 2. *p53* germline mutations in members of nine families with Li-Fraumeni syndrome [21–25]

Family	DNA source	Codon	Base change	Amino acid change
1	Fibroblasts Lymphocytes	248	C to T	Arginine to tryptophan
2	Lymphocytes	258	G to A	Glutamic acid to lysine
3	Fibroblasts	245	C to T	Glycine to cysteine
4	Lymphocytes	248	C to T	Arginine to tryptophan
5	Fibroblasts	252	T to C	Leucine to proline
6	Fibroblasts	245	G to A	Glycine to aspartic acid
7	Lymphocytes	248	G to A	Arginine to glutamine
8	Lymphocytes Fixed tissue	248	C to T	Arginine to tryptophan
9	Lymphocytes	133	T to C	Threonine to methionine

mutations in LFS might be as diverse in nature and gene location as those that are quite often seen in sporadic tumors [26].

In summary, *p53* germline mutations are frequently detected in LFS family members and might be responsible (or contribute) for the high incidence of cancer in this disease. Mutations of the gene are not limited to a specific region, but have been observed from codon 133 to codon 258; finally, available evidence suggests that there are families with LFS but without germline *p53* mutations, and that in single patients *p53* may appear normal even if closely related family members show various types of genetic changes. Table 2 summarizes the spectrum of *p53* germline mutations in LFS reported in references [21–25].

Germline Mutations of **p53** *in Clinical Conditions Related to Li-Fraumeni Syndrome*

As could reasonably be expected, the detection of germline *p53* mutations in LFS prompted various investigators to analyze the gene sequence in other clinical conditions, especially if these could appear somehow related to LFS. The high frequency of breast carcinoma and its tendency to "run in families" (see chapter on "Hereditary and Familial Breast Cancer") rendered this neoplasm a natural candidate for the search for such mutations. However, at least four different studies reported that germline changes of the gene are extremely rare in breast cancer patients who do not show a family history suggestive of LFS. Thus, Prosser et al. [27] were unable to detect *p53* mutations in constitutional DNA from various members of five families with hereditary breast cancer. Similarly, Sidranski et al. [28] examined 126 consecutive patients with mammary tumors diagnosed before the age of 40 years; DNA was isolated from peripheral blood lymphocytes and a portion of the *p53* gene, including exons 5–8, was amplified, and sequenced. Point mutation of the gene was found only in one individual who had a marked family history of breast and other tumors, though the cluster was not consistent with LFS. Moreover, Warren et al. [29] did not find constitutional *p53* mutations among members of 25 families with positive histories of breast cancer, and concluded that mutations of the gene were unlikely to account for the majority of familial/hereditary mammary tumors. Finally, Borresen et al. [30] screened 237 women with breast carcinoma for germline *p53* mutations; two patients only showed alterations of the gene (point mutations at codons 181 or 245); interestingly, for both patients there was a striking cluster of cancers among close relatives, which was highly suggestive of LFS (early onset breast cancer and leiomyosarcoma in both pedigrees).

Besides early onset breast cancer, other features of LFS include multiple tumors in children or young adults, and soft tissue sarcoma. Malkin et al. [31] analyzed genomic DNA from peripheral lymphocytes of 59 children (or young adults) with multiple primaries but without clinical histories indicative of LFS. Missense mutations of *p53* were found in 6.8% of patients (4 out of 59); three of these mutations were detected in exons 7 or 8, while the fourth was found in exon 9 (codon 324), a region which is conserved in mammals but not in lower vertebrates. Moreover, analysis of constitutional DNA from close relatives of these patients showed that in three cases one of the parents was carrier of the same mutation, thus suggesting that the genetic abnormalities were inherited, and that cancer may develop in children before a tumor arises in their parents (or other relatives) who presumably remain at risk because of the mutations. These findings therefore expand the subgroups of individuals who are prone to cancer development in relation to point mutations of *p53*, and pose the practical problem of dealing with asymptomatic relatives who are carriers of these mutations. Toguchida et al. [32] analyzed constitutional DNA from 196 patients with various types of sarcoma; *p53* changes were found in five patients with a family history of cancer and in three without any cancer aggregation among relatives, but in none of the 200 controls. These mutations (four missense and four causing stop codons) were located in various regions of the gene; moreover, three occurred outside the highly conserved domains. The authors concluded that germline mutations of *p53* occur both in families which meet the commonly accepted definition of LFS [8] and in families that do not show all the criteria featuring the syndrome; it follows that the tumor spectrum associated with germline *p53* mutations is probably broader and more complex than that defined in the initial reports [21, 33, 34]. In accordance with this contention, Prosser et al. [35] recently reported the presence of a constitutional *p53* mutation (exon 8, codon 267) in an extended breast/ovary cancer family without the tumor spectrum of LFS and in which cancers did not develop at an early age.

Biological and Clinical Problems of Germline **p53** *Mutations*

From the above discussion, it is clear that germline *p53* mutations have been detected in at least nine families with LFS [21–25] and in various other related conditions, including multiple tumors of childhood, sarcomas, and spurious aggregates of breast/ovarian cancer [27–35]. These findings pose a number of difficult biological and clinical questions, which should be addressed in future investigations.

Li-Fraumeni syndrome seems to be genetically heterogeneous, since only part of the affected families show germline *p53* mutations; it follows that at a molecular level the syndrome remains to be fully elucidated, and that additional studies are needed on both *p53* and, presumably, other cancer-related genes. Despite these uncertainties, there is a general consensus that germline *p53* mutations in LFS family members, and in closely related clinical conditions, should be considered as biomarkers of increased susceptibility to cancer [36]. But what is the role of such mutations in inducing a more general predisposition to neoplasms? Initial reports showed only a specific region of the gene (exon 7, codon 245, and a few others) to be mutated in a well-defined clinical setting (i.e., LFS); subsequent observations showed a gradual broadening of the problem, with genetic alterations in a much larger region of the gene (exons 4–9), and the involvement of clinical conditions which appear rather distant from LFS [32, 35]; are we simply looking at the tip of an iceberg?

Since germline *p53* mutations seem to be a biomarker of increased susceptibility to specific cancers, a further problem is the definition of those individuals who should be screened for the presence of these genetic alterations. Several important aspects need to be considered. First, the prevalence of *p53* mutations in the population is still poorly defined; consequently, sensitivity, specificity, and predictive value of *p53* testing are unknown [11, 26]. Second, since the tumor spectrum in LFS is very wide, developing an effective screening program, with the purpose of early detection, is a difficult if not impossible task. Third, if radiologic investigations are used for screening, we should not forget the susceptibility of these individuals to tumor development, and the carcinogenic effect of radiation. For these and other reasons, most of the participants to a recent workshop favored the restriction of screening procedures to high-risk relatives of cancer patients with germline *p53* mutations [37].

One should also consider the potential benefits and risks of *p53* predictive testing. Those who are found not to be carriers of the mutated gene can be reassured and would obtain some relief from the adverse emotional effects of a family history of cancer; but the real problem regards asymptomatic individuals in whom a positive test (for mutations) is detected. These subjects – who cannot be labeled as "patients" – should be advised to undergo periodic investigations for early detection of tumors, although it is clear that this type of surveillance is complex, and there is still no evidence of its effectiveness in reducing cancer mortality. In addition, these high-risk individuals should be encouraged to adopt a "healthier" lifestyle, thus avoiding cigarette smoking, alcohol, dietary excess, and exposure to other carcinogens. Similarly, they should be alerted towards various signs or symptoms of cancer, and chemoprevention might be offered, with the aims of preventing or delaying tumor occurrence [38–40]. Despite all these preventive approaches, it is quite possible that a positive p53 test would generate anxiety and/or depression in carriers of the mutated gene; moreover, several social discrimination (i.e., difficulty obtaining life insurance or a mortgage, problems with career or occupation) can be expected. It was partially reassuring, however, that during a recent symposium [11] a patient with LFS, operated on for three primaries, claimed that she wanted her family to be tested for *p53* mutations, and that the possible presence of constitutional changes in one of her children would not render her more anxious; moreover, she did not complain of any social discrimination because of her medical and family history of cancer.

Other Biomolecular Changes in Li-Fraumeni Syndrome

Evidence that other cancer-related genes can be involved in the pathogenesis of LFS is scanty. Altered expression and various structural alterations of the retinoblastoma (*Rb*) gene have been reported in a large fraction of patients with bone and soft tissue sarcomas (see chapter on "Retinoblastoma"); it is therefore not surprising that Lee et al. [41, 42] suggested that the *Rb* gene might be related to cancer susceptibility in LFS; on the other hand, retinoblastomas are not part of the tumor spectrum of the syndrome, and this observation renders the *Rb* gene an unlikely candidate for mutations in LFS. Similarly, other tumor suppressor genes located on chromosome 11p have also been taken into consideration [43, 44] because of their frequent implication in sarcomas and other rare tumors. Finally, although several oncogenes can be mutated or overexpressed in breast tumors (see chapter on "Hereditary and Familial Breast Cancer"), there is no evidence that these dominantly acting genes are somehow related to tumor development in LFS.

References

1. Bottomley RH, Condit PT (1968) Cancer families. Cancer Bull 20:22–24
2. Bottomley RH, Trainer AL, Condit PT (1971) Chromosome studies in a cancer family. Cancer 28:519–528
3. Li FP, Fraumeni JF Jr (1969) Soft-tissue sarcomas, breast cancer, and other neoplasms. A familial syndrome? Ann Intern Med 71:747–752
4. Li FP, Fraumeni JF Jr (1969) Rhabdomyosarcoma in children: epidemiologic study and identification of a familial cancer syndrome. JNCI 43:1365–1373
5. Malkin D (1993) p53 and the Li-Fraumeni syndrome. Cancer Genet Cytogenet 66:83–92
6. Lynch HT, Krush AJ, Harlan WL et al. (1973) Association of soft tissue sarcoma, leukemia, and brain tumors in families affected with breast cancer. Am Surg 39:199–206
7. Lynch HT, Mulcahy GM, Harris RE et al. (1978) Genetic and pathologic findings in a kindred with hereditary sarcoma, breast cancer, brain tumors, leukemia lung, laryngeal and adrenal cortical carcinoma. Cancer 41:2055–2064
8. Li FP, Fraumeni JF Jr, Mulvihill JJ et al. (1988) A cancer family syndrome in 24 kindreds. Cancer Res 48:5358–5362
9. Birch JM, Hartley AL, Blair V et al. (1990) Cancer in the families of children with soft tissue sarcoma. Cancer 66:2239–2248
10. Hartley AL, Birch JM, Val Blair BA et al. (1993) Patterns of cancer in the families of children with soft tissue sarcoma. Cancer 72:923–930
11. Li FP, Correa P, Fraumeni JF Jr (1991) Testing for germ line p53 mutations in cancer families. Cancer Epidemiol Biomark Preven 1:91–94

12. Mulvihill JJ, Gralnick HR, Whang-Peng J et al. (1977) Multiple childhood osteosarcomas in an American Indian family with erythroid macrocytosis and skeletal anomalies. Cancer 40:3115–3122
13. Hartley AL, Birch JM, Kelsey AM et al. (1989) Are germ cell tumors part of the Li-Fraumeni cancer family syndrome? Cancer Genet Cytogenet 42:221–226
14. Birch JM, Hartley AH, Marsden HB et al. (1984) Excess risk of breast cancer in the mothers of children with soft tissue sarcomas. Br J Cancer 49:325–331
15. Strong LC, Stine M, Norsted TL (1987) Cancer in survivors of childhood soft tissue sarcoma and their relatives. JNCI 79:1213–1200
16. Li FP, Fraumeni JF Jr (1982) Prospective study of a cancer family syndrome. JAMA 247:2692–2694
17. Garber JE, Goldstein AM, Kantor AF et al. (1991) Follow-up study of 22 families with Li-Fraumeni syndrome. Cancer Res 51:6094–6097
18. Williams WR, Strong LC (1985) Genetic epidemiology of soft tissue sarcomas in children. In: Muller HR, Weber W (eds) Familial cancer. Karger, Basel, pp 151–153
19. Romano JW, Ehrhart JC, Duthu A et al. (1989) Identification and characterization of a p53 gene mutation in a human osteosarcoma cell line. Oncogene 4:1483–1488
20. Coles C, Condie A, Chetty U et al. (1992) p53 mutations in breast cancer. Cancer Res 52:5291–5298
21. Malkin D, Li FP, Strong LC et al. (1990) Germ line p53 mutations in a familial syndrome of breast cancer, sarcomas and other neoplasms. Science 250: 1233–1238
22. Srivastava S, Zou Z, Pirollo K et al. (1990) Germ-line transmission of a mutated p53 gene in a cancer-prone family with Li-Fraumeni syndrome. Nature 348: 747–749
23. Li FP (1993) Molecular epidemiology studies of cancer in families. Br J Cancer 68:217–219
24. Santibanez-Koref MF, Birch JM, Harley AL et al. (1991) p53 germline mutations in Li-Fraumeni syndrome. Lancet 338:1490–1491
25. Law JC, Strong LC, Chidambaram A et al. (1991) A germ line mutation in exon 5 of the p53 gene in an extended cancer family. Cancer Res 51:6385–6387
26. Eeles RA (1993) Predictive testing for germline mutations in the p53 gene: are all the questions answered? Eur J Cancer 29A:1361–1365
27. Prosser J, Elder PA, Condie A et al. (1991) Mutations in the p53 do not account for heritable breast cancer: a study in 5 affected families. Br J Cancer 63: 181–184
28. Sidranski D, Tokino T, Helzlsouer K et al. (1992) Inherited p53 gene mutations in breast cancer. Cancer Res 52:2984–2986
29. Warren W, Eeles RA, Ponder BAJ et al. (1992) No evidence for germline mutations in exons 5–9 of the p53 gene in 25 breast cancer families. Oncogene 7:1043–1046
30. Boressen AL, Andersen TI, Barber J et al. (1992) Screening for germ line TP53 mutations in breast cancer patients. Cancer Res 52:3234–3236
31. Malkin D, Jolly KW, Barbier N et al. (1992) Germline mutations of the p53 tumor-suppressor gene in children and young adults with second malignant neoplasms. N Engl J Med 326:1309–1315
32. Toguchida J, Yamaguchi T, Dayton SH et al. (1992) Prevalence and spectrum of germline mutations of the p53 gene among patients with sarcoma. N Engl J Med 326:1301–1308
33. Eeles RA, Warren W, Knee G et al. (1993) Constitutional mutaton in exon 8 of the p53 gene in a patient with multiple primary tumours. Oncogene 8:1269–1276

34. Brugieres L, Gardes M, Moutou C et al. (1993) Screening for germ line p53 mutations in children with malignant tumors and a family history of cancer. Cancer Res 53:452–455
35. Prosser J, Ported D, Coles C et al. (1992) Constitutional p53 mutations in a non-Li-Fraumeni cancer family. Br J Cancer 65:527–528
36. Strong LC, Williams WR, Tainsky MA et al. (1992) The Li-Fraumeni syndrome: from clinical epidemiology to molecular genetics. Am J Epidemiol 135:190–199
37. Li FP, Fraumeni JF Jr (1992) Predictive testing for inherited mutations in cancer susceptibility genes. J Clin Oncol 10:1203–1204
38. Henson DE, Block G, Levine M (1991) Ascorbic acid: biologic function and relation to cancer JNCI 83:547–550
39. Smith MA, Parkinson DR, Cheson BD et al. (1992) Retinoids in cancer therapy. J Clin Oncol 10:839–864
40. Nayfield SG, Karp JE, Ford LG et al. (1991) Potential role of Tamoxifen in prevention of breast cancer. JNCI 83:1450–1459
41. Lee EY-HP, To H, Shew JY et al. (1988) Inactivation of the retinoblastoma susceptibility gene in human breast cancers. Science 241:218–221
42. Birch JM (1990) The Li-Fraumeni cancer family syndrome. J Pathol 161:1–2
43. Koufos A, Hansen MF, Copelanf NG et al. (1985) Loss of heterozygosity in 3 embryonal tumours suggest a common pathogenetic mechanism. Nature 316: 330–334
44. Scrable HJ, Witte DP, Lampkin BC et al. (1987) Chromosomal localization of the human rhabdomyosarcoma locus by mitotic recombination mapping. Nature 329:645–647

Genetic Factors in Leukemia and Lymphoma

. . . Leukemia as a whole shows a genuinely increased familial incidence, and this is more marked in chronic lymphocytic leukemia, less so in acute leukemia, and probably absent in chronic granulocytic leukemia. . . . It is more likely that, as in the experimental model, leukemia is determined by the action of multiple genes which, in certain families, have the effect of increasing the predisposition to the disease.

(F.W. GUNZ et al. 1975)

Introduction

Leukemias are neoplastic proliferations of hematopoietic cells, while lymphomas arise from the malignant transformation of cells residing predominantly in the lymphoid tissues. The former is a heterogeneous group of neoplasms including acute lymphocytic leukemia (ALL), acute myelogenous leukemia (AML), chronic lymphocytic leukemia (CLL), chronic myelogenous leukemia (CML), and hairy cell leukemia (HCL), in relation to the cell types involved and the clinical course. Lymphomas are usually subdivided into non-Hodgkin's lymphoma (NHL) and Hodgkin's disease (HD); although both types of lymphomas infiltrate reticuloendothelial organs, differences in their clinical and biological behavior suggest that NHL and HD are probably unrelated entities.

Although leukemias and lymphomas are less frequent than many solid tumors, they have been the subject of detailed studies because of the insights that they give into the etiology, pathogenesis, and treatment of human neoplasms. Thus, for example, the Philadelphia chromosome was the first cytogenetic abnormality specifically associated with cancer (i.e., CML); moreover, the role of retroviruses in inducing leukemia has been investigated in animal models for many years, and recently a viral etiology was established for a rare form of human leukemia (adult T-cell leukemia-lymphoma). Finally, the intensive polychemotherapy which has been responsible for the remarkable improvement or the cure of some leukemias and lymphomas served as an example for the treatment of other neoplasms; similarly, bone marrow transplantation was found to be an effective therapy for both ALL and AML, and is at present under investigation for the treatment of other malignancies.

The possible role of genetic background in leukemia and lymphoma stems from various clinical and biological observations. First, familial aggregations of both diseases have frequently been reported, though no specific mode of genetic transmission has been so far identified. Second, there is an increased likelihood of leukemia developing in monozygotic twins, with a concordance rate – at least in some studies – as high as 17%. Third, there is a significant increase in the incidence of leukemia in children with chromosomal abnormalities or with genetic diseases. Finally, studies on the molecular basis of Philadelphia chromosome showed that this is formed by a reciprocal translocation between chromosomes 9 and 22, which results in fusion of the *abl* and *bcr* genes, production of *abl-bcr* fusion mRNA, and expression of a chimeric protein whose presence in hematopoietic stem cells might be associated with the development of CML (and probably other leukemias). A similar chain of cytogenetic and molecular events seems to be involved in the pathogenesis of Burkitt's lymphoma.

Detailed descriptions of histopathology, biological characterization, classification, clinical aspects, and treatment of leukemias and lymphomas would require a much longer chapter and are beyond the objectives of this book. Thus, after a concise discussion of the main clinical and epidemiologic features, familial aspects of the diseases will be focused upon. Finally, the main highlights of the cellular and molecular genetics of lymphohematoproliferative disorders will be mentioned, referring the reader to several excellent reviews for a detailed analysis of the chromosomal basis and the molecular biology of these diseases.

Clinical and Epidemiologic Characteristics

Acute and Chronic Leukemias

The incidence of all leukemias is in the order of 10–15 new cases/100000 per year in most Western countries; ALL is basically a disease of children and young adults, while age-specific incidence rates of other leukemias peak around age 60–80 years [1]. The main etiologic factors implicated in human leukemias include (a) ionizing irradiation (survivors of the atomic explosions during the Second World War have a dose-related increased risk of leukemia; patients receiving radiation therapy and subjects with occupational X-ray exposure are similarly at increased risk); (b) cytotoxic drugs, such as the alkylating agents frequently used for treatment of solid tumors; (c) human retroviruses (adult T-cell leukemia, a severe malignancy characterized by mature T-lymphoid cells, has been etiologically related to a retrovirus referred to as human T-cell leukemia virus, or HTLV-I) [2]; and (d) chemical compounds (such as benzene and other aromatic hydrocarbons).

Acute lymphocytic leukemia and AML are characterized by proliferation and defective terminal differentiation of lymphoid or myeloid cells, respectively, which accumulate initially in the bone marrow, circulate in the peripheral blood, and then invade other organs (especially lymph nodes, spleen, liver, and central nervous system). CLL is characterized by the accumulation of apparently normal lymphocytes (B cells in the majority of cases) in the peripheral blood, lymph nodes, spleen, and bone marrow, while in CML an increase in all stages of the granulocytic series is usually seen. In HCL, the lymphocyte count may be normal; however, typical "hairy cells" (i.e., large B lymphocytes with an eccentric nucleus, foamy cytoplasm, and unusual cytoplasmic villi) can be observed. The main clinical and morphologic features of the most frequent types of leukemia are summarized in Table 1 [3–8].

The diagnosis of leukemia is essentially based on peripheral blood and bone marrow examinations, with cytochemical and immunologic studies. In acute leukemias, a lumbar puncture may show leukemic cells in the liquor, even without evidence of disease in the central nervous system; in CLL, if the diagnosis is in doubt a lymph node biopsy may show diffuse infiltration with small and well-differentiated lymphocytes. Finally, in CML cultured marrow cells should be analyzed for the cytogenetic determination of Philadelphia chromosome; it has been shown that in patients who are negative for this chromosomal abnormality the disease runs a less favorable course [8].

Prognosis of ALL and AML has improved dramatically over the last 20–30 years because of intensive chemotherapy, radiotherapy, and bone marrow transplantation [9]; thus, 50%–70% of children with ALL between the ages of 3 and 9 years and with a low white blood cell count may achieve long-term survival (and perhaps cure) with the available treatments. Age and chromosomal abnormalities are also of prognostic value in AML; in the most favorable cases (i.e., children with few cytogenetic changes) complete remission and long-term survival can be observed [10]. In CLL, the current treatment (Table 1) improves symptoms by reducing lymphocyte count and lymphadenopathy, but is ineffective in eradicating leukemic cells and in inducing complete remission; a median survival of 5 years has been reported in various studies [6], and there is little evidence that prognosis is improving. Moreover, second malignancies can be observed in CLL. At variance with CLL, the evolution of CML is characterized by the development of a particularly aggressive acute leukemia usually resistant to treatment and followed by a fatal outcome in a few months. Rather interestingly, the final step from CML to acute leukemia does not necessarily involve the transformation into AML; indeed, in approximately 20% of cases an ALL develops, in which blast cells are positive for Philadelphia chromosome. This observation strongly suggests that in leukemias the malignant phenotype develops in a very early progenitor cell. Finally, the clinical course of HCL is usually slow, and a broad spectrum of severity and rate of progression among patients can be observed; about one-half of the affected individuals

Table 1. Clinical features of leukemias

Leukemias	Clinical symptoms	Histopathology	Chemotherapy	Prognostic factors	Ref.
ALL	Bleeding, infections, hepatosplenomegaly, bone pain	Leukemic lymphoblasts with various immunologic features	Vincristine Doxorubicin Asparaginase Prednisolone	Age, leukocyte count, cytogenetic abnormalities	[3, 67]
AML	Bleeding, infections, hepatosplenomegaly, bone pain	Leukemic myeloblasts with abnormal granules (Auer rods) in the cytoplasm	Cytosine arabinoside Daunorubicin 6-Thioguanine Mitoxantrone	Age, chromosomal abnormalities	[4, 66]
CLL	Anemia, splenomegaly, adenopathy, infections	Normal-appearing lymphocytes expressing immunoglobulins on cell surface	Chlorambucil Cyclophosphamide Prednisolone	Stage	[6, 68]
HCL	Splenomegaly, infections, erythema nodosum, cutaneous nodules	Hairy cells, expressing monoclonal immunoglobulins (i.e., activated clonal B lymphocytes)	Splenectomy Interferon Pentostatin	–	[5, 11]
CML	Anemia, weight loss, splenomegaly, bleeding, abdominal pain	Granulocytes (40%), metamyelocytes (10%), myelocytes (30%), promyelocytes and myeloblasts, Philadelphia chromosome in cultured marrow cells	Busulfan 6-Thioguanine Hydroxyurea	Philadelphia chromosome	[7, 72]

ALL, acute lymphocytic leukemia; AML, acute myelogenous leukemia; CLL, chronic myelogenous leukemia; HCL, hairy cell leukemia; CML, chronic myelogenous leukemia.

survive more than 8 years from diagnosis, and there is evidence that the most recent treatments (i.e., interferon and others) have further improved these figures [5, 11].

Non-Hodgkin's Lymphomas

Incidence of NHL ranges between 11.4 new cases/100 000 per year in Switzerland to 1.5 cases in India [1]. Although the frequency of NHL rises with age, these tumors are the most common malignancy of patients between the ages of 20 and 40 years, at least in Western countries. Moreover, observations from cancer registries indicate that the incidence of NHL is increasing in North America (by 57%, according to the Surveillance, Epidemiology, End Results – SEER – study, between 1973 and 1988) as well as Europe [9, 12].

Besides genetic alterations, which will be discussed later, viruses and conditions associated with depressed immunity seem to be the main etiologic factors in NHL. The possible role of viruses is supported by several observations. First, herpesviruses and retroviruses have been isolated in various animals with lymphocytic lymphoma. Second, a strong association was found between serologic evidence of Epstein-Barr virus (EBV) and Burkitt's lymphoma (in countries where Burkitt's lymphoma is endemic most children have evidence of past infection with EBV; the majority of these children, however, will not develop the disease, thus suggesting that other factors are required for inducing malignancy). Third, HTLV-1, a retrovirus implicated in the pathogenesis of adult T-cell leukemia, was isolated from T-cell lymphomas [13, 14]; moreover, antibodies to HTLV-1 are often present in patients with this type of lymphoma [13, 14]. Similarly, the importance of depressed or deregulated immunity stems from (a) the frequent occurrence of NHL in AIDS and in autoimmune diseases; (b) the possible occurrence of NHL in patients on long-term immunosuppressive treatment (for autoimmune diseases or to prevent rejection of transplantations); and (c) the risk of lymphoma in individuals with congenital immunodeficiency and in patients with Hodgkin's disease treated with radiation and polychemotherapy [13, 15]. Finally, immunosuppression might be carcinogenic not by itself, but by allowing the activity of other oncogenic agents, such as HTLV-1 or EBV.

The first attempt to classify lymphomas is attributed to Conheim, in 1865 [16]; since then things have become more complex and various histologic classifications of NHL have been proposed. Although the histologic type (or subtype) is probably the most important factor for therapeutic strategies, it is also possible – and probably more useful – to classify NHL on the basis of their immunologic properties. Thus, B-cell lymphomas can be identified and categorized by the expression of specific immunoglobulins on the cell surface or cytoplasm, and for their capacity to produce immunoglobulins; similarly, monoclonal antibodies directed against T-cell surface molecules may allow a detailed classification of T-cell lymphomas. Recently, a panel of experts proposed a new scheme – termed the Working Formulation [17] – which incorporates the most important biological and clinical features of the previous systems. According to this classification, there are three main types of NHL – low-, intermediate-, and high-grade lymphomas – which are further subdivided into several subgroups (roughly corresponding to the previously used Rappaport's classification). Low-grade lymphomas show a slowly progressive clinical course, and their natural history is virtually unaffected by therapy. Intermediate- and high-grade lymphomas are much more aggressive diseases associated with a poor prognosis, although for some the clinical outcome has improved remarkably with chemotherapy [13]. Table 2 outlines the main clinical and morphologic features of NHL [8, 13].

The diagnosis of NHL is usually made by lymph node or tissue biopsy followed by a precise determination of the immunologic subtype of lymphoma. Chest X-ray, computed tomography, magnetic resonance imaging, abdominal ultrasounds, radionuclide scan, and lymphography (for the detection of infiltrated but normal-sized lymph nodes) are extremely useful for the presence of disease staging. The same (Ann Arbor) staging notation is used for both HNL and HD; in stage I, there is the involvement of a single lymph node region or single extralymphatic site, while in stage II two or more regions on the same side of the diaphragm are involved. In more advanced stages (III and IV) the disease spreads to lymph nodes on both sides of the diaphragm and infiltrates extralymphatic organs [8, 13]. At variance with HD, the great majority of patients with NHL usually show stage. III and IV disease at presentation. This is probably one of the reasons why prognosis is less favorable in NHL than in HD; however, the course of NHL is quite variable in relation – besides stage at diagnosis – to the marked morphologic and immunologic heterogeneity of the disease. Similarly, the impact of chemotherapy on the prognosis of NHL has been extremely variable [13, 18]: thus, if the effect of treatment in low-grade lymphoma is still uncertain, complete remission and long-term disease-free survival can be obtained, with modern polychemotherapy, in 50%–80% of patients with some types of intermediate-grade lymphoma ("diffuse large cell lymphoma"); moreover, promising results can also be observed in high-grade lymphoma, usually treated more aggressively than the other lymphomas owing to its rapid clinical course. According to the SEER study, overall 5-year survival of NHL has shown a definite increase over the last 20 years, from 31% in 1960–1963 to 51% in 1985–1987 [9].

Hodgkin's Disease

Hodgkin's disease was identified by Thomas Hodgkin in 1832 [19]; many years later C. Sternberg gave a detailed histopathologic description of the

Table 2. Clinical features and classification of non-Hodgkin's lymphomas

Lymphomas	Main clinical characteristics	Histopathology (working formulation)	Chemotherapy	References
Low grade	Peripheral adenopathy, generalized lymphoadenopathy and/or abdominal masses	Small lymphocytic cells Follicular (predominantly small cleaved cells) Follicular mixed	Cyclophosphamide Vincristine Adriamycin Prednisolone (CHOP)	[13, 17, 18]
Intermediate grade	Peripheral adenopathy, infiltration of spleen, liver, and bone marrow. Possible lung and kidney involvement (in diffuse large cell type)	Follicular, predominantly large cells Diffuse small cleaved cells Diffuse mixed Diffuse large cells	Cyclophosphamide Vincristine Adriamycin Bleomycin Methotrexate Procarbazine Cytosine arabinoside Etoposide (MOPP, BACOD, and others)	[13, 17, 18]
High grade	Anemia, lymphopenia, high serum gamma-globulin levels (immunoblastic type), peripheral adenopathy or mediastinal masses, extranodal involvement (testis, bones, and others)	Large cells (immunoblastic) Lymphoblastic Small noncleaved cells	Cyclophosphamide Vincristine Adriamycin Bleomycin Methotrexate Procarbazine Cytosine arabinoside Etoposide (MOPP, BACOD, and others)	[13, 17, 18]
Burkitt's	1. Jaw tumor which spreads to bone marrow and nervous system (African type) 2. Abdominal masses, with involvement of extranodal organs (Western type)	Small noncleaved cells expressing pan-B cell antigens	Cyclophosphamide Vincristine Methotrexate Prednisolone (COMP)	[13, 49]

disease, which could be classified as a distinct nosologic entity [20]. Age-standardized incidence of HD is approximately three to five new cases/100 000 per year in most Western countries, with a certain preponderance of the male sex [1]. Age-specific incidence shows a typical bimodal pattern, with a first peak in young adults (15–30 years) and a second after the fifties.

No firm etiologic factor was associated with the development of HD, although various putative risk factors have been identified [21]; these include socioeconomic class, altered immune response, HLA antigens, and many others. Individuals infected with EBV seem to run an increased risk of developing HD, and this has led to the hypothesis that the disease might be related to an oncogenic virus whose deleterious effect (a) seems to be relatively low, (b) presumably requires various cofactors to become manifest, and (c) increases with age at the time of infection.

The majority of patients with HD present with cervical and/or mediastinal adenopathy; these lesions may remain stable for a long time, and temporary regression is not infrequent. Symptoms of HD are rather vague and aspecific, but the most frequent include night sweat, weight loss, fluctuating fever, and generalized pruritus. The diagnosis of HD is usually based on lymph node biopsy and the histologic identification of the Reed-Sternberg cells, though these cells are not specific for HD but can occasionally be found in other clinical conditions, such as infectious mononucleosis and some non-Hodgkin's lymphomas. HD is usually subdivided into four main histologic types ("lymphocyte-predominant," "nodular sclerosis," "mixed cellularity," and "lymphocyte-depleted"), which are associated with different natural histories [22]. Accurate staging of HD is based on the already discussed Ann Arbor system, and requires the same investigations as NHL.

Treatment of HD represents one of the major achievements of radiation therapy [22] and modern polychemotherapy [23, 24]. According to the SEER data, 5-year survival was around 40% in 1960–1963 but increased to 77% during the period 1981–1986 [9], mostly because of the beneficial effects of the new therapeutic regimens (mechlorethamine, vincristine, procarbazine, and prednisolone – MOPP; doxorubicin, bleomycin, vinblastine, and dacarbazine – ABVD; and others) for advanced disease, and of radiotherapy for localized HD. In a recent editorial [25], DeVita and Hubbard claimed that "Radiotherapy is curative for localized Hodgkin's disease, and there is now general agreement that advanced Hodgkin's disease can be cured by chemotherapy."

Familial Aspects

At variance with many solid tumors, hereditary factors seem to play a lesser role in the pathogenesis of lymphohematopoietic malignancies, and much more attention has been given to the possible etiologic role of other (environmental) factors, such as viruses, chemical compounds, ionizing radiation, and altered immunity. However, a careful review of the available literature reveals several reports on the familial aggregation of some types of leukemia and lymphoma, thus suggesting a possible multifactorial origin for some of these neoplasms.

"Familiality" in Leukemias

One of the first observations on the role of familial factors in leukemia was reported by Videbaek in 1947 [26]. According to the author, a family history of other cases of leukemia was found in 17 out of 209 (8.1%) leukemic patients, while the incidence of the disease among control families was only 0.5%. An increased incidence of leukemia among first-degree relatives of affected individuals was also reported in several investigations by Gunz et al. [27–31]. In one of these studies [31], the authors evaluated family history of cancer in 909 patients with leukemia of all types, with the specific objective of establishing the frequency of other cases of the disease among relatives. Seventy-two patients had one or more relatives with leukemia, an incidence which was three times the number of first-degree relatives with the disease that would have been expected in a control population matched for age and sex. By examining each specific type of leukemia, it was found that this increased familial incidence was much more marked in CLL than in acute leukemias, while CML showed no tendency toward familial aggregation. With the possible exception of a few families, the occurrence of leukemia among family members did not show features of monogenic transmission; the authors, therefore, suggested that polygenic inheritance was the most plausible cause of the heightened susceptibility to leukemia observed in these families.

A further element supporting a possible genetic basis of leukemia is the high concordance rate among identical twins. Thus, MacMahon and Levi [32] showed that in 5 out of 72 sets of twins both members were affected by childhood leukemia; similarly, in his series of identical twin pairs, Miller [33] found concordance for leukemia in 7 out of 42 cases, which was much greater than the frequency among nontwin sib pairs, and confirmed the concordance rate of approximately 17% for leukemia among presumably identical twins in the United States.

An interesting cluster of acute leukemia was recently described by Leverger et al. [34]. In the investigated family, three cousins of the same generation were affected by ALL within a period of 14 years (at the ages of 2, 3, and 5 years, respectively); two of these patients shared the same rare haplotype which had previously been reported in a pair of siblings with ALL [35]. It was proposed that the rarity of this haplotype in the caucasian population could be consistent with the existence of a high susceptibility-to-leukemia gene linked to HLA in some familial cases of ALL.

Segregation and consanguinity analysis, together with genetic marker studies (i.e., HLA and dermatoglyphic pattern) and cytogenetic analysis, were carried out by Hafez et al. [36] in 162 patients (age range, 2 months – 15 years) will ALL. While HLA frequencies did not show appreciable differences from those of 234 normal controls (with the exception of A2 antigen), the results of segregation analysis strongly supported the multifactorial model of inheritance, thus leading further support to previous observations [31]. Finally, Linet et al. [37] investigated the frequency of cancers among relatives of CLL patients in a population-based case-control study which included 342 affected individuals, 342 matched cancer controls, and 342 matched controls without cancer. Information was obtained from 2985 first-degree relatives of the case group versus 2714 and 2923 relatives in the two control groups. Twenty-three siblings of patients had a previous diagnosis of leukemia or lymphoma, as opposed to four and ten siblings in cancer controls and in noncancer controls respectively; moreover, breast and kidney tumors were similarly reported to occur more often among case relatives than in control relatives. The authors concluded that close relatives of patients with CLL are at a higher risk of developing leukemia as well as other lymphoproliferative malignancies, and breast and renal carcinoma; in addition, the observed findings were consistent with the presence of a strong genetic susceptibility to cancer (especially leukemia) in a few high-risk families, while the majority of affected patients presumably represent sporadic cases.

"Familiality" in Lymphomas

Familial aggregation of lymphoma is rare, and its real incidence remains to be determined; moreover, clinical studies on this topic are often controversial, and it has also been suggested that our limited knowledge on "familiality" of lymphomas might partially be attributed to the insufficient attention frequently given to the family history of cancer [38]. These concepts apply to both HD and NHL.

There are various clinical reports of NHL occurring in blood relatives [39–42], suggesting that besides environmental agents (especially viruses) genetic factors might also play a role in the etiology of these diseases. This concept is further reinforced by a report of 38 multiple case families, for a total of 111 individuals with diagnosis of NHL and an average of 3 cases per family, with approximately the same male: female ratio (=1.8) as is observed for sporadic cases [43]. However, when Heim and coworkers [44] assessed the statistical significance of the occurrence of lymphoma among first-degree relatives of 532 patients with NHL, no increased risk for the disease could be detected (at variance with HD patients). In 1987, Clark et al. [45] described a family in which three sisters developed NHL in the age range 55–65 years; in addition, in the extended pedigree 13 maternal relatives showed tumors of various types, but mostly breast and colorectal carcinoma. The interest of these observations was that various immunologic abnormalities (i.e., elevated titers of antibodies against EBV, decreased percentage of T cells, and others) were observed in some family members, thus supporting the view that subtle alterations of the immune system might be implicated in familial clustering of NHL. Similar conclusions were drawn by Lynch and coworkers [38], who studied a large family with seven cases of malignant lymphoma (six NHL and one HD) spanning three generations; immunologic abnormalities included low serum IgG3 levels (in four family members), and altered responses to pokeweed and concanavalin A stimulation. Two more aspects should be considered in this interesting kindred. First, a family member was considered an "obligate carrier "of a putative susceptibility-to-lymphoma gene, since her mother died of lymphoma and her daughter had already expressed the disease; indeed, 6 months after genetic counselling this individual developed a diffuse mixed lymphocytic lymphoma at the base of the tongue. Second, the striking aggregation of lymphomas, together with the apparent verticality and the identification of an obligate carrier, strongly suggest that in this family the disease was transmitted through an autosomal dominant type of inheritance.

Finally, familial aggregations of Burkitt's lymphoma have been reported not only in African series but also in American and European kindreds [46–49]. In two of these families [48, 49], some healthy family members showed various immunologic alterations, such as decreased helper:suppressor T-cell ratio, low total T cells, and abnormal antibody response to EBV infection; however, it is still unclear whether these subtle changes are somehow implicated in inducing an increased susceptibility to this rare disease.

Familial aggregations of HD have frequently been reported [50–52], and more often related to common environmental rather than to genetic factors [53, 54]. Quantitative estimation of the relative risk of HD among blood relatives was attempted by Razis et al. [53], who found 13 patients with verified HD among first-degree relatives of more than 1000 probands with the same disease; on the basis of these figures and the prevalence of HD in the general population, the authors suggested that family members of HD patients have an approximately threefold increased risk of the disease. An even higher risk (sevenfold) was reported by Grufferman et al. [50], who found five sibling pairs against an expected value of 0.7. Similarly, four pairs of close relatives with HD were seen by Haim and coworkers [44] among 183 patients diagnosed during a 20-year period versus an expected value of 0.45; these findings correspond to a ninefold increased risk of developing HD for close family members of affected individuals. These studies, however, did not allow any interpretation of the genetic mechanisms presumably implicated in the increased predisposition to HD observed in some families. Hefer et al. [55] carried out segregation analysis on 140 histologically verified cases of HD (males, 94; females, 46) in the age range 3–49 years. The results of this analysis fulfilled the criteria of the multifactorial type of transmission, since (a) the frequency of HD among close relatives equals the square root of the frequency of the disease in the general population and (b) the observed frequency in siblings is almost equal to that expected for multifactorial inheritance. These findings provide further elements favoring the hypothesis that genetic and environmental factors may be associated with the development of HD.

Finally, "familiality" has also been investigated in multiple myeloma (MM); several studies showed the occurrence of families with two or more individuals affected by this disease [56–59], thus raising the possibility of a genetic component in the pathogenesis of MM. However, more recent studies failed to confirm the existence of an increased risk of MM among close relatives of affected patients [60].

Cytogenetics and Molecular Genetics

Over the last 20 years there has been a real explosion of investigations on chromosomal and biomolecular alterations in lymphohematoproliferative disorders. These have been favored by the accessibility of material for studies (i.e., blood samples, bone marrow aspiration biopsy, superficial lymph node examination), the development of new chromosomal banding techniques, and the availability of well-characterized monoclonal antibodies against B- and T-cell surface molecules. There is little doubt that the main insights into the etiopathogenesis and management of human tumors largely depended on clinical observations and laboratory investigations carried out in leukemias and lymphomas. In general terms, the results of these studies can be summarized by stating that chromosomal rearrangements in leukemic and lymphomatous cells may alter the structure or the function of cellular oncogenes, thus inducing quantitative or qualitative changes in their gene products which seem to play a relevant role in initiating or maintaining the neoplastic state.

Acute and Chronic Leukemias

With the most recent techniques, chromosomal alterations can be detected in most (if not all) patients with leukemia [61–65]. The most frequent of these are (a) deletions of chromosomal regions, (b) reciprocal translocations between two chromosomes in which one breaks at a specific site (donor chromosome) while the other may vary (receptor chromosome), and (c) occurrence of chromosomes in triplicate (trisomy). Thus, a translocation involving chromosomes 15 and 17 has been detected in acute promyelocytic leukemia, a subtype of AML. Other chromosomal abnormalities frequently observed in this type of leukemia include t(8;21), t(9;11), t(6;9), deletion of

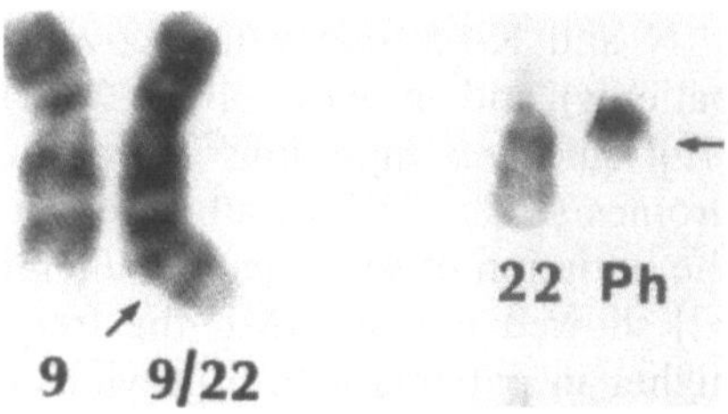

Fig. 1. Reciprocal translocation involving the long arms of chromosomes 9 and 22, and the Philadelphia (*Ph*) chromosome, in a patient with chronic myelogenous leukemia

5q or 7q, and inversion of chromosome 16; finally, of particular interest (see later) is the observation of t(9;22) in a small proportion of AML [61, 66]. In ALL, t(8;14); t(4;11), and deletion of 6q have been reported; moreover, in approximately 30% of adult patients with ALL, t(9;22) can be observed. Abnormalities of chromosome 12 and t(11;14) are not rare in CLL [68–70]; in addition, structural alterations of chromosome 13q14 have been reported in a fraction of patients with B-cell CLL. Since the retinoblastoma (*Rb*) gene has been mapped on this chromosomal region, these observations raise the possibility that loss or rearrangements of *Rb* might be implicated in leukemogenesis (at least in CLL), although the possible role of other genes located in close proximity to *Rb* cannot be excluded [71].

Over 90% of patients with CML show the Philadelphia chromosome (Fig. 1), which is the result of a reciprocal translocation involving the long arms of chromosomes 9 and 22 (i.e., 22q- – the Philadelphia chromosome – and 9+ chromosome) [61–63, 72]. At a molecular level, this alteration is characterized by a translocation of the c-*abl* protooncogene from chromosome 9 to within the *bcr* region on chromosome 22 [73]. Although the breakpoints on both chromosomes may be variable, the *bcr-abl* fusion gene produces an 8-kilobase fusion mRNA, containing *bcr* sequences upstream of the breakpoint and c-*abl* sequences downstream, that is translated into a chimeric phosphoprotein of 210 kDa, called p210, with high levels of tyrosine kinase activity [74]. The presence of this chimeric protein in a pluripotent hematopoietic cell stem is usually considered to be closely associated with the development of CML, and probably with a relevant proportion of adult-type ALL [75]. However, while there is convincing evidence that the chronic phase of CML is related to rearrangements of the *abl* gene and formation of the *bcr-abl* oncogene, no consistent alterations were found in the blastic crisis, although the frequent chromosomal changes observed during disease progression suggest that additional genetic events may occur. Thus, alterations of the *ras* genes [76], amplification of c-*myc* [77], and, more recently, rearrangements in the *p53* gene [78] have been reported in the acute phase of CML, and might play a certain role in development of the blastic crisis.

N and K-*ras* oncogene activation is also seen in AML (15%–30% of patients) and in ALL (10%–20%), but only rarely in chronic leukemias [79]; since *ras* mutations are particularly frequent in myelodysplastic syndromes (60%–70% of all cases), it is likely that these genes play a role in the initiation of some acute leukemias [80]. Interestingly, recent studies [81, 82] showed that in AML the frequency of *ras* mutations was significantly higher in patients with a previous occupational exposure to chemicals of a various nature than in patients without a history of an occupation associated with an elevated risk of leukemia. These findings, therefore, suggest that mutational activation of the *ras* oncogenes might identify a subgroup of patients with AML in whom chronic exposure to chemical compounds might play an etiologic role.

Lymphomas

Several cytogenetic abnormalities have been documented in NHL of various degrees of differentiation [61–63]. These include trisomy of chromosomes 3, 7, 8, and 12, and a number of well-characterized translocations; in many cases, genes of possible relevance in tumorigenesis have been localized at specific chromosomal breakpoints. Thus, t(11;14) seems to involve the *bcl-1* gene in some B-cell neoplasms, while t(4;18) is associated with the *bcl-2* gene in follicular lymphomas, and other translocations frequently observed in T-cell malignancies involve genes of the *tcl* class [83–85]. Owing to these cytogenetic alterations, *bcl* and *tcl* (for B-cell lymphoma and T-cell lymphoma, respectively) oncogenes are brought into close proximity to either the *Ig* genes (in B-cell malignancies) or to T-cell receptor genes (in T-cell lymphoma). Thus, what became clear from these and other studies [13, 63, 86, 87] was that genes regulating immunoglobulin synthesis were juxtaposed with genes which normally regulate cell proliferation and differentiation; a further biomolecular definition of these events was made through detailed investigations on the 8;14 translocation in Burkitt's lymphoma (BL).

In patients with BL, malignant cells show a chromosomal translocation involving chromosomes 8 and 14, with breakpoints at subbands q24 and q32, respectively [13, 62]; subsequent studies revealed that the c-*myc* oncogene is located on chromosome 8q24, while the genes for heavy chain immunoglobulins were identified on 14q32. Thus, the main effect of 8;14 translocation is to join the c-*myc* oncogene to the immunoglobulin heavy chain locus [62, 63], with the result that in BL c-*myc* transcription may increase several times over normal levels [61]. Despite the several possible rearrangements ot BL cells, it was found that the protein produced by the c-*myc* gene was qualitatively normal; thus, the cancerous effect of t(8;14) does not seem to be due to abnormalities within the gene, but rather should be attributed to an altered expression. It is likely, therefore, that the c-*myc* gene which is translocated to the immunoglobulin locus on chromosome 14q32 escapes the mechanisms that normally control transcription; in other words, there is evidence that *c-myc* becomes deregulated following its new location in proximity to genes that code for heavy chain immunoglobulins [63]. This conclusion is further reinforced by the observation that the *c-myc* gene can be activated by other translocations – such at t(2;8) or t(8;22) – in which the oncogene is joined to sequences encoding antibody production (lambda or kappa light chains). It has been suggested that *c-myc* deregulation in t(8;14) might be due to the juxtaposition of the oncogene to "enhancers" (i.e., sequences of DNA that increase the level of transcription of certain genes, as in the case of immunoglobulins) within the immunoglobulin locus; consequently, the *c-myc* gene would be expressed in the same way as immunoglobulin genes are expressed in normal B cells [88]. Finally, besides the interest in characterizing the genetic basis of a rare neoplasm (BL), it is likely that the translocation and the biomolecular abnormalities characterizing BL may provide a general model for understanding tumorigenesis in human B-cell malignancies.

At variance with NHL, no cytogenetic alterations have been consistently demonstrated in HD. The main obstacles in elucidating the biology of HD remain the relative paucity of Reed-Sternberg cells (the real neoplastic elements) and the difficulty of their isolation. In accordance with epidemiologic observations, in situ hybridization showed the presence of the EBV genome in Reed-Sternberg cells of approximately one-third of patients with HD [89, 90]. Recent studies [91, 92] showed the frequent immunohistochemical detection of mutated p53 protein in HD; positive immunoreactivity localized to the Reed-Sternberg cells was observed in the majority of patients with nodular sclerosing and mixed cellularity histologic subtypes (86% and 57% of the cases, respectively), while no positive staining was detected in the nodular lymphocyte predominant type of HD. These findings (a) confirm the common belief that Reed-Sternberg cells are the neoplastic elements of HD, (b) provide some evidence of the possible different origin of the lymphocyte predominant nodular HD, and (c) seem to suggest that p53 mutations might have a role in HD development and progression.

References

1. Muir C, Waterhouse J, Mack T et al. (1987) Cancer incidence in five continents, vol 5. Lyon, France (IARC scientific publication, no 8)
2. Wong-Staal F, Gallo RC (1985) The family of human T-lymphotropic leukemia viruses: HTLV-I as the cause of adult T cell leukemia and HTLV-III as the cause of AIDS. Blood 65:253–258
3. Hoelzer D (1988) Prognostic factors in a multicentric study for treatment of acute lymphoblastic leukemia in adult. Blood 71:120–131
4. Weinstein HJ (1983) Chemotherapy for acute myelogenous leukemia in children and adults. Blood 62:315–322
5. Bergsagel DE, Haas RH, Messner HA (1986) Interferon alpha-2 in treatment of chronic granulocytic leukemia. Semin Oncol 13:29–35

6. Foon K, Gale RP (1987) Staging and therapy of chronic lymphocytic leukemia. Semin Hematol 24:264–271
7. Talpaz M, Kurzrock R, Kamtarjian HM et al. (1988) Recent advances in the treatment of chronic myelogenous leukemia. In: DeVita VT, Hellman S, Rosenberg SA (eds) Important advances in oncology. Lippincott, Philadelphia, pp 297–321
8. Polliack A (1992) Leukaemia and lymphoma: reviews 1. Harwood Academic
9. Ries L, Hankey BF, Miller BA et al. (1991) Cancer statistics review 1973–1988. NCI publication no 91, p 2789
10. Preisler HD (1987) The treatment of acute nonlymphocytic leukemia. Blood Rev 1:97–108
11. Jaiyesimi I, Kantarjian HM, Estey EH (1993) Advances in therapy for hairy cell leukemia. Cancer 72:5–16
12. Barnes N, Cartwright RA, O'Brien C et al. (1986) Rising incidence of lymphoid malignancies: true or false? Br J Cancer 53:393–398
13. DeVita VT (1989) Lymphocytic leukemia. In: DeVita VT, Hellman S, Rosenberg SA (eds) Cancer: principles and practice of oncology, 3rd edn. Lippincott, Philadelphia, pp 1741–1798
14. Epstein MA, Achong BG, Barr YM (1964) Virus particles in cultured lymphoblasts from Burkitt's lymphoma. Lancet 1:202–203
15. Biggar RJ, Horm J, Goedart JJ et al. (1987) Cancer in a group at risk of AIDS through 1984. Am J Epidemiol 126:578–586
16. Cohnheim J (1865) Ein Fall von Pseudoleukemie. Arch Pathol Anat 33:451
17. Classification of non-Hodgkin's lymphomas (1982) Summary and description of a "Working Formulation" for clinical usage. Cancer 49:2112–2120
18. Canellos GP (1988) Advances in chemotherapy for Hodgkin's and non-Hodgkin's lymphomas. Semin Hematol 25(2):1–15
19. Hodgkin T (1832) On some morbid appearances of absorbent glands and spleen. Med Chir Ter 17:68
20. Sternberg C (1898) Uber eine Eigenartice unter dem bilderer Pseudoleukemie verlaufende Tuberkulose des lympatischen Apparates. Z Heilkd 19:21–26
21. Grufferman S, Delzell E (1984) Epidemiology of Hodgkin's disease. Epidemiol Rev 6:76–106
22. Hellman S, Jaffe ES, DeVita VT (1989) Hodgkin's disease. In: DeVita VT, Hellman S, Rosenberg SA (eds) Principles and practice of oncology, 3rd edn. Lippincott, Philadelphia, pp 1696–1740
23. Longo DL, Young RC, Welsey M et al. (1986) Twenty years of MOPP therapy for Hodgkin's disease. J Clin Oncol 4:1295–1306
24. Bonadonna G, Valagussa P, Santoro A (1986) Alternating non-cross-resistant combination chemotherapy or MOPP in stage IV Hodgkin's disease: a report of a 8-year study. Ann Intern Med 104:739–746
25. DeVita VT, Hubbard SM (1993) Hodgkin's disease. N Engl J Med 328:560–565
26. Videbaek A (1947) Heredity in human leukemia and its relation to cancer. Einar Munksgaard, Copenhagen, Denmark
27. Gunz FW (1964) Leukaemia in New Zealand and Australia Pathol Microbiol 27:697–704
28. Gunz FW, Dameshek W (1956) Chronic lymphocytic leukemia in a family, including twin brothers and a son. JAMA 164:1323–1325
29. Gunz FW, Veale AMO (1969) Leukemia in close relatives – accident or predisposition? JNCI 42:517–524
30. Gunz FW (1977) The epidemiology and genetics of the chronic leukemias. Clin Haematol 6:3–20
31. Gunz FW, Gunz JP, Veale AMO et al. (1975) Familial leukemia: a study of 909 families. Scand J Haematol 15:117–131

32. MacMahon B, Levy MA (1964) Prenatal origin of childhood leukemia. N Engl J Med 270:1082–1085
33. Miller RW (1971) Death from childhood leukemia and solid tumors among twins and other sibs in the USA, 1960–67. JNCI 46:203–209
34. Leverger G, Tourani JM, Schaison G et al. (1985) HLA haplotypes in a family with three cases of acute lymphoblastic leukemia. In: Muller HJ, Weber W (eds) Familial canncer. Karger, Basel, pp 167–171
35. Blattner WA, Naiman JL, Mann DL et al. (1978) Immunogenetic determinants of familial acute lymphocytic leukemia. Ann Intern Med 89:173–176
36. Hafez M, El-Tahan H, El-Morsi Z et al. (1985) Genetic-environmental interaction in acute lymphocytic leukemia. In: Muller HJ, Weber W (eds) Familial cancer. Karger, Basel, pp 161–166
37. Linet MS, van Natta ML, Brookmeyer R et al. (1989) Familial cancer history and chronic lymphocytic leukemia. Am J Epidemiol 130:655–664
38. Lynch HT, Marcus JN, Weisenburger DD et al. (1989) Genetic and immunopathological findings in a lymphoma family. Br J Cancer 59:622–626
39. Johnson MJE, Peters CH (1957) Ten lymphomas in four siblings. JAMA 163: 20–25
40. Miller RW (1968) Death from childhood cancer in sibs. N Engl J Med 279:122–126
41. Scolozzi R, Boccafogli A, Cereri C et al. (1979) Malignant lymphoma present almost simultaneously in two brothers. Tumori 65:455–458
42. Laurence RP (1979) Familial gastric lymphoma. J Maine Med Assoc 70:456–457
43. Greene MH (1982) Non-Hodgkin's lymphoma and mycosis fungoides. In: Schottenfeld D, Fraumeni JF (eds) Cancer epidemiology and prevention. Saunders, Philadelphia, pp 754–778
44. Haim N, Cohen Y, Robinson E (1982) Malignant lymphoma in first-degree blood relatives. Cancer 49:2197–2200
45. Clark JW, Tucker MA, Greene MH (1987) Clinical and laboratory observations in a lymphoma-prone family. Cancer 60:864–869
46. Purtilo DT, DeFlorio D Jr, Hutt LM et al. (1977) Variable phenotypic expression of an X-linked recessive lymphoproliferative syndrome. N Engl J Med 297: 1077–1081
47. Stevens DA, O'Conor GT, Levine PH et al. (1972) Acute leukemia with "Burkitt's lymphoma cells" and Burkitt's lymphoma. Ann Intern Med 76: 967–973
48. Anderson KC, Jamison DS, Peters WP et al. (1986) Familial Burkitt's lymphoma. Am J Med 81:158–162
49. Poulsen LO, Christensen JH, Sorensen B et al. (1991) Immunologic observations in close relatives of two sisters with mammary Burkitt's lymphoma. Cancer 68:1031–1034
50. Grufferman S, Cole P, Smith PG et al. (1977) Hodgkin's disease in siblings. N Engl J Med 296:248–252
51. Maldonado JE, Taswell HF, Kiely JM (1972) Familial Hodgkin's disease. Lancet 2:1259–1263
52. Grufferman S (1977) Clustering and aggregation of exposures in Hodgkin's disease. Cancer 39:1829–1833
53. Rezis DV, Diamond HD, Craver LF (1959) Familial Hodgkin's disease: its significance and implications. Ann Intern Med 51:933–971
54. Vianna NJ, Davies JNP, Polan AK et al. (1974) Familial Hodgkin's disease: an environmental and genetic disorder. Lancet 2:854–857
55. Hafez M, El-Tahan H, El-Morsi Z et al. (1985) Genetic susceptibility in Hodgkin's lymphoma. In: Muller HJ, Weber W (eds) Familial cancer. Karger, Basel, pp 175–179

56. Mandema E, Wildervanck LS (1954) La maladie de Kahler (myelomes multiples) chez deux soeurs. J Genet Hum 3:170–175
57. Boga M, Jako J, Doman J et al. (1973) Familial myeloma. Folia Haematol (Leipz) 3:201–212
58. Shoenfield Y, Shaklay M, Berliner S et al. (1982) Familial multiple myeloma. Postgrad Med J 58:12–16
59. Maldonado JE, Kyle RA (1974) Familial myeloma: report of 8 families and a study of serum proteins in their relatives. Am J Med 57:875–884
60. Bourguet CC, Grufferman S, Delzell E et al. (1985) Multiple myeloma and family history of cancer. Cancer 56:2133–2139
61. Yunis JJ (1983) The chromosomal basis of human neoplasia. Science 221: 227–236
62. Cline MJ (1989) Biology of disease: molecular diagnosis of human cancer. Lab Invest 61:368–380
63. Solomon E, Borrow J, Goddard AD (1991) Chromosome aberrations in cancer. Science 254:1153–1160
64. Thirman MJ, Gill HJ, Burnett RC et al. (1993) Rearrangement of the MLL gene in acute lymphoblastic and acute myeloid leukemias with 11q23 chromosomal translocation. N Engl J Med 329:909–914
65. Heyman M, Grandèr D, Brondum-Nielsen K et al. (1993) Deletions of the short arm of chromosome 9, including the interferon genes, in acute lymphocytic leukemia. Int J Cancer 54:748–753
66. Kizrock R, Gutterman JU, Talpaz M (1988) The molecular genetics of Philadelphia chromosome-positive leukemias. N Engl J Med 319:990–998
67. Hooberman AL, Westbrook CA, Heisterkamp N et al. (1989) Molecular diagnosis of Philadelphia chromosome in acute lymphoblastic leukemia. Leuk Lymph 1:3–10
68. Einhorn S, Burvall K, Juliusson G et al. (1989) Molecular analyses of chromosome 12 in chronic lymphocytic leukemia. Leukemia 3:871–874
69. Einhorn S, Meeker T, Juliusson G et al. (1990) No evidence of trisomy 12 or t(11;14) by molecular genetic techniques in chronic lymphocytic leukemia cells with a normal karyotype. Cancer Genet Cytogenet 48:183–192
70. Lo Coco F, Mandelli F, Breccia M et al. (1993) Southern blot analysis of ALL-1 rearrangements at chromosome 11q23 in acute leukemia. Cancer Res 53:3800–3803
71. Liu Y, Grandèr D, Soderhall S et al. (1992) Betinoblastoma gene deletions in B-cell chronic lympocytic leukemia. Gener Chromos Cancer 4:250–256
72. Swolin B, Weinfeld A, Westin J (1985) Karyotypic evolution in Ph-positive chronic myeloid leukemia in relation to management and disease progression. Cancer Genet Cytogenet 18:65–72
73. Groffen J, Stephenson JR, Heisterkamp N et al. (1984) Philadelphia chromosome breakpoints are clustered within a limited region, bcr, on chromosome 22. Cell 36:93–101
74. Dreazen O, Cannani E, Gale RP (1988) Molecular biology of chronic myelogenous leukemia. Semin Hematol 25:35–44
75. Witte ON (1993) Role of the BCR-ABL oncogene in human leukemia. Cancer Res 53:485–489
76. Liu E, Hjelle B, Bishop GM (1988) Transforming genes in chronic myelogenous leukemia. Proc Natl Acad Sic USA 85:1952–1956
77. McCarthy DM, Rassool F, Glodman J et al. (1984) Genomic alterations involving the c-myc proto-oncogene locus during the evolution of a case of chronic granulocytic leukemia. Lancet 2:1362–1364

78. Kelman Z, Prokocimer M, Peller S et al. (1989) Rearrangements in the p53 gene in Philadelphia chromosome positive chronic myelogenous leukemia. Blood 74:2318–2324
79. Needleman SW (1991) ras protooncogene activation in acute myeloid leukemia and related disorders. Leuk Lymph 5:85–91
80. Liu et (1990) ras gene mutations in acute myelogenous leukemia. In: Gale RP (ed) Acute myelogenous leukemia: progress and controversies. Wiley-Liss, New York, pp 107–115
81. Taylor JA, Sandler DP, Bloomfield CD et al. (1992) ras oncogene activation and occupatione exposure in acute myeloid leukemia. JNCI 84:1626–1632
82. Smith MT, Wiemels J, Rothman N et al. (1992) Chemical exposure, ras oncogene activation and acute myeloid leukemia. JNCI 84:1614–1615
83. Tsujimoto Y, Yumis J, Onorato-Showe L et al. (1984) Molecular cloning of the chromosomal breakpoint of B-cell lymphomas and leukemias with the t(11;14) translocation. Science 224:1403–1405
84. Tsujimoto Y, Finger LR, Yunis J et al. (1985) Cloning of the chromosome breakpoint of t(11;18) human lymphomas: clustering around JH on chromosome 14 and near a transcriptional unit on 18. Cell 41:899–910
85. Reynolds TC, Smith SD, Sklar J (1987) Analysis of DNA surrounding the breakpoint of chromosomal translocations involving the beta T-cell receptor gene in human lymphoblastic neoplasms. Cell 50:107–116
86. Morton CC, Duby AD, Eddy RL et al. (1985) Genes for beta gene for human T cell antigen receptor map to regions of chromosomal rearrangement in T cells. Science 228:582–584
87. Ye BH, Rao PH, Chaganti RSK et al. (1993) Cloning of bcl-6, the locus involved in chromosome translocations affecting band 3q27 in B-cell lymphoma. Cancer Res 53:2732–2735
88. Croce CM (1987) Role of chromosome translocations in human neoplasia. Cell 49:155–164
89. Wiess LM, Movahed LA, Warnke RA et al. (1989) Detection of Epstein-Barr viral genome in Reed-Sternberg cells of Hodgkin's disease. N Engl J Med 320:502–506
90. Khan G, Coates PJ, Gupta RK et al. (1992) Presence of Epstein-Barr virus in Hodgkin's disease is not exclusive to Reed-Sternberg cells. Am J Pathol 140:757–762
91. Gupta RK, Norton AJ, Thompson IW et al. (1992) p53 expression in Reed-Sternberg cells of Hodgkin's disease. Br J Cancer 66:649–652
92. Doussis IA, Pezzella F, Lane DP et al. (1993) An immunocytochemical study of p53 and bcl-2 protein expression in Hodgkin's disease. Am J Clin Pathol 99:663–667

Familial Factors in Cancer of the Genitourinary Tract

When the DNA from the human EJ bladder cancer cell line was introduced into mouse 3T3 cells and the cultures observed, foci of transformed mouse cells appeared. No such foci appeared when DNA from a non-malignant source was used. This strongly supported the notion that the bladder cancer DNA contained a dominantly acting cancer gene, which was promptly named as oncogene.

(T.D. Gelehrter and F.S. Collins 1990)

Introduction

Cancer of the genitourinary tract includes tumors of the kidney, bladder, prostate, and testis; together these neoplasms represent approximately 25% of all malignancies in the male sex. Ovarian tumors have already been described in the chapter on "Hereditary and Familial Ovarian Cancer," and endometrial carcinoma in the chapter on "Hereditary and Familial Colorectal Cancer," as part of Lynch syndrome II. Wilms' tumor – undoubtedly the most interesting tumor of the genitourinary tract, for its genetic implications – has already been considered in the chapter on "Genetic Factors in Solid Tumors of Childhood," together with other malignancies of childhood.

Despite the frequency of prostatic cancer, there have been few observations on the familial aspects of the disease, and these tumors have been more often related to environmental factors. In contrast, aggregation of cancers among family members and increased risk of tumor development in close relatives have been reported more frequently for neoplasms of the bladder and testis, although no clear pattern of inheritance has been defined. Clusters of renal tumors have also been described; in addition, some of these familial aggregates are characterized by a balanced translocation between chromosomes 3 and 8 in the germline cells of many affected individuals. Finally, alterations in various oncogenes and tumor suppressor genes (in particular, *p53* and *ras*, together with allele losses at chromosomes 3, 5, 6, 10, 17, and others) have been found by many authors, thus suggesting that various genetic events might contribute to the development of urogenital neoplasms.

General Aspects

Incidence and Etiologic Factors

Incidence rates of prostatic cancer show wide geographic and racial variation, from less than one case/100 000 inhabitants per year in the Chinese population to more than 100 in black Americans [1]. The disease does not seem to be related to diet, cigarette smoking, or occupation, while some studies indicate that the risk of this tumor can be somehow related to serum testosterone levels [1, 2]. The fact that circulating androgenic hormones are higher in black men than in white individuals lends further support to this interpretation [3]. Mortality rates for this tumor appear to have stabilized during the last 30 years [4].

In Western countries, incidence rates of bladder cancer are in the order of 15–20 new cases/100 000 per year in men and about five in women, with peak values in the age group 60–70 years [5, 6]. Since the beginning of this century, clinical observations showed that workers in the aniline dye industry had incidence rates of bladder carcinoma higher than expected; the carcinogen to which they were exposed was subsequently identified as β-naphthalene [7]. More recent studies indicated that cigarette smoking, chronic infections of the urinary tract (especially schistosomiasis), and excessive ingestion of analgesics containing phenacetin may increase the risk of bladder carcinoma, whereas the role of other hypothetical etiologic agents (i.e., coffee, saccharin) remains uncertain [8, 9].

Testicular cancers are relatively rare, with incidence rates of approximately 1–3 new cases/100 000 per year and a peak of incidence between the ages of 25 and 35 years [10]. The disease does not seem to be related to well-defined risk factors, with the exception of cryptorchidism, which is associated with a tenfold increase in the frequency of these tumors [11]. Similarly, little is known of the etiology of renal carcinoma, though there is some evidence that cigarette smoking increases the risk of the disease [12]. Cancer of the kidney shows incidence rates of about 10–15 new cases/100 000 per year and is more frequent in the male sex [4, 13].

Clinical and Biological Features

Cancers of the prostate are usually well to moderately differentiated adenocarcinomas. The disease is frequently asymptomatic, though many patients may complain of urinary infections or obstruction, stranguria, and/or nycturia; on rectal palpation the gland is usually firm, enlarged, and indurated. Tumors tend to invade the surrounding organs, more often the seminal vescicles and the neck of the bladder. TNM staging includes four main categories [2]; in stage I, only microscopic tumors (not detectable by palpation) can be detected; in stage II, tumors appear as well-defined nodules confined to the gland on rectal examination; in stage III cancer there is a local spread beyond the confines of the prostate (to seminal vescicles, bladder, or other organs) but no distant metastases; finally, stage IV tumors manifest with nodal involvement or hematogenous dissemination (especially to the bones, liver, and lung). Autoptic studies showed an extremely high frequency of microadenocarcinonas in the prostate of normal individuals older than 50 years, and every decade of ageing doubles the incidence of these "in situ" lesions [14, 15]. These unexpected findings strongly suggest that only a small fraction of prostate tumors become clinically manifest, whereas the majority presumably remain undetected for decades in a latent state. A similar phenomenon was recently observed for breast carcinoma (see the chapter on "Hereditary and Familial Breast Cancer," [20, 21]). Besides rectal examination, diagnosis and preoperative staging of prostate cancer are based on transrectal ultrasonography, bone scintiscan, computed tomography, nuclear magnetic imaging, thin-needle biopsy, and serum determination of prostate specific antigen or acid phosphatase [2, 16, 17]. Ultrasonography and prostate-specific antigen are also widely used with the purpose of screening for prostate carcinoma, though this is controversial [2, 18–20].

Most bladder tumors are transitional cell carcinomas, while less common histologic types include leiomyosarcoma, squamous cell carcinoma (particularly frequent in areas where schistosomiasis is endemic), and adenocarcinoma. The disease usually becomes manifest with hematuria or, more rarely, with dysuria and back pain. Intravenous urogram, cystoscopy, and endoscopic biopsy are the most common diagnostic procedures, whereas lymphography and computed tomography are of great value for preoperative assessment of local spread. TNM staging is mainly based on the degree of local invasion at presentation [21]; superficial tumors usually remain confined to the mucosa and submucosa (Tis, Ta, T1) through most of their natural history; in contrast, tumors infiltrating the bladder wall (T2–T4) are frequently associated with local recurrences and/or distant metastasis [9].

The large majority of testicular tumors are of germ cell origin, and can be classified into seminomas, teratomas, and mixed forms; non-germ cell neoplasms include Sertoli cell tumors, lymphomas, and Leydig cell tumors. The disease progresses though the invasion of various lymph node groups (iliac, paraaortic, mediastinal, and supraclavicular) and with hematogenous metastases (mostly in the lung). The main symptom is a painless swelling of the testis, while the occasional presence of pain usually indicates rapidly growing tumors. The diagnosis is based on biopsy of the testicular mass; in addition, lymphography and computed tomography are essential for a proper assessment of tumor extension, and have been of great value in elucidating the natural history of these neoplasms. Serum levels of two tumor markers (alpha-fetoprotein and beta-chorionic gonadotropin) are elevated in 50%–70% of patients with teratomas [22]. Besides their help in diagnosis, the basal levels of these markers seem to be of prognostic relevance; in addition, repeated measurements of their values give useful indications as to the response to treatment, and become an essential part for the clinical management of these neoplasms [23]. Testicular tumors are usually staged with the TNM system, and are grouped into four main categories [21].

Tumors of the kidney are mostly hypernephromas (renal cell carcinoma) which originate from the epithelium of the renal tubules, while tumors of the pelvis are relatively uncommon. Local spread into the perirenal tissues is frequent and closely related to the degree of differentiation; commonly affected lymph nodes include perirenal, iliac, and paraaortic groups; hematogenous metastases are particularly frequent in the lung, bones, and brain [24]. Renal tumors can remain symptomless for a long time, and then become clinically manifest with hematuria, loin pain, or symptoms related to metastasis (bone fractures, cough, or dyspnea). Ultrasonography, intravenous pyelography, and computed tomography are the techniques of choice for a proper diagnosis, and their combined use – together with fine-needle, ultrasound-guided biopsy, and aspiration cytology – has consistently reduced the need for renal arteriography. Computed tomography of the lung and isotope bone scintiscan are valuable techniques for identifying unsuspected distant deposits. Renal tumors are classified into four main categories according to the TNM system: in stage I, tumors are confined to the kidney, which may appear slightly enlarged; stage II tumors are associated with deformities and enlargement of the kidney, but without evidence of extrarenal disease; in stage III, the disease spreads to the perirenal tissues or renal vein; in addition, ipsilateral lymph nodes can be involved; finally, stage IV neoplasms invade the diaphragm, the abdominal wall, or other surrounding organs, with or without lymph node or hematogenous metastasis [21]. Renal tumors can be associated with paraneoplastic syndromes (arterial hypertension, polycytemia, hypercalcemia, and several others, due to the production of hormones or hormone-like substances) in approximately 5% of all affected patients [25].

Management and Prognosis

As for most tumors, survival of patients with prostate cancer is closely related to stage at diagnosis [2, 26]. Prognostic indicators include degree of differentiation, nuclear ploidy, tumor size, levels of prostate-specific antigen, and presence of pelvic lymph node metastasis [27–30]. In stage I–II prostate cancer, either radical prostatectomy or radiotherapy can be proposed as curative treatments [2]; impotence was a common consequence of the surgical approach, but new techniques have been developed which spare the nerves required for normal erection, so that in the majority of patients potency returns to normal after operation [31]. In locally advanced (stage III) or metastatic disease, orchiectomy and/or hormonal therapy which suppresses testosterone activity (estrogens, or analogues of hypothalamic luteinizing hormone-releasing factor) are the treatments of choice [32, 33], while conventional chemotherapy does not seem to be effective.

Prognosis of bladder carcinoma is closely dependent on stage at diagnosis; for Tis to T1 tumors (i.e., those limited to the lamina propria) 5-year survival is in the order of 75%–80% with surgery alone; in tumors with superficial or deep muscular involvement (T2–T3) survival at 5 years is 30%–40%, whereas the outcome is extremely poor for patients with more advanced disease [9]. One of the main objectives in the treatment of superficial bladder carcinoma is the identification of tumors which are likely to relapse or to assume a locally invasive or metastatic pattern of growth; for this purpose, besides staging, many biological indicators of clinical outcome have been defined or are under active investigation. Thus, progression and recurrences seem to correlate with nuclear DNA aneuploidy and with a high proliferative rate [34]; similarly, degree of differentiation, pattern of growth (papillary versus solid), and chromosomal abnormalities appear to be independent prognostic indicators [9, 35–37]. Treatment of superficial bladder cancer is based on endoscopic resection (or electrocauterization) or cystectomy; more recent photodynamic techniques can be used for visualizing, by fluorescence, "in situ" carcinomas, after intravenous injection of hematoporphyrin derivatives [38]. In addition, it has been shown that intravescical administration of either chemotherapeutic agents or bacille Calmette-Guérin significantly reduces relapse rate and increases disease-free survival [39, 40]. Treatment of invasive bladder cancer is more controversial; either radical surgery or radiation therapy (or both) have been proposed with comparable survival and recurrence rates, while the role of adjuvant chemotherapy is still undefined [9, 41]. In relapsing or metastatic disease encouraging results have been obtained with various combinations of chemotherapeutic agents (especially cisplatin, doxorubicin, cyclophosphamide, and methotrexate), though long-term survival usually does not exceed 10%–15% [42, 43].

One of the main features of testicular tumors is their sensitivity to various chemotherapeutic agents and to radiation, so that the majority of these neoplasms are now curable even in advanced stages, with overall response rates and 5-year survivals of approximately 80%. In particular, in patients with seminoma, radiotherapy – at a dose of 30–40 Gy over a period of 4 weeks – seems to be effective in inducing complete response even with diffuse lymph node involvement; in addition, these tumors are highly sensitive to various combination chemotherapies [44, 45]. The initial treatment of malignant teratoma can be "debulking" surgery (which often requires retroperitoneal lymphadenectomy) or radiotherapy (usually at doses higher than for seminoma), both associated with chemotherapy; in the most recent protocols, combination chemotherapy is often used before surgery. Testicular teratomas are remarkably sensitive to polychemotherapy (especially the association of cisplatin, vinblastine, and bleomycin), though toxicity and side effects remain a serious problem [46, 47].

The clinical outcome of patients with renal cancer is closely dependent on staging and degree of differentiation. In localized disease (stage I–II), 5-year survival can be more than 60%, but it drops to 20%–40% if regional lymph nodes are involved, whereas there are virtually no long-term survivors in locally advanced or metastatic disease. Surgery remains the treatment of choice (usually "en bloc" resection of the kidney with wide dissection of regional lymph nodes), although one-third of these neoplasms are technically unresectable [48]. While radiotherapy and conventional chemotherapy are only marginally effective, encouraging results have recently been obtained with immunotherapy (interferon, interleukin 2, and/or lymphokine-activated killer cells) [49].

Neoplastic "Familiality"

Although "familiality" has not been extensively investigated in prostate cancer, familial clusters of prostate and other urologic tumors have been reported [50–52]. In addition, individuals with first-degree relatives affected by prostate cancer seem to be at higher risk for the disease than the general population, and the risk increases proportionally with the number of affected family members [53–55]. Finally, recent studies showed that a small proportion of prostate cancers can be transmitted through a Mendelian (autosomal dominant) type of inheritance, and suggested that this mode of transmission might account for a significant fraction of early onset prostate carcinomas [56], thus further emphasizing that the early occurrence of neoplasms is a constant feature of hereditary tumors.

Familial aggregations of bladder carcinomas have frequently been reported. In 1967, Fraumeni and Thomas [57] described a family in which the father and his three sons were all affected by this tumor; similarly, McCullough et al. [58] reported the occurrence of bladder cancer in six members from two generations of a large American family of Western European descent, and hypothesized that tumors in this kindred could be inherited through an autosomal dominant gene. Families with a striking aggregation of bladder carcinomas, often associated with other tumors of the urinary tract, have been described by several other authors [59–61]. In 1983, Marchetto et al. [62] evaluated a family in which three closely related women had transitional cell carcinoma of the ureter associated with other neoplasms of the genitourinary tract, including bladder carcinoma (one case), well-differentiated renal cell cancer (one case), and endometrial carcinoma (two cases); moreover, other family members died of breast cancer, brain tumor, and liver or lung carcinoma. The authors interpreted this unusual aggregation of multiple tumors as due to interaction between a genetic susceptibility to cancer and the exposure to common environmental factors (i.e., cigarette smoking, excessive coffee consumption, and artificial sweeteners). More recent studies showed that both endometrial and transitional cell carcinoma of the ureter are among the neoplasms featuring the tumor spectrum of Lynch syndrome II [50, 51]. However, the absence of documented colorectal carcinomas (in a total of more than 50 individuals spanning 3 generations) and the late onset of most tumors do not favor the hypothesis of an anomalous Lynch syndrome. In addition, familial aggregation of ureteral carcinoma has also been described [63]. Two case control studies [64, 65] assessed the frequency of urinary tract cancer among first-degree relatives of patients with bladder carcinoma. Both investigations showed an elevated risk of bladder tumors associated with a positive family history; the overall increased risk was about 45% (RR, 1.5; CI, 1.2–1.8), which is undoubtedly less than the risk observed for other common carcinomas (see the chapters on "Familial and Hereditary Breast Cancer," "Genetic Factors in Lung Cancer," and "Hereditary and Familial Colorectal Cancer"). Rather interestingly, the familial risk was higher (RR, 2.7; CI, 0.8–8.9) for individuals below the age of 45 years, which is consistent with similar observations in other types of tumors. Finally, the risk of bladder carcinoma rose sharply (RR up to 28) in various subgroups of patients with a positive family history for the disease and who were also currently cigarette smoking (from less than one to more than three packs/day), thus suggesting that for these tumors, in analogy with breast or lung carcinoma [66], a close interaction between environmental factors and genetic predisposition is presumably required for the induction and progression of malignancy.

Despite their relative rarity, there are several reports indicating a possible contribution of genetic factors in testicular cancer; most of these studies concern pairs of identical twins, or aggregation of two (or more) cases of germ cell tumors of the testis in brothers or in father-son pairs [67–70]. In one of these families, five close relatives were affected by the disease [71], while in another testicular cancer developed in four brothers [72]. Moreover, by analyzing clinical data of more than 200 individuals affected by cancer of the testis, Tollerud et al. [73] found that the presence of a first-degree relative with this type of tumor was associated with a sixfold increase of the risk for the disease. The existence of a registry for testicular cancer enabled Forman and colleagues [74] to assess "familiality" for this type of tumor in a large series of patients diagnosed in the United Kingdom between 1984 and 1986. Among 794 patients with cancer of the testis, eight individuals (1%) had a brother and four (0.5%) had the father with a previous diagnosis of the same disease; in the control group, only two subjects (out of 794) reported a family history of testicular cancer among first-degree relatives (0.3%). The authors estimated that the cumulative risk for brothers of affected individuals developing a testicular tumor by the age of 50 years was in the order of 2%, and that the relative risk versus the general population was 9.8 (CI, 2.8–16.7). Moreover, in a subset of 22 nonidentical affected twins the HLA haplotype distribution did not differ from the expected proportions. Thus, at variance with previous investigations – which showed a different distribution of HLA in patients with testicular cancer as compared to the general population – these observations do not suggest the existence of a major gene localized on chromosome 6, near the *HLA* gene locus, and associated with the susceptibility to testicular cancer. In accordance with many other observations on hereditary and familial tumors, in this English series familial cases were diagnosed at a significantly younger age than the apparently sporadic neoplasms. Finally, Hartley et al. [75] recently described the occurrence of five cases of testicular germline tumors among family members of children with soft tissue sarcomas; since in three of these families cancer aggregation was consistent with Li-Fraumeni syndrome (see chapter on 'Li-Fraumeni Syndrome"), the authors suggested that cancer of the testis might be an uncommon clinical manifestation of this genetically determined disease.

Renal carcinomas are frequent in von Hippel-Lindau syndrome, a genetically determined disease characterized by hemangioblastomas of the retina, cerebellum, and spinal cord, pancreatic malignancies, pheochromocytomas, and epididymal cysts (see the chapter on "Hereditary Tumors of the Nervous System"). In addition, several familial aggregates of renal tumors have been described. Thus, Franksson et al. [76] reported the occurrence of renal cell carcinomas in five siblings, while in another family four closely related members were affected by the disease, which tended to appear at an earlier age than that of the usual diagnosis [77]. In 1979, Cohen et al. [78] described a large family in which ten members (of both sexes) in two successive generations developed renal cell carcinomas. Age at diagnosis ranged between 37 and 59 years, with a mean of 46 years, which is markedly lower than the average age of onset of renal cancer; moreover, six out of ten patients had bilateral disease (three men and three women). Besides renal cancer, no other neoplasm occurred in this family; in addition, accurate clinical examination did not reveal signs suggestive of Hippel-Lindau disease. Finally, karyotype analysis of peripheral blood lymphocytes showed the presence of a balanced reciprocal translocation between chromosomes 3 and 8 in 10 out of 22 family members; of these, five were survivors of renal cancer, one had a renal cyst, and four had no renal disease (though three were under the age of 35 years). The authors hypothesized that the chromosomal rearrangement might induce gene alterations (deletion, point mutation, or others) which eventually result in an increased susceptibility to renal carcinoma. Moreover, clinical and genetic analysis in this family support the two-mutation model proposed by Knudson (see the chapter on "Retinoblastoma"), and this might provide a further explanation for early onset and frequent bilateral occurrence of tumors.

Molecular Biology and Cytogenetics

Despite the significant impact of prostate cancer in the Western world (in many countries these tumors represent the second leading cause of cancer-related mortality, in men, after lung carcinoma), little is known of its genetic determinants [79, 80]. Carter et al. [81] reported the frequent loss of heterozygosity on chromosomes 16q and 10q in human prostate carcinoma; moreover, in 20% of these tumors allelic losses on chromosome 17p were also seen, suggesting a possible role of the *p53* gene in tumor development. Following this line of evidence, Isaacs et al. [82] carried out detailed investigations of the *p53* gene in prostate cancer cell lines and in two primary tumors; sequence analysis of exons 5–8 showed point mutations in three out of five cell lines and in one carcinoma; moreover, transfection of the wild-type gene into cell lines carrying *p53* mutations resulted in reduced colony formation. These observations may indicate a possible role of *p53* in prostatic tumorigenesis, and add further evidence to the tumor suppressor function of this gene in another common malignancy [83]. Finally, recent studies showed frequent alterations of other putative tumor suppressor genes in prostate cancer [84, 85].

Several cytogenetic abnormalities, including monosomy 9 and deletion of chromosome 11p, have been reported in human bladder carcinoma, though their biological meaning remains undefined [86–88]. Biomolecular changes in these tumors include activation of the *ras* oncogene [89, 90] and increased expression of epidermal growth factor receptor [91, 92]; it is noteworthy that the first evidence of *ras* oncogene activation was obtained in a bladder carcinoma cell line [93]. Restriction fragment length polymorphism analysis revealed frequent loss of heterozygosity at chromosomes 9q, 11p, and 17p in human bladder cancer, thus suggesting the presence of putative tumor suppressor genes within the deleted chromosomal regions [94–97]. Moreover, cloning and sequencing analysis of the *p53* gene showed alterations (more often point mutations, usually associated with allele deletion) in the evolutionary conserved region of the gene in a large fraction of bladder tumors [98, 99]; rather interestingly for the possible practical implications, *p53* mutations were also detected in cells of the urine sediment of three patients. In a subsequent study [100], *p53* mutations were found more frequently in invasive and poorly differentiated bladder carcinomas than in superficial and well-differentiated neoplasms, raising the suspicion that these mutations represent a late event in tumor progression. Finally, the retinoblastoma gene – a tumor suppressor gene frequently lost in human cancer (see the chapters on "Oncogenes and Tumor Suppressor Genes" and "Retinoblastoma") – has also been found to be altered in bladder cancer cell lines and in advanced tumors, although the meaning of these observations remains unclear [101].

Bartkova et al. [102] used a new monoclonal antibody to examine *p53* expression in a large series of patients with testicular cancer of various histologic types. Positive immunostaining, indicative of an altered gene product, was observed in 77% (36 out of 47) of seminomas and in 92% (24 of 26) of teratocarcinomas; in the whole series of 107 tumors, 84% showed a positive immunoreaction, while normal tissues were constantly negative.

Moreover, an altered gene expression was seen in a high proportion (59%) of the preinvasive tumors, suggesting that changes in the *p53* gene might be an early event in testicular germline tumorigenesis; these data seem to be at variance with those observed in other tumors [103, 104], in which *p53* changes are usually detected in the late stages of the disease. However, neither constitutional nor somatic *p53* mutations were detected in familial testicular cancer [105].

Genetic abnormalities in renal cell carcinoma are much more complex than initially believed, and it is now evident that multiple genetic defects are prerequisite for the full development of the malignant phenotype. The story began in 1979, when Cohen et al. [78] described a family with a striking aggregation of early onset and frequently multifocal renal carcinoma; karyotype analysis showed the presence of a balanced translocation between chromosomes 3 and 8 in peripheral blood leukocytes of five affected and five unaffected members of this family. Several years later, Pathak et al. [106] described another family with renal cancer aggregation and a 3;11 translocation in tumor cells. Subsequent studies showed that the specific breakpoint of the 3;8 reciprocal translocation was at p14.2;q24.1 [107]; moreover, restriction fragment length polymorphism analysis showed frequent loss of alleles at loci on the short arm of chromosome 3 also in patients with sporadic renal cell carcinoma [108–110]. Taken together, these observations might indicate the presence of a tumor suppressor gene, located on chromosome 3p, which is involved in the pathogenesis of renal carcinoma. Things became more complex when evidence was provided that besides 3p loss of heterozygosity was frequent also at various other chromosomal loci, such as 5q, 6q, 10q, 11q, 13q, and 17p, thus suggesting the involvement of several recessive oncogenes in renal tumorigenesis [111, 112]. In particular, allele losses were common at chromosome 5q21, a region in which various genes closely related to colonic cancer and adenomatosis coli have recently been mapped [113]. Since chromosome 3p alterations were not seen in all patients with renal tumors, it is also possible that alternative pathways exist for the development of these neoplasms which may or may not require the involvement of chromosome 3. Finally, unbalanced translocations between chromosomes 3p and 5q have also been reported [114, 115].

A further element favoring the view that chromosome 3 may play a role in the origin of renal cancer stems from the fact that in von Hippel-Lindau disease, in which patients are highly predisposed to neoplasms, loss of alleles on chromosome 3 has been reported [116], and the gene responsible for the disease has been mapped at 3p [117]. Thus, in summary, losses of genetic material from chromosome 3p seem to be of relevance for initiation of many sporadic and familial renal carcinomas, although it is well known that abnormalities at this region are also frequently seen in other human tumors (such as lung and cervix) [118–120]. Little is known of the progression of these tumors, but several chromosomal loci other than 3p might be involved [111–121]. Finally, it is likely that further human investigations and detailed genetic amalysis on a strain of rats genetically susceptible to renal carcinoma [122–123] will provide new insight into the pathogenesis of this insidious malignancy.

References

1. Zaridze DG, Boyle P (1987) Cancer of the prostate: epidemiology and etiology. Br J Urol 59:493–502
2. Gittes RF (1991) Carcinoma of the prostate. N Engl J Med 324:236–245
3. Ross RK, Bernstein L, Judd H et al. (1986) Serum testosterone levels in healthy young black and white men. JNCI 76:45–48
4. Silverberg E, Lebera JA (1989) Cancer Statistics 1989. CA 39:3–21
5. King H, Bailar JC III (1966) Epidemiology of urinary bladder cancer: a review of selected literature. J Chronic Dis 19:735–772
6. Wynder EL, Goldsmith R (1977) The epidemiology of bladder cancer: a second look. Cancer 40:1246–1268
7. Hueper WC, Wiley PH, Wolfe HD (1938) Experimental production of bladder tumors in dogs by administration of beta-naphthylamine. J Industr Hyg Toxicol 20:46–53
8. McCredie M, Stewart JH, Ford JM et al. (1983) Phenacetin-containing analgesics and cancer of the bladder or renal pelvis in women. Br J Urol 55:220–225
9. Raghavan D, Shipley WU, Garnick MB et al. (1990) Biology and management of bladder cancer. N Engl J Med 322:1129–1137
10. Zanetti R, Crosignani P (1992) Cancer in Italy: incidence data from cancer registries 1983–1987. Lega Italiana Lotta contro i Tumori, Torino
11. Devesa SS, Silverman DT, Young LY et al. (1987) Cancer incidence and mortality trends among whites in the United States. JNCI 79:701–770
12. Doll R, Peto R (1981) The causes of cancer. JNCI 66:1191–1308
13. Byrne J, Kessler LG, Devesa SS (1992) The prevalence of cancer among adults in USA. Cancer 69:2154–2159
14. Scott R, Mutchnik DL, Laskowski TZ et al. (1969) Carcinoma of the prostate in elderly men: incidence, growth characteristics and clinical significance. J Urol 101:602–607
15. Pienta KJ, Esper PS (1993) Risk factors for prostate cancer. Ann Intern Med 118:793–803
16. Stamey TA (1989) Prostate specific antigen in the diagnosis and treatment of adenocarcinoma of the prostate. Urol Monogr 10:50–64
17. Hudson MA, Bahanson RR, Catalona WJ (1989) Clinical use of prostate specific antigen in patients with prostate cancer. J Urol 142:1011–1017
18. Chodak GW (1989) Screening for prostate cancer: role of ultrasonography. Urol Clin North Am 16:657–661
19. Lange PH, Brawer MK (1989) Serum prostate-specific antigen: its use in diagnosis and management of prostate cancer. Urology 33[Suppl 6]:13–17
20. Stamey TA, Yang N, Hay AR et al. (1987) Prostate specific antigen as a serum marker for adenocarcinoma of the prostate. N Engl J Med 317:1916–1920
21. International Union against cancer (1982) TNM classification of malignant tumors, 3rd edn. Springer, Berlin Heidelberg New York
22. Lange PH, McIntire KR, Waldmann TA et al. (1976) Serum alpha-fetoprotein and human chorionic gonadotrophin in the diagnosis and management of non-seminomatous germ cell testicular cancer. N Engl J Med 295:1237–1240

23. Birch R, Williams S, Cone A et al. (1986) Prognostic factors for favorable outcome in disseminated germ cell tumors. J Clin Oncol 4:400–407
24. Hricak H (1988) Detection and staging of renal neoplasms. Radiology 166:643–649
25. Chisholm GD, Roy RR (1971) The systemic effect of malignant renal tumors. Br J Urol 43:687–693
26. National Institute of Health Consensus Conference (1987) The management of clinically localized prostate cancer. J Urol 138:1369–1375
27. Gleason DF (1977) The veterans administration cooperative urologic research group: histologic grading and clinical staging of prostatic carcinoma. In: Tannenbaumm M (ed) Urologic pathology: the prostate. Lea and Febiger, Philadelphia, pp 171–198
28. Paulson D, Piserchia PV, Gardner W (1980) Prediction of lymphatic spread in prostatic adenocarcinoma: uro-oncology research group study. J Urol 123:697–699
29. Oesterling JE, Brendler CB, Epstein JL et al. (1987) Correlation of clinical stage, serum prostatic acid phosphatase, and preoperative Gleason grade with final pathologic stage in 275 patients with clinically localized adenocarcinoma of the prostate. J Urol 138:92–98
30. Tinari N, Natoli C, Angelucci D et al. (1993) DNA and S-phase fraction analysis by flow cytometry in prostate cancer. Cancer 71:1289–1296
31. Walsh PC, Epstein JL, Lowe FC (1987) Potency following radical prostatectomy with wide unilateral excision of the neurovascular bundle. J Urol 138:823–827
32. de Voogt HJ, Smith PH, Pavone-Macaluso M et al. (1986) Cardiovascular side effects of ethylstilbestrol, cyproterone acetate, medroxyprogesterone acetate and estramustrine phosphate used for the treatment of advanced prostatic cancer. J Urol 135:303–307
33. Schally AV, Redding TW, Comaru-Schally AM (1983) Inhibition of prostate tumors by agonistic and antagonistic analogues of LH-RH. Prostate 4:545–552
34. Bretton PR, Herr HW, Kimmel M et al. (1989) Flow cytometry as a predictor of response and progression in patients with superficial bladder cancer treated with bacillus Calmette-Guerìn. J Urol 141:1332–1336
35. Slack NH, Prout GR Jr (1980) The heterogeneity of invasive bladder carcinoma and different response to treatment. J Urol 123:644–652
36. Torti FM, Lum BL (1983) The biology and treatment of superficial bladder cancer. J Clin Oncol 2:505–531
37. Wijkstrom H, Granberg-Ohman I, Tribukait B (1984) Chromosomal and DNA pattern in transitional cell bladder carcinoma. Cancer 53:1718–1723
38. Prout GR Jr, Lin CW, Benson R Jr et al. (1987) Photodynamic therapy with hematoporphyrin derivative in the treatment of superficial transition-cell carcinoma of the bladder. N Engl J Med 317:1251–1255
39. Kalish LA, Garnick MB, Richie JP (1987) Appropriate endpoints for superficial bladder cancer clinical trials. J Clin Oncol 5:2004–2008
40. Herr HW, Badalament RA, Amato DA et al. (1989) Superficial bladder cancer treated with bacillus Calmette-Guerìn. J Urol 141:22–29
41. Raghavan D, Wallace DMA, Sandeman T et al. (1989) First randomized trial of pre-emptive intravenous cisplatin for invasive transitional cell carcinoma of the bladder. Proc Am Soc Clin Oncol 8:133 (abstract)
42. Khanderan JD, Esson PJ, Dewys WD et al. (1985) Comparative activity and toxicity of DDP and a combination of doxorubicin, cyclophosphamide and DDP in disseminated transitional cell carcinoma of the urinary tract. J Clin Oncol 3:539–545

43. Hillcoat BL, Raghavan D, Matthews J et al. (1989) A randomized trial of cisplatin or cisplatin plus methotrexate in advanced cancer of the urothelial tract. J Clin Oncol 7:706–709
44. Vugrin D, Whitmore W, Cvitkovic E et al. (1981) Adjuvant chemotherapy with VAB-3 of stage II-B testicular cancer. Cancer 48:233–237
45. Williams SD, Birch R, Einhorn LH et al. (1987) Treatment of disseminated germ cell tumors with cisplatin, bleomycin, and either vinblastine or etoposide. N Engl J Med 316:1435–1440
46. Bredael JJ, Vugrin D, Whitmore WF et al. (1983) Selective experience with surgery and combination chemotherapy in the treatment of nonseminomatous testis tumors. J Urol 129:985–988
47. Williams SD, Stablein DM, Einhorn LH et al. (1987) Immediate adjuvant chemotherapy versus observation with treatment at relapse in pathological stage II testicular cancer. N Engl J Med 317:1433–1438
48. Skinner DG, Colvin RB, Vermillon CD et al. (1971) Diagnosis and management of renal cell carcinoma. Cancer 28:1165–1174
49. Waxman J, Thomas H (1990) Is the outlook changing for patients with renal cell carcinoma? Eur J Cancer 26:860–862
50. Lynch HT, Ens JA, Lynch JF et al. (1990) The Lynch syndrome II and urological malignancies. J Urol 143:24–28
51. Lynch HT, Richardson JD, Mohammad Amin MD et al. (1991) Variable gastrointestinal and urologic cancers in a Lynch syndrome II kindred. Dis Colon Rectum 34:891–895
52. Cannon-Albright L, Bishop TD, Skolnick M et al. (1982) Genetic epidemiology of prostate cancer in the Utah Mormon genealogy. Cancer Surv 1:47–69
53. Spitz MR, Currier RD, Fueger JJ et al. (1991) Familial pattern of prostate cancer. J Urol 146:1305–1307
54. Steinberg GD, Carter BS, Beaty Th et al. (1990) Family history of the risk of prostate cancer. Prostate 17:337–347
55. Carter BS, Carter HB, Isaacs JT (1990) Epidemiologic evidence regarding predisposing factors to prostate cancer. Prostate 16:187–197
56. Carter BS, Beaty TH, Steinberg GD et al. (1992) Mendelian inheritance of familial prostate cancer. Proc Natl Acad Sci USA 89:3367–3371
57. Fraumeni JF Jr, Thomas LB (1967) Malignant bladder tumors in a man and his three sons. JAMA 201:507–509
58. McCullough DL, Lamm DL, McLaughlin AP III et al. (1975) Familial transitional cell carcinoma of the bladder. J Urol 113:629–633
59. Lynch HT, Walzak MP, Fried R et al. (1979) Familial factors in bladder carcinoma. J Urol 122:458–461
60. Najem GR, Louria DB, Seebode JJ et al. (1982) Lifetime occupation, smoking, caffeine, saccharine, hair dyes and bladder carcinogenesis. Int J Epidemiol 11:212–217
61. Petrova-Bocharova T, Chernozemsky IN, Nikolov IG et al. (1977) Families with multiple cases of urinary system tumors. JNCI 59:1419–1421
62. Marchetto D, Li FP, Henson DE (1983) Familial carcinoma of ureters and other genitourinary organs. J Urol 130:772–773
63. Burland CE, Juzek RH (1966) Familial occurrence of carcinoma of the ureter. J Urol 96:697–700
64. Cartwright RA (1979) Genetic association with bladder cancer. Br Med J 2:798
65. Kantor AF, Hartge P, Hoover RN et al. (1985) Familial and environmental interactions in bladder cancer risk. Int J Cancer 35:703–706
66. Sellers TA, Kushi LH, Potter JD et al. (1992) Effect of family history, body-fat distribution, and reproductive factors on the risk of post-menopausal breast cancer. N Engl J Med 326:1323–1329

67. Dieckmann KP, Boeckmann W, Brosig W et al. (1986) Bilateral testicular germ cell tumors. Report of nine cases and review of the literature. Cancer 57:1254–1259
68. Dieckmann KP, Becker T, Jonas D et al. (1987) Inheritance of testicular cancer. Arguments based on a report of 3 cases and review of the literature. Oncology 44:367–373
69. Weissbach L, Widmann T (1986) Familial tumor of the testis. Eur Urol 12:104–109
70. Patel SR, Kvols LK, Richardson RL (1990) Familial testicular cancer: report of 6 cases and review of the literature. Mayo Clin Proc 65:585–591
71. Goss PE, Bulbul MA (1990) Familial testicular cancer in 5 members of a cancer-prone kindred. Cancer 66:2044–2049
72. Gedde Dahl T, Hannisdal E, Klepp OH et al. (1985) Testicular neoplasms occurring in 4 brothers: a search for a genetic predisposition. Cancer 55:2005–2011
73. Tollerud DJ, Blattner WA, Fraser MC et al. (1985) Familial testicular cancer and urogenital developmental anomalies. Cancer 55:1849–1856
74. Forman D, Oliver RTD, Brett AR et al. (1992) Familial testicular cancer: a report of the U.K. family register, estimation of risk and HLA class 1 sib-pair analysis. Br J Cancer 65:255–262
75. Hartley AL, Birch JM, Kelsey AM et al. (1989) Are germ cell tumors part of the Li-Fraumeni cancer family syndrome? Cancer Genet Cytogenet 42:221–226
76. Franksson C, Bergstrand A, Ljundhal I et al. (1972) Renal carcinoma occurring in 5 siblings. J Urol 108:58–61
77. Guirguis AB (1973) Renal-cell carcinoma: unusual occurrence in four members of one family. Urology 2:283–285
78. Cohen AJ, Li FP, Berg S et al. (1979) Hereditary renal-cell carcinoma associated with a chromosomal translocation. N Engl J Med 301:592–595
79. Arps S, Rodewald A, Schmalenberger B et al. (1993) Cytogenetic survey of 32 cancers of the prostate. Cancer Genet Cytogenet 66:93–99
80. Peehl DM (1993) Oncogenes in prostate cancer: an update. Cancer 71:1159–1164
81. Carter BS, Ewing CM, Ward WS et al. (1990) Allelic loss of chromosome 16q and 10q in human prostate cancer. Proc Natl Acad Sci USA 87:8751–8755
82. Isaacs WB, Carter BS, Ewing CM (1991) Wild-type p53 suppresses growth of human prostate cancer cells containing mutant p53 alleles. Cancer Res 51:4716–4720
83. Bookstein R, MacGrogan D, Hilsenbeck SG et al. (1993) p53 is mutated in a subset of advanced-stage prostate cancers. Cancer Res 53:3369–3373
84. Gao X, Honn KV, Grignon D et al. (1993) Frequent loss of expression and LOH of the putative tumor suppressor gene DCC in prostatic carcinoma. Cancer Res 53:2723–2727
85. Bova GS, Carter BS, Bussemakers MJG et al. (1993) Homozygous deletion and frequent allelic loss of chromosome 8p22 loci in human prostate cancer. Cancer Res 53:3869–3873
86. Gibas Z, Prout GR, Pontes JE et al. (1986) A possible specific chromosomal change in transitional cell carcinoma of the bladder. Cancer Genet Cytogenet 19:229–238
87. Smeets W, Pauwels R, Laarakkers L et al. (1987) Chromosomal analysis of bladder cancer. Cancer Genet Cytogenet 29:29–41
88. Babu VR, Lutz M, Miles BJ et al. (1987) Tumor behavior in transitional cell carcinoma of the bladder in relation to chromosomal markers and histopathology. Cancer Res 47:6800–6805

89. Fujita J, Srivastava SK, Kraus M et al. (1985) Frequency of molecular alterations affecting ras protooncogene in human urinary tract tumors. Proc Natl Acad Sci USA 82:3849–3853
90. Meyers FJ, Gumerlock PH, Kokoris SP et al. (1989) Human bladder and colon carcinomas contain activated ras p21. Cancer 63:2177–2181
91. Neal DE, Marsh C, Bennet MK (1985) Epidermal growth factor receptors in human bladder cancer. Lancet I:366–368
92. Berger MS, Greefielg G, Gullick WJ et al. (1987) Evaluation of epidermal growth factor receptors in human bladder tumours. Br J Cancer 56:533–537
93. Reddy EP, Reynolds RK, Santos E et al. (1982) A point mutation is responsible for the acquisition of transforming properties by the T24 human bladder carcinoma oncogene. Nature 300:149–152
94. Fearon ER, Feinberg AP, Hamilton SH et al. (1985) Loss of genes on the short arm of chromosome 11 in bladder cancer. Nature 318:377–380
95. Olumi AF, Tsay YC, Jones P et al. (1990) Allelic loss of chromosome 17p distinguishes high grade from low grade transitional cell carcinoma of the bladder. Cancer Res 50:7081–7083
96. Cairns P, Shaw ME, Knowles MA (1993) Initiation of bladder cancer may involve deletion of a tumour suppressor gene on chromosome 9. Oncogene 8:1083–1085
97. Miyao N, Tsai YC, Lerner SP et al. (1993) Role of chromosome 9 in human bladder cancer. Cancer Res 53:4066–4070
98. Sidranski D, von Eschenbach A, Tsay YC et al. (1991) Identification of p53 mutations in bladder cancers and urine samples. Science 252:706–709
99. Lipponen PK (1993) Overexpression of p53 in transitional bladder cancer and its prognostic value. Int J Cancer 53:365–370
100. Fujimoto K, Yamada Y, Okajima E et al. (1992) Frequent association of p53 gene mutation in invasive bladder cancer. Cancer Res 52:1393–1398
101. Logothetis CJ, Xu HJ, Ro JY et al. (1992) Altered expression of retinoblastoma protein and known prognostic variables in locally advanced bladder cancer. JNCI 84:1256–1261
102. Bàrtkovà J, Bàrtek J, Lukàs J et al. (1991) p53 protein alterations in human testicular cancer including pre-invasive intratubular germ-cell neoplasia. Int J Cancer 49:196–202
103. Baker SJ, Fearon AR, Nigro JM et al. (1989) Chromosome 17 deletions and p53 mutations in colorectal carcinomas. Science 244:217–221
104. Baker SJ, Preisinger AC, Jessup JM et al. (1990) p53 mutations occur in combination with 17p allelic deletions as late events in colorectal tumorigenesis. Cancer Res 50:7717–7722
105. Heimdal K, Lothe RA, Lystad S et al. (1993) No germline p53 mutations detected in familial and bilateral testicular cancer. Genes Chromos Cancer 6:92–97
106. Pathak S, Strong LC, Ferrell RE et al. (1982) Familial renal cell carcinoma with a 3; 11 chromosome translocation limited to tumor cells. Science 217:939–940
107. Wang N, Perkins KL (1984) Involvement of band 3p14 in t(3;8) hereditary renal carcinoma. Cancer Genet Cytogenet 11:479–481
108. Zbar B, Brauch H, Talmadge C et al. (1987) Loss of alleles of loci on the short arm of chromosome 3 in renal cell carcinoma. Nature 327:721–724
109. LaForgia S, Lasota J, Latif F et al. (1993) Detailed genetic and physical map of the 3p chromosome region surrounding the familial renal cell carcinoma chromosome translocation, t(3;8) (p14.2;q24.1). Cancer Res 53:3118–3124
110. Yamakawa K, Morita R, Takahashi E et al. (1991) A detailed deletion mapping of the short arm of chromosome 3 in sporadic renal cell carcinoma. Cancer Res 51:4707–4711

111. Morita R, Ishikawa J, Tsutsumi M et al. (1991) Allelotype of renal cell carcinoma. Cancer Res 51:820–823
112. Reiter RE, Anglard P, Liu S et al. (1993) Chromosome 17p deletions and p53 mutations in renal cell carcinoma. Cancer Res 53:3092–3097
113. Morita R, Saito S, Ishikawa J et al. (1991) Common regions of deletion on chromosomes 5q, 6q and 10q in renal cell carcinoma. Cancer Res 51:5817–5820
114. Kovacs G, Szucs S, DeRiese W et al. (1987) Specific chromosome aberration in human renal cell carcinoma. Cancer Res 40:171–178
115. Presti JC, Rao P, Chen Q et al. (1991) Histopathological, cytogenetic, and molecular characterization of renal cortical tumors. Cancer Res 51:1544–1552
116. Tory K, Brauch H, Lineham M et al. (1989) Specific genetic change in tumors associated with von Hippel-Lindau disease. JNCI 1097–1101
117. Latif F, Tory K, Gnarra J et al. (1993) Identification of the von Hippel-Lindau disease tumor suppressor gene. Science 270:1317–1320
118. Naylor SL, Johnson BE, Minna JD et al. (1987) Loss of heterozygosity of chromosome 3p markers in small-cell lung cancer. Nature 329:451–454
119. Yokota J, Tsukada Y, Nakajima et al. (1989) Loss of heterozygosity on the short arm of chromosome 3 in carcinoma of the uterine cervix. Cancer Res 49:3598–3601
120. Mori N, Yokota J, Oshimura M et al. (1989) Concordant deletions of chromosome 3p and loss of heterozygosity for chromosome 13 and 17 in small cell lung carcinoma. Cancer Res 49:5130–5135
121. Decker HJH, Wullich B, Whaley JM et al. (1992) Cytogenetic and molecular studies of a familial renal cell carcinoma. Cancer Genet Cytogenet 63:25–31
122. Walker C, Goldsworthy TL, Wolf DC et al. (1992) Predisposition to renal cell carcinoma due to alteration of a cancer susceptibility gene. Science 255:1693–1695
123. Funaki K, Evnritt J, Oshimura M et al. (1991) Hereditary renal cell carcinoma in the rat associated with nonrandom loss of chromosomes 5 and 6. Cancer Res 51:4415–4422

Cancer-Prone Hereditary Diseases Associated with Abnormalities of DNA Repair

It is possible that, in the human population, there are individuals with various degrees of defective DNA-repair system. That is, some persns may be slightly defective in one DNA-repair mechanism of another, and others, more severely defective. If this is the case, then affected individuals, after exposure to enviromental mutagens, may acquire more mutations than persons with efficient DNA-repair mechanisms; thus, affected individuals more easily accumulate genetic damage and develop cancer.

(T.C. Hsu 1986)

Introduction

In 1968, Cleaver [1] was able to establish a direct correlation between defective DNA repair and carcinogenesis. The author showed that normal skin fibroblasts could repair ultraviolet radiation-induced DNA damage by inserting new bases into DNA, while in fibroblasts from patients with xeroderma pigmentosum DNA repair occurred at a much reduced level, or it was completely absent. Since patients with xeroderma pigmentosum are particularly susceptible to skin cancer occurrence when exposed to sunlight, it was speculated that the inability to repair DNA in the skin cells as efficiently as normal individuals might be somehow related to cancer development. In the following years, besides xeroderma pigmentosum, other diseases were identified in which a particular predisposition to cancer could be associated with alterations in processing the damaged DNA. The most widely investigated of these clinical conditions include ataxia telangiectasia, Bloom's syndrome, Cockayne's syndrome, and Fanconi's anemia, all inherited diseases characterized by an autosomal recessive type of transmission.

Although all these syndromes or conditions are extremely rare, nonetheless they represent an interesting "alternative" model of carcinogenesis; in fact, while in most human malignancies the development of cancer has been associated with chromosomal alterations, oncogene activation or amplification, and/or inactivation of tumor suppressor genes, in diseases with DNA processing abnormalities the main defect seems to be a reduced capacity of cells to maintain the integrity of their DNA or, in other words, a defective "cellular adaptation" [2]. One of the main objectives of basic research for these diseases, therefore, should be the identification and characterization of the genes involved in DNA repair processes.

General Aspects

As already discussed in the chapter on "Biomarkers of Increased Susceptibility to Cancer," the human genome is continually subjected to structural alterations caused by a myriad of environmental factors with cancer-inducing activity. These include (a) ultraviolet and ionizing radiation, (b) foreign bodies, such as asbestos fibers, (c) chemical compounds (i.e., alkylating agents, nitrosamines, polycyclic hydrocarbons, and others), and (d) biological factors (i.e., free radicals). A crucial point is the site of these genomic lesions; in fact, DNA damage might lead to mutation and/or activation of protooncogenes, or to various abnormalities in tumor suppressor genes, which would mean a high risk of tumor development; alternatively, the damage might also occur in DNA sequences not strictly implicated in the process of cell replication and differentiation, with a consequent lesser risk of neoplasia [3, 4]. Considering the importance of DNA integrity for living organisms, it is rather obvious that cells possess a variety of enzymatic activities for repairing or tolerating DNA damage, thus allowing cellular survival. Several DNA repair systems have been described in humans and in various animal species [3]; in the "direct reversal" process, the altered sequence of DNA is simply returned to normality in situ, without any further modification of the nucleic acid. The "excision repair" is the most versatile system, and is effective against a large variety of DNA lesions, such as those induced by ultraviolet radiation or alkylating agents; the various steps of this process have been discussed in detail in the chapter on "Biomarkers of Increased Susceptibility to Cancer." A third more complex and still poorly understood system is called "postreplication repair" [3].

Direct measurement of DNA repair and, thus, evaluation of defects of this process is usually carried out with rather sophisticated techniques that may require the incorporation of radioactive nucleotides. However, in some of the syndromes characterized by alterations of the DNA repair processes (i.e., Bloom's syndrome, ataxia telangiectasia), chromosomal aberrations can be observed spontaneously, or can be induced with specific treatments; it follows that these diseases have also been designated as "chromosomal breakage syndromes" [4]. Thus, relatively simple cytogenetic analysis can provide – at least in some instances – an acceptable estimate of the defective DNA repair, since chromosomes may show DNA damage induced by various agents if there is no adequate repair. In other words, the number of chromosomal breaks can be considered a measure of the DNA repair capacity, in the sense that a high number of breaks will indicate a more marked impairment of the repair mechanisms. The method has been used by Hsu et al. [5], who cultured peripheral lymphocytes in the presence of bleomycin (a mutagen), and then counted the number of chromosomal breaks at metaphase.

Cancer-associated genetic diseases with defects in DNA repair, or with chromosome instability, have been considered "rare mistakes of nature" [3]. Their rarity, however, should not obscure the scientific relevance of these syndromes, which represent an interesting and original model of tumorigenesis. Three more aspects deserve some comment. First, diseases related to alterations of DNA repair are a further demonstration that cancer development often requires a complex and still incompletely understood interplay between environmental determinants (radiations, chemical compounds, other physical or biological factors) and constitutional alterations (in this case inborn errors of DNA metabolism) [3]. Second, some of these syndromes (i.e., ataxia telangiectasia, Fanconi's anemia) show evidence of immunologic defects together with an increased frequency of lymphoid tumors; this presumably indicates that the immune system is somehow vulnerable to failure to maintain DNA integrity. In this context, it is worth noting (a) that accelerating ageing is a feature of some of these rare diseases associated with DNA repair alterations, (b) that lymphocytes from aged individuals frequently show an impairment of DNA repair synthesis, and (c) that various immunologic changes and autoimmune manifestations usually accompany ageing [6, 7]. Finally, recent studies [8] indicate that a few genes are presumably involved in the pathogenesis of some of these diseases (especially xeroderma pigmentosum and Cockayne's syndrome); more specifically, preliminary observations seem to suggest that helicases and transcriptional regulators might be the products of genes implicated in DNA repair processes.

Xeroderma Pigmentosum

Xeroderma pigmentosum (XP) is a rare, autosomal recessive, multisystem disease in which the skin is the major target organ; XP occurs worldwide in all ethnic groups, and its frequency is in the order of one to ten patients per million. The main clinical manifestations are acute sensitivity to sunlight and damage to exposed areas of the skin surface. Symptoms start early in life with freckling, hypo- or hyperpigmentation, actinic keratosis, and multiple skin tumors [3, 6]. These include squamous and basal cell carcinomas, occurring virtually in all these patients at a very early age, and malignant melanomas [9]; severe ocular defects and neurologic abnormalities are also frequently observed in XP. The available evidence suggests that the disease develops owing to a striking interaction between an environmental agent (i.e., ultraviolet radiation) and a constitutional abnormality of DNA repair [1].

At a molecular level, it has been shown that fibroblasts or lymphocytes cultured from patients with XP have a partial or total defect in their ability to repair DNA damage induced by ultraviolet light or by some chemical carcinogens; it follows that XP cells are particularly sensitive to the lethal action of ultraviolet light [10]. Variants with normal excision repair of DNA have been described, thus suggesting that various DNA repair mechanisms may be defective in XP. Moreover, the disease shows a marked genetic complexity and heterogeneity, since at least nine complementation groups have been identified [11], mostly on the basis of biochemical features (i.e., degree of repair defect, kinetics of recovery after fusion with normal cells, association with Cockayne's syndrome, and other criteria).

Since XP patients have a constitutional abnormality of DNA repair processes, one should expect an increased frequency of internal malignancies in these individuals, owing to the constant exposure of certain organs (lung, gastroenteric mucosa, urothelial tract) to various chemical carcinogens capable of inducing the formation of DNA adducts. Moreover, besides the homozygote (i.e., the affected patient) an increased risk of cancer might also be expected for heterozygotes (i.e., many of the first-degree relatives). Rather surprisingly, non-skin tumors were reported only occasionally in XP patients, and systematic studies failed to show an excess mortality for internal neoplasms, either in XP patients or in their close relatives [12, 13], with the possible exception of brain tumors [14]. In addition, there are reports indicating that various immunologic abnormalities (impaired cell-mediated immunity, presence of antibodies to ultraviolet-irradiated DNA) may be frequent in XP patients [15].

Despite the extremely high risk of skin cancer in XP, surveillance and control programs can be planned and carried out. Thus, Lynch and coworkers [16] described two identical twins in whom a detailed program of protection from sunlight exposure was started virtually at birth. The program was based on the topical use of photoprotective substances (esters of parabenzoic acid); moreover, the twins usually wore long trousers, long-sleeved shirts, hats, and dark glasses; the home and the classroom had fluorescent lights with plastic covers, while physical activity (swimming, tennis) was usually performed at night, under artificial light. During an 8-year period of observation, the two patients appeared healthy, were able to attend high school regularly, and accepted without apparent problems their rather peculiar life style; even more importantly, no skin cancer developed in the two twins.

Several genes (*ERCC2*, *ERCC3*, *XPAC*) are under investigation for their possible role in the pathogenesis of XP and Cockayne's disease [8]. The available evidence suggests that these genes encode for enzymes involved in the regulation of transcription or translation, and for multiple helicases. However, the majority of these investigations have been carried out in animal models; consequently, there is still limited information on the precise role of these genes in the regulation of DNA repair in human cells. Finally, recent studies [17, 18] showed point mutations of the *ras* or *p53* genes in over 50% of skin tumors from XP patients, as opposed to 22%–40% observed in tumors from normal individuals; the findings, therefore, suggest a possible involvement of these genes in ultraviolet-induced tumorigenesis.

Ataxia Telangiectasia

Ataxia telangiectasia (AT) is an autosomal recessive disorder characterized by progressive loss of muscular coordination (ataxia), permanent dilation of the small blood vessels of the eyes and face, deficient humoral and cell-mediated immunity, and increased risk of cancer [3, 6]. Clinical manifestations of the disease usually occur in infancy and are progressive; death generally results from infections during the first 2 decades of life or from malignancies (more often lymphomas or lymphocytic leukemias) in the 3rd or 4th decade. Immunodeficiency may become manifest by recurrent lung infections leading to bronchiectasis; other immunologic defects include reduced levels of IgA, IgE, and low molecular weight IgM, lymphocytopenia, and skin hyporesponsiveness to several antigens. Various types of autoantibodies have been observed with increased frequency in AT, and insulin-dependent diabetes mellitus is rather frequent. These immunologic abnormalities have been related to an altered development of the thymus, which in these patients is usually hypoplastic and similar to the embryonic thymus.

One of the main features of AT patients is their extreme sensitivity to ionizing radiation. Thus, there are reports of subjects who underwent radiotherapy and subsequently died within a short time from the radiation [6]. Moreover, this in vivo hypersensitivity is also present at the cellular level; in fact, spontaneous as well as X-ray-induced cytogenetic abnormalities are a constant feature of cultured lymphocytes or fibroblasts from AT patients [19]; these include chromatid gaps, and nonrandom rearrangements, with a preferred breakpoint on 14q12 [3]. In contrast, the response of AT cells to ultraviolet radiation and to various chemical compounds (i.e., those mutagens to which XP cells appear hypersensitive) seems to be normal. It follows that AT cells have an alteration in a repair process acting on some type of DNA damage specifically induced by ionizing radiation, but not by many other mutagens. However, unlike the situation for XP, no clearly defined DNA repair deficiency has been identified in AT patients, although several lines of evidence favor the existence of a constitutional alteration in DNA metabolism as the most plausible explanation for the abnormal cellular and cytogenetic response to radiation in cultured AT cells [3, 20, 21]. Finally, AT cells are not sensitive only to ionizing radiation; recent studies showed an increased frequency of chromosomal aberrations in cultured AT cells also after treatment with chemotherapeutic agents, such as bleomycin, neocarzinostatin, and etoposide [21–23]. Moreover, AT cells showed a certain heterogeneity either in initial chromosome break sensitivity or in the rate of break repair (19); these observations are consistent with the existence of at least five complementation groups [3] which can be assessed using various end points, such as the frequency of cytogenetic alterations, DNA repair synthesis, and radioresistant DNA synthesis [20, 24, 25].

The presence of defective DNA repair mechanisms may account for the high frequency of malignancies in this syndrome. Patients with AT have an unusually high incidence of neoplasms; of these, lymphomas and lymphocytic leukemias are undoubtedly the most frequent, but several other solid tumors – including carcinoma of the gastrointestinal tract, liver, breast, ovary, and salivary glands – have also been reported [26–28]. Indeed, the risk of cancer among AT patients was estimated to be 61–184 times higher than that in the general population [28]. Moreover, Swift and coworkers [29–31] evaluated on various occasions the risk of cancer among close relatives of patients with AT, many of whom are heterozygotes for the deleterious gene. Their initial study included 27 families [29], while in the latest study [31] they were able to gather information on 161 families with AT, for a total of 1931 first-degree relatives prospectively evaluated together with 824 spouses. The observed rates of cancer of all sites were significantly higher in the group of relatives of AT patients than in their spouses; the estimated relative risks among heterozygotes were 3.8 in men and 3.5 in women, while the risk of breast cancer in the female sex was 5.1. Moreover, in the blood relative group, women with a diagnosis of breast neoplasms were more likely to have been exposed to ionizing radiation than controls without cancer, an observation which is consistent with the characteristic sensitivity to X-rays associated with the *AT* gene. The authors concluded that the *AT* gene, even in the heterozygous state, predisposes to an increased risk of neoplasia, and in particular breast tumors; these findings may have clinical relevance for the increased risk of cancer related to radiologic examinations in the 1.4% of the general population who are heterozygotes for the *AT* gene.

Finally, recent studies [32, 33] suggest that *p53* and other genes are presumably involved in a signal transduction pathway controlling cell cycle arrest after DNA damage; it is possibile that alterations in this pathway might play some role in tumor development associated with AT. More recent studies revealed elevated spontaneous rates of mitotic recombination in AT fibroblast lines, and suggested that this defect might contribute to the increased cancer risk reported in these patients [34].

Fanconi's Anemia

Fanconi's anemia (FA) is a rare genetic disease in which the main manifestations consist of progressive hypoplastic pancytopenia of the bone marrow, short stature, dark pigmentation of the skin, and skeletal abnormalities, especially of the radius and thumb [6, 35, 36]. The immune status of FA patients has not been well documented, though there is evidence of some defects of cell-mediated immunity and serum IgA depression. Cultured cells from patients with FA are particularly sensitive to the lethal and chromosome-damaging effects of chemical mutagens – such as mitomycin C, nitrogen mustards, and psoralens – which introduce various cross-links into cellular DNA [37]; these findings led to the hypothesis that cells in FA might have a defect in their ability to remove interstrand cross-links from the DNA. Individuals affected by FA have a slightly higher than expected incidence of malignancies, and in particular lymphocytic leukemia. Thus, although our limited knowledge of the metabolic defects of this disease does not favor speculation as to the possible association between cellular abnormalities and clinical manifestations, it is likely that the marked sensitivity to the damaging effect of chemical compounds, together with the increased risk of tumors, reflects the existence of an underlying disorder of DNA repair.

Cockayne's Syndrome

Cockayne's syndrome (CS) is an autosomal recessive disease sharing some biological and clinical features with XP. The syndrome is characterized by progressive neurologic disease and growth failure. Patients are usually normal at birth, but subsequently show severe impairment of physical and mental development, which results in cachectic dwarfism, microcephaly, and loss of adipose tissue and skeletal abnormalities [6, 38]. Premature ageing and severe photosensitivity are also part of the syndrome, whereas rather surprisingly these individuals are not abnormally susceptible to cancer of the skin or other organs [39]. A characteristic of CS is the extreme sensitivity of cultured cells to both ultraviolet radiation and some chemical mutagens, but without any obvious abnormality in DNA excision repair; however, CS cells seem unable to recover from blockage of nucleic acid synthesis induced by these treatments [6, 40], thus suggesting the possible existence of an incompletely characterized defect in DNA repair. CS is genetically complex, and at least three different complementation groups have been detected using the recovery of DNA synthesis in damaged cells as the screening procedure [41]. As already discussed, several genes have been characterized which might be implicated in the etiopathogenesis of both XP and CS [8].

Bloom's Syndrome

Sensitivity to sunlight, telangiectatic erythema, and stunted growth are the main clinical manifestations of Bloom's syndrome (BS). Patients with this disease show a defective cell-mediated immunity with increased susceptibility to infections. Photosensitivity is also a feature of BS, although cells from these individuals are not excessively sensitive to ultraviolet light and may show normal or even enhanced unscheduled DNA synthesis. Leukemia seems to occur with increased frequency in BS patients [42]. Spontaneous sister chromatid exchange and chromosome aberrations can be found virtually in all patients with BS, and clearly indicate that some undefined alteration of DNA repair should play some role in the clinical and biological manifestations of this syndrome. This contention is further reinforced by the recent observation of reduced levels of DNA ligase in BS cells [43]; in addition, subsequent studies suggested that the molecular alteration in BS might be a missense mutation in a specific region of the gene for DNA ligase I [44]. Finally, *p53* mutations are frequent in transformed cells from patients with BS [45].

References

1. Cleaver JE (1968) Defective repair replication of DNA in xeroderma pigmentosum. Nature 218:652–656
2. Tonini GP (1988) Molecular mechanisms involved in DNA repair, in gene rearrangement and gene amplification may be considered as an integrated system in maintaining cellular homeostasis and cell survival. Anticancer Res 8:881–884
3. Paterson MC, Gentner NE, Middlestadt et al. (1984) Cancer predisposition, carcinogen hypersensitivity, and aberrant DNA metabolism. J Cell Physiol [Suppl] 3:45–62
4. Hsu TC (1986) Genetic susceptibility to carcinogenesis. Cancer Bull 38:125–128
5. Hsu HT, Cherry LM, Samaan NA (1985) Differential mutagen susceptibility in cultured lymphocytes of normal individuals and cancer patients. Cancer Genet Cytogenet 17:307–313
6. Lehmann AR (1981) Cancer-associated human genetic diseases with defects in DNA repair. J Cancer Res Clin Oncol 100:117–124
7. Licastro F, Franceschi C, Chiricolo M et al. (1982) DNA repair after gamma radiation and superoxide dismutase activity in lymphocytes from subjects of far advanced age. Carcinogenesis 3:45–48
8. Friedberg EC (1992) Xeroderma pigmentosum, Cockayne's syndrome, helicases, and DNA repair: what's the relationship? Cell 71:887–889
9. Robbins JH, Kraemer KH, Lutzner MA et al. (1974) Xeroderma pigmentosum. An inherited disease with sun sensitivity, multiple cutaneous neoplasms, and abnormal DNA repair. Ann Intern Med 80:221–248
10. Cleaver JE, Bootsma D (1975) Xeroderma pigmentosum: biochemical and genetic characteristics. Annu Rev Genet 9:19–38
11. Bohr VA, Phillips DH, Hanawalt PC (1987) Heterogeneous DNA damage and repair in the mammalian genoma. Cancer Res 47:6426–6436
12. Cairns J (1981) The origin of human cancer. Nature 289:353–357
13. Pippard EC, Hall AJ, Barker DJP et al. (1988) Cancer in homozygotes and heterozygotes of ataxia-telangiectasia and xeroderma pigmentosum in Britain. Cancer Res 48:2929–2932
14. Kraemer KH, Lee MM, Scotto J (1984) DNA repair protects against cutaneous and internal neoplasms: evidence from XP. Carcinogenesis 5:511–541
15. Dupuy JM, Lafforet D (1974) A defect of cellular immunity on xeroderma pigmentosum. Clin Immunol Immunopathol 3:52–58

16. Lynch HT, Lynch J, Lynch P (1977) Management and control of familial cancer. In: Mulvihill JJ, Miller RW, Fraumeni JF (eds) Genetics of human cancer. Raven, New York, pp 235–256
17. Daya-Grosjean L, Robert C, Drougart C et al. (1993) High mutation frequency in ras genes of skin tumors isolated from DNA repair deficient XP patients. Cancer Res 53:1625–1629
18. Sato M, Nishigori C, Zghal M et al. (1993) Ultraviolet-specific mutations in p53 gene in skin tumors in XP patients. Cancer Res 53:2944–2946
19. Taylor AMR (1982) Cytogenetics of ataxia-telangiectasia. In: Bridges BA, Harnden DG (eds) AT – a cellular and molecular link between cancer, neuropathology and immune deficiency. Wiley, Chichester, pp 53–81
20. Murname JP, Painter RB (1982) Complementation of the defects in DNA synthesis in irradiated and unirradiated AT cells. Proc Natl Acad Sci USA 79:1960–1963
21. Hittelman WN, Sen P (1988) Heterogeneity in chromosome damage and repair rates after bleomycin in AT cells. Cancer Res 48:276–279
22. Cohen MM, Simpson SJ (1983) Increased clastogenicity and decreased inhibition of DNA synthesis by neocarzinostatin and tallyomycin in AT lymphoid cells. Mutat Res 112:119–128
23. Henner WD, Blazka ME (1986) Hypersensitivity of cultured AT cells to etoposide. JNCI 76:1007–1011
24. Inoue T, Yokoiyama A, Kada T (1981) DNA repair enzyme deficiency and in vitro complementation of the enzyme activity in cell-free extracts from AT fibroblasts. Biochim Biophys Acta 655:49–53
25. Inoue T, Aikawa K, Tezuka H et al. (1986) Effect of DNA-damaging agents on isolated spleen and lung fibroblasts from the mouse mutant "wasted", a putative animal model for AT. Cancer Res 46:3979–3982
26. Narita T, Takagi K (1984) AT with dysgerminoma of right ovary, papillary carcinoma of the thyroid, and adenocarcinoma of pancreas. Cancer 54:1113–1116
27. Lambert WC, Kolber LR, Gorelli LA et al. (1982) Epidermoid carcinoma of the oral cavity following diagnostic roentgenographic examination in a patient with AT. Clin Prev Dent 4:3–8
28. Morrell D, Cromartie E, Swift M (1986) Mortality and cancer incidence in 263 patients with AT. JNCI 77:89–92
29. Swift M, Sholman L, Perry M et al. (1976) Malignant neoplasms in the families of patients with AT. Cancer Res 36:209–215
30. Swift M, Reitnauer PJ, Morrell D et al. (1987) Breast and other cancers in families with AT. N Engl J Med 316:1289–1294
31. Swift M, Morrell D, Massey RB et al. (1991) Incidence of cancer in 161 families affected by AT. N Engl J Med 325:1831–1836
32. Kastan MB, Onyekwere O, Sidransky D et al. (1991) Participation of p53 protein in the cellular response to DNA damage. Cancer Res 51:6304–6311
33. Kastan MB, Zhan Q, El-Deiry WS et al. (1992) A mammalian cell cycle checkpoint pathway utilizing p53 and GADD45 is defective in AT. Cell 71:587–597
34. Meyn MS (1993) High spontaneous intrachromosomal recombination rates in ataxia-teleangiectasia. Science 260:1327–1330
35. Beard MEJ (1976) Fanconi anemia. Ciba Found Symp 37:103–114
36. Swift M (1971) Fanconi's anemia in the genetics of neoplasia. Nature 230:370–373
37. Sasaki MS (1978) Fanconi's anemia. A condition possibly associated with a defective DNA repair. In: Hanawalt PC, Friedberg EC, Fox CF (eds) DNA repair mechanisms. Academic, New York, pp 675–684

38. Nance MA, Berry SA (1992) Cockayne syndrome: review of 140 cases. Am J Med Genet 42:68–84
39. Guzetta F (1972) Cockayne-Neill-Dingwall syndrome. In: Vinken PJ, Bruyn GW (eds) Handbook of clinical neurology, vol 13. North Holland, Amsterdam, pp 431–440
40. Wade MH, Chu EHY (1979) Effects of DNA damaging agents on cultured fibroblasts derived from patients with Cockayne syndrome. Mutat Res 59:49–60
41. Hoeijmakers JHJ, Bootsma D (1990) Molecular genetics of eukaryotic excision repair. Cancer Cell 2:311–320
42. German J (1977) Boom's syndrome IV. Sister-chromatid exchange in lymphocytes. Am J Hum Genet 29:248–255
43. Lindahl T (1987) Regulation and deficiencies in DNA repair. Br J Cancer 56:91–95
44. Willis AE, Lindahl T (1987) DNA ligase I deficiency in Bloom's syndrome. Nature 325:355–357
45. Shiraishi Y (1993) p53 mutation in fresh lymphocytes, B-lymphoblastoid cell lines and their trnsformed cell lines originating from Bloom syndrome patients. Cancer Genet Cytogenet 58:70–73

Familial Tumors of Other Organs

It is imperative that physicians and surgeons have a more profound knowledge of the growth pattern and mode of spreading of salivary gland tumors. Although it is a rare type of carcinoma, the salivary gland undifferentiated carcinoma gives an excellent opportunity for further studies because of its unique ethnic and geographic distribution.

(Y. Merrick et al. 1986)

Introduction

In the previous chapters the main elements in favor of the genetic basis of the most common malignancies have been discussed; moreover, emphasis has been given to the possible interaction between genetic and environmental factors in the pathogenesis of many tumors, as in the case of esophageal, gastric, or mammary carcinogenesis. In addition, rare neoplasms or conditions (retinoblastoma, Wilms' tumor, Li-Fraumeni syndrome, and others) have also been discussed, especially because they provide interesting models or clues towards a more complete understanding of the molecular basis of cancer genetics.

This final chapter will briefly summarize the evidence of "familiality" in other tumors not yet considered. In some cases the evidence is limited to a few familial reports, but it is likely that the increased alertness of many physicians towards these problems will, in future years, increase the number of reports on the familial aggregation of neoplasms in disorders for which a possible genetic basis was unsuspected or escaped detection. It is beyond our scope to analyze all the occasional or anecdotal reports of cancer aggregation which have appeared in the literature; instead, we have focused our attention on four cancer types – nonmelanoma skin cancer, nasopharyngeal carcinoma, salivary gland tumors, and pleural mesothelioma – for which there is sufficient evidence to hypothesize a strict interrelationship between the environmental and genetic factors in tumor development.

"Familiality" in Nonmelanoma Skin Cancer

Although rarely invasive, nonmelanoma skin cancer is the most common neoplasm, and is consequently a major health problem in many countries. The situation is particularly alarming in Australia, which shows the highest incidence rates in the world; in this country a gradient has been observed from the more temperate areas (in the south) to the subtropical northern regions, where rates as high as 1500 new cases/100 000 per year have been recorded [1]. These figures apply only to the white population, and can be explained by the fact that the ultraviolet component of sunlight represents the most important environmental factor associated with the development of skin cancer in general [2, 3]. Thus, we can hypothesize that individuals who lived for many generations in north European countries, where sun exposure is relatively low, acquired a substantial risk of the disease after they left their country of origin and moved to other regions of the world, where they were exposed to a much stronger sunlight. The fact that white individuals with light eye color and fair complexion are at even higher risk lends further support to this contention.

The role of hereditary factors in nonmelanoma skin cancer is still undefined, although it is generally acknowledged that the genetic background does not represent a major component of the disease as in the case of melanoma. Despite this, there are reports in the literature indicating that more than one member of a family can be affected by this cancer type [4, 5]. Most recently, Czarnecki et al. [6] reported their experience on the detection and occurrence of familial nonmelanoma skin cancer in the state of Victoria, Australia. The investigation included 1108 patients with either basal cell or squamous cell carcinomas diagnosed during a 18-month period; of these, 12 families were found in which two or more members had nonmelanoma skin cancer. In all but one family at least two generations were affected, and in nine families multiple skin cancers were detected. Although both sexes were affected, men were slightly more frequent than women (26 versus 17). The frequency of nonmelanoma skin cancer in these 12 families was 18 times higher than that expected in the general population; moreover, among relatively young individuals (age range, 15–39 years) the occurrence of skin cancer was several times higher than the expected prevalence. Finally, the risk of multiple cancer was also markedly increased among affected members of these families.

According to these data, therefore, it seems that these highly selected families are characterized by all the clinical elements which are usually seen in the most common types of hereditary cancers; more specifically, (a) aggregation of tumors, with apparent vertical transmission; (b) early age of onset of many cases; and (c) high frequency of multiple tumors. The authors concluded that although the large majority of nonmelanoma skin cancers are sporadic, in a subset of cases there is evidence suggesting that heritable factors might play a definite role, a situation which is analogous not only to melanoma but also to many other common neoplasms. Moreover, the susceptibility to the development of skin cancer seems to be inherited through an autosomal dominant type of transmission, though exposure to ultraviolet light is probably necessary for the full manifestation of the malignant phenotype.

Finally, two recent studies further emphasize the possible interaction between exposure to the ultraviolet portion of the solar spectrum and genetic changes in the pathogenesis of basal cell and squamous cell carcinoma [7, 8]. Thus, DNA from 14 basal cell cancers was analyzed for the presence of *p53* mutations; these could be detected in 50% of the samples and were mostly G:C – A:T transitions at codon 248 or 273. Interestingly, the observed mutations were similar to the alterations of *p53* induced by ultraviolet radiation in studies of experimental mutagenesis in human cells [7, 9]. Moreover, *p53* mutations within the region of exons 5–8 were found in the large majority (14 out of 15) of squamous cell carcinomas of the oral cavity, thus suggesting that alterations of this tumor suppressor gene are presumably implicated in the pathogenesis of other types of squamous cell neoplasm [8].

Familial Clusters of Salivary Gland Tumors and of Nasopharyngeal Carcinoma

Nasopharyngeal carcinoma (NPC) and salivary gland tumors (SGT) are two rare neoplasms which share some biological aspects. Thus, both tumors are relatively rare in Western populations (around 1 case/100 000 inhabitants per year, for both tumors) [10–13], but occur at an increased frequency in some particular populations, such as the Eskimos and Cantonese Chinese [13–17]. Moreover, various studies suggested an association between the Epstein-Barr virus (the causative agent of infectious mononucleosis) and both NPC and SGT [18–21]; thus, almost 100% of Eskimo children are infected with the Epstein-Barr virus by the age of 3 years, as opposed to 20%–60% of Danish children of the same age [22]; similarly, a high frequency and elevated levels of antibodies to this virus have been reported in patients with NPC [20, 21], especially in those with less differentiated tumors [23]. It has been suggested that excessive exposure to Epstein-Barr virus, together with the natural presence of this infectious agent in the larynx and salivary glands, might induce with time (and possibly with other exogenous factors, or in the presence of a genetic background) the development of the malignant phenotype [24]. Finally, the histologic features of SGT and NPC are often very similar.

Besides the histopathologic and epidemiologic characteristics, familial aspects are also of interest in both SGT and NPC. Thus, Newman et al. [25] reported the occurrence of SGT in two siblings from Bolivia who were affected by submandibular cancer (a moderately differentiated and a mucoepidermoid carcinoma) at a very early age of onset (33 and 32 years, respectively). Similarly, aggregates of SGT were also described in Eskimo families [11, 24, 26]; in one of these, SGT were present in three sisters who developed cancer at the age of 31, 34, and 50 years. Rather interestingly, two other malignancies developed in this sibship, and one of these was a nasopharyngeal carcinoma; moreover, the family history showed that the maternal grandfather had a mass in the neck, which was of a probable malignant nature. In another family two sisters developed SGT at the age of 37 and 44 years, respectively.

The aggregation of more than two cases of NPC among close relatives was reported by several authors in various races and populations. Thus, the occurrence of NPC in two or more siblings has been described by Stinson [27], Bell et al. [28], and Fisher et al. [29], while Poletti et al. [30] reported the simultaneous development of this type of tumor in a mother and her son, and Nevo et al. showed the appearance of NPC in twins [31]. In addition, familial aggregates of NPC have been observed in several countries, including Canada [32], Italy [30], Alaska [33], and Bermuda [34]. More recently, Coffin et al. [35] reported a remarkable American family of Scandinavian origin in which NPC developed in five individuals of three different generations; moreover, six other family members exhibited a broad spectrum of malignancies, including melanoma, lymphoma, cancer of the tongue, and colorectal and breast carcinoma. Segregation analysis showed that the particular susceptibility to cancer observed in this family was inherited through an autosomal dominant type of genetic transmission; moreover, the mean age of onset of NPC was 50 years (range 40–62 years), which is appreciably lower than the peak age of incidence for this tumor in the general population. Finally, numerical and structural abnormalities involving group C chromosomes and a certain association with a specific haplotype were also observed in affected members, whereas various tests did not show significantly increased levels of antibodies to the Epstein-Barr virus. The authors concluded by emphasizing the role of autosomal codominant inheritance in this family; however, the data clearly indicated that other (environmental) factors could influence tumor development, thus lending further support to the existence of a close interaction between environment and genes in the pathogenesis of this uncommon neoplasm. Another interesting cluster of NPC was recently described by Levine et al. [36]; in this family, the disease developed in three siblings at the ages of 42, 46, and 53 years, respectively, and the neoplastic spectrum also included melanoma (the father of the three siblings) and basal cell carcinoma (the proband). Interestingly, an X-linked genetic disease (hemophilia) was also present in this family. Finally, evidence of an interaction between genetic and exogenous factors in the origin of NPC has also been documented in some provinces of China (Canton) with incidence rates of NPC much higher than those seen in Western populations [17, 37].

Familial Mesothelioma

Mesothelioma of the pleura and peritoneum, with its strong and largely documented association with asbestos exposure, provides a final example of the way in which an exogenous agent and an underlying genetic predisposition may both contribute to the development of neoplasia.

Clinical and Familial Aspects

Several lines of evidence showed a close association between asbestos exposure and cancer of different organs, such as lung, larynx, kidney, but especially mesothelioma of the pleura and peritoneum [38, 39]. The commercial production of asbestos started at the end of the last century and since then this mineral has been extremely useful in many fields (i.e., pipe insulation, protective clothes, ship building, and others), playing a relevant role in the industrial revolution of this century. Asbestos workers are directly exposed to the carcinogenic effect of this mineral, and in many cases confirmation of this exposure can be obtained by the observation of asbestos fibers in lung tissue, or by assessing the lung mineral fiber content with more sophisticated techniques [40]. However, asbestos can be much more insidious, and it has been documented that household contact (for example, washing the dusty clothes of workers) over the course of many years may lead to a substantial exposure to the mineral, with a consequent increased risk of mesothelioma and other tumors [41, 42].

Familial aggregates of mesothelioma have frequently been reported; thus, Krousel et al. [43] and Munoz et al. [44] described kindreds with mesothelioma in three family members, while Li et al. [45] gave a detailed description of a family with early onset mesothelioma in a mother and a daughter whose husband (or father) had been exposed to asbestos (he was a pipe insulator) for more than 20 years, so that indirect exposure from the husband's clothes was considered highly probable. Malignant mesothelioma was also reported by Risbert et al. [46] in a father and four siblings, all in the age range 48–61 years. Similarly, De Giovanni et al. [47] described a small family in which this cancer type occurred in a mother and a daughter (age 66 and 32 years, respectively), while three other first-degree relatives died of "presumable lung carcinoma"; again, a strong and prolonged exposure to asbestos was suspected in some members of this family. The occurrence of malignant pleural mesothelioma in two brothers (aged 78 and 54 years, after a prolonged exposure to asbestos) was described by Lynch and collaborators [48, 49]; interestingly, two other siblings of the same sibship developed tumors, though apparently unrelated to asbestos (prostate and skin cancer in a brother, carcinoma of the cervix in a sister). Finally, Dawson et al. [40], recently updated their original report of three families [39], and gave additional information on four more kindreds with pleural or peritoneal mesothelioma in various family members. Again, occupational exposure to asbestos was not only suspected by the clinical history, but also documented with transmission electron microscopy and energy-dispersive X-ray analysis in four cases. The onset of the disease was below the age of 50 years in 7 out of 17 individuals, with an average age of diagnosis of 54 years, which is appreciably lower than that reported in nonfamilial mesothelioma; in contrast, histologic features seem to be similar to those usually observed in sporadic cases.

In summary, owing to the excessive exposure to asbestos in recent years and the very long latency period between this exposure and clinical manifestation of the disease, it is likely that morbidity and mortality for mesothelioma and other neoplasms related to asbestos will remain clinically relevant for many years [49]. On the other hand, the available evidence suggests that familial predisposition might play a role in the development of these tumors among family members of exposed individuals; thus, although the chances of early diagnosis and successful management of mesothelioma are rather low, close surveillance of individuals at risk in families with two or more affected patients seems justifiable.

Genetic Alterations

Various cytogenetic abnormalities have been described in human mesothelioma, the most frequent being deletions of 3p [50], structural or numerical abnormalities of chromosome 1 and 22 [51], and losses on the short arm of chromosome 17 [52]. Restriction fragment length polymorphism analysis confirmed loss of heterozygosity at specific loci on chromosome 17 and 22, and disclosed alterations of chromosome 7 which were not detected by cytogenetic investigations [53–55]. Of particular interest was the loss of heterozygosity on 17p13, where the *p53* gene has been localized; indeed, sequence analysis of *p53* from mesothelioma cell lines showed point mutations at codons 175 and 245, both in the evolutionary conserved region of the gene [53]. The strict concordance between karyotype changes (deletion of 17p), restriction fragment length polymorphism analysis (loss of heterozygosity at 17p), and sequencing analysis (point mutations, with consequent amino acid substitution at positions 175 and 245) led the authors to speculate that alterations of *p53* could be pathogenetically relevant in malignant mesothelioma, and that asbestos might exert its deleterious effect through the inactivation of a tumor suppressor gene [53]. More recent studies, however, failed to show *p53* mutations in the large majority of cell lines established from human mesotheliomas [56]; similarly, no mutation of K-*ras* gene could be detected, thus suggesting that alterations of these two genes frequently involved in human neoplasia do not seem to represent a critical step in the development of human mesothelioma [56].

References

1. Kricker A, English DR, Randell PL et al. (1990) Skin cancer in Geraldton, West Australia. Med J Aus 152:399–407
2. Strickland PT, Vitassa BC, West SK (1989) Quantitative carcinogenesis in man: solar ultraviolet-B dose-dependence of skin cancer in Maryland watermen. JNCI 81:1910–1913
3. Kaldor J, Shugg D, Young B et al. (1993) Non-melanoma skin cancer: ten years of cancer-registry based surveillance. Int J Cancer 53:886–891
4. Hall AF (1946) Relationship of sunlight, complexion and heredity to skin carcinogenesis. Arch Dermatol 48:589–610
5. Elliott JA, Welton DG (1946) Epithelioma. Arch Dermatol Syphilol 53:307–329
6. Czarnecki D, Zalcberg J, Meehan C et al. (1992) Familial occurrence of multiple non-melanoma skin cancer. Cancer Genet Cytogenet 61:1–5
7. Rady P, Scinicariello F, Wagner RF et al. (1992) p53 mutations in basal cell carcinomas. Cancer Res 52:3804–3806
8. Sakai E, Tsuchida N (1992) Most human squamous cell carcinomas in the oral cavity contain mutated p53 tumor suppressor gene. Oncogene 7:927–933
9. Bredberg A, Kraemer KH, Seidmen MM (1986) Restricted ultraviolet mutational spectrum in a shuttle vector propagated in xeroderma pigmentosum cells. Proc Natl Acad Sci USA 83:8273–8277
10. Wallace AC, McDougall JT, Hildes JA et al. (1963) Salivary gland tumors in Canadian Eskimos. Cancer 16:1338–1353
11. Nielsen NH, Mikkelsen F, Hansen JPH (1978) Incidence of salivary gland neoplasms in Greenland with special reference to an anaplastic carcinoma. Acta Pathol Microbiol Scand [A] 86:185–193
12. Fedder M, Gonzales RF (1985) Nasopharyngeal carcinoma: brief review. Am J Med 79:365–369
13. Levine PH, Connelly RR (1985) Epidemiology of nasopharyngeal cancer. In: Wittes RE (ed) Head and neck cancer. Wiley, Sussex, pp 13–34
14. Lanier AP, Bender TR, Blot WJ et al. (1976) Cancer incidence in Alaskan natives. Int J Cancer 18:409–412
15. Nielsen NH, Mikkelsen F, Hansen JPH (1977) Nasopharyngeal cancer in Greenland: the incidence in an arctic Eskimo population. Acta Pathol Microbiol Scand [A] 85:850–858
16. Ho JHC (1972) Nasopharyngeal carcinoma. In: Klein G, Weinhouse S, Haddow A (eds) Advances in cancer research. Academic, New York, pp 57–92
17. Chan SH, Day NE, Kunaratnam N et al. (1983) HLA and nasopharyngeal carcinoma in Chinese. Int J Cancer 32:171–176
18. Lanier AP, Bender TR, Talbot M et al. (1980) Nasopharyngeal carcinoma in Alaskan Eskimos, Indian and Aleuts. Cancer 46:2100–2106
19. Smith TF (1989) Nasopharyngeal carcinoma due to Epstein-Barr Virus: serologic tests. Mayo Clin Proc 60:205–206
20. Neel HB, Pearson GR, Taylor WF (1984) Antibodies to Epstein-Barr virus in patients with nasopharyngeal carcinoma and in comparison groups. Ann Otol Rhinol Laryngol 93:477–482
21. Sam CK, Brooks LA, Niedobitek G et al. (1993) Analysis of Epstein-Barr virus infection in nasopharyngeal biopsies from a group at high risk of nasopharyngeal carcinoma. Int J Cancer 53:957–962
22. Ebbesen P, Melbye M, Levine PH et al. (1983) Danish children in Greenland have high Epstein-Barr virus titer. Infect Immunol 41:418–419
23. Easton JM, Levine PH, Hyams VJ (1980) Nasopharyngeal carcinoma in the USA: a pathologic study of 177 U.S. and 30 foreign cases. Arch Otolaryngol 106:88–91

24. Merrick Y, Albeck H, Nielsen NH et al. (1986) Familial clustering of salivary gland carcinoma in Greenland. Cancer 57:2097–2102
25. Newman AN, Calcaterra TC, Bhuta S (1981) Familial carcinoma of the submandibular gland. Arch Otolaryngol 107:169–171
26. Albeck H, Bentzen J, Ockelmann HH et al. (1993) Familial clusters of nasopharyngeal carcinoma and salivary gland carcinomas in Greenland natives. Cancer 72:196–200
27. Stinson W (1940) Epidermoid carcinoma of the nasopharynx occurring in two young brothers. Ann Otol Rhinol Laryngol 49:536–539
28. Bell RB, Maguda TA (1970) Nasopharyngeal carcinoma in Caucasian siblings: report of two cases. J Tenn Med Assoc 63:753–754
29. Fischer RA, Wharam MD, Kashima HK (1979) Nasopharyngeal carcinoma in siblings. Ear Nose Throat J 58:72–77
30. Poletti T, Capaldi E (1965) Neoplasia maligna del rinofaringe ad insorgenza clinica contemporanea in madre e figlio. Cancro 18:132–139
31. Nevo S, Meyer W, Altman M (1971) Carcinoma of nasopharynx in twins. Cancer 28:807–809
32. Joncas JH, Rioux E, Wastiaux JP et al. (1976) Nasopharyngeal carcinoma and Burkitt's lymphoma in a Canadian family. Can Med Assoc J 115:858–860
33. Lanier AP, Bender TR, Tschopp CF et al. (1979) Nasopharyngeal carcinoma in an Alaskan Eskimo family: report of 3 cases. JNCI 62:1121–1124
34. Brown TH, Heath CW, Land RM et al. (1976) Nasopharyngeal cancer in Bermuda. Cancer 37:1464–1468
35. Coffin CM, Rich SS, Dehner LP (1992) Familial aggregation of nasopharyngeal carcinoma and other malignancies. Cancer 68:1323–1328
36. Levine PH, Pocinki AG, Madigan P et al. (1992) Familial nasopharyngeal carcinoma in patients who are not Chinese. Cancer 70:1024–1029
37. Yu MC, Ho JHC, Ross RK et al. (1981) Nasopharyngeal carcinoma in Chinese-salted fish or inhaled smoke. Prev Med 10:15–24
38. Seilikoff IJ, Churg J, Hammond EC (1964) Asbestos exposure and neoplasis. JAMA 22:188–195
39. Browne K (1983) Asbestos related mesothelioma: epidemiological evidence for asbestos as a promoter. Arch Environ Health 38:261–266
40. Dawson A, Gibbs A, Browne K et al. (1992) Familial mesothelioma. Cancer 70:1183–1187
41. Ferguson GC, Watson H (1984) Mesothelioma due to domestic exposure to asbestos. BMJ 288:1654
42. Lillington GA, Jamplis RW, Differding JR (1974) Conjugal malignant mesothelioma. N Engl J Med 291:583–584
43. Krousel T, Garcas N, Rothschild H (1986) Familial clustering of mesothelioma. Am J Prev Med 2:186–188
44. Munoz L, Guzman J, Ponce de Leon S et al. (1988) Familial malignant pleural mesothelioma. Rev Invest Clin 40:413–417
45. Li FP, Dreyfus MG, Antman KH (1989) Asbestos contaminated nappies and familial mesothelioma. Lancet 1:909–910
46. Risberg B, Nickels J, Wagermark J (1980) Familial clustering of malignant mesothelioma. Cancer 45:2422–2427
47. Degiovanni D, Botta M, Castagneto B et al. (1989) Un cluster di tumori delle vie respiratorie nella famiglia di un dirigente di un'industria del cemento-amianto. Acta Oncol 10(4):299–301
48. Lynch HT, Katz D, Markvicka SE (1985) Familial mesothelioma: review and family study. Cancer Genet Cytogenet 15:25–35
49. Lynch HT, Lynch JF (1989) Familial mesothelioma. In: Lynch HT, Hirayama T (eds) Genetic epidemiology of cancer. CRC Press, Boca Raton, pp 333–342

50. Gibas Z, Li FP, Antman KH et al. (1986) Chromosome changes in malignant mesothelioma. Cancer Genet Cytogenet 20:191–201
51. Flejter WL, Li FP, Antman KH et al. (1989) Recurring loss involving chromosomes 1, 3 and 22 in malignant mesothelioma. Genes Chromosomes Cancer 1:148–154
52. Popescu NC, Chainian AP, DiPaolo JA (1988) Nonrandom chromosome alterations in human malignant mesothelioma. Cancer Res 48:142–147
53. Cote RJ, Jhanwar SC, Novick S et al. (1991) Genetic alterations of the p53 gene are a feature of malignant mesothelioma. Cancer Res 51:5410–5416
54. Tiainen M, Kere J, Tammilehto L et al. (1992) Abnormalities of chromosomes 7 and 22 in human malignant pleural mesothelioma. Genes Chromos Cancer 4:176–182
55. Taguchi T, Jhanwar SC, Siegfried JM et al. (1993) Recurrent deletions of specific chromosomal sites in 1p, 3p, 6q, and 9p in human malignant mesothelioma. Cancer Res 53:4349–4355
56. Metcalf RA, Welsh JA, Bennet WP et al. (1992) p53 and K-ras mutations in human mesothelioma cell lines. Cancer Res 52:2610–2615

Subject Index

Springer-Verlag and the Environment

We at Springer-Verlag firmly believe that an international science publisher has a special obligation to the environment, and our corporate policies consistently reflect this conviction.

We also expect our business partners – paper mills, printers, packaging manufacturers, etc. – to commit themselves to using environmentally friendly materials and production processes.

The paper in this book is made from low- or no-chlorine pulp and is acid free, in conformance with international standards for paper permanency.

MIX
Papier aus verantwortungsvollen Quellen
Paper from responsible sources
FSC® C105338

If you have any concerns about our products,
you can contact us on
ProductSafety@springernature.com

In case Publisher is established outside the EU,
the EU authorized representative is:
Springer Nature Customer Service Center GmbH
Europaplatz 3, 69115 Heidelberg, Germany

Printed by Libri Plureos GmbH
in Hamburg, Germany